T0186592

The Abnormal Menstrual Cycle

The Abnormal Menstrual Cycle

Edited by

Margaret Rees
Nuffield Department of Obstetrics and Gynaecology
University of Oxford
Oxford, UK

Sally Hope
Park Lane Surgery
Woodstock, Oxfordshire, UK

and

Veronica Ravnikar
Department of Obstetrics and Gynecology
St Barnabas Medical Center
Livingston, NJ, USA

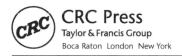

CRC Press
Taylor & Francis Group
Boca Raton London New York

CRC Press is an imprint of the
Taylor & Francis Group, an **informa** business

CRC Press
Taylor & Francis Group
6000 Broken Sound Parkway NW, Suite 300
Boca Raton, FL 33487-2742

First issued in paperback 2019

© 2005 by Taylor & Francis Group, LLC
CRC Press is an imprint of Taylor & Francis Group, an Informa business

No claim to original U.S. Government works

ISBN-13: 978-1-84214-212-7 (hbk)
ISBN-13: 978-0-367-39227-7 (pbk)

This book contains information obtained from authentic and highly regarded sources. Reasonable efforts have been made to publish reliable data and information, but the author and publisher cannot assume responsibility for the validity of all materials or the consequences of their use. The authors and publishers have attempted to trace the copyright holders of all material reproduced in this publication and apologize to copyright holders if permission to publish in this form has not been obtained. If any copyright material has not been acknowledged please write and let us know so we may rectify in any future reprint.

Except as permitted under U.S. Copyright Law, no part of this book may be reprinted, reproduced, transmitted, or utilized in any form by any electronic, mechanical, or other means, now known or hereafter invented, including photocopying, microfilming, and recording, or in any information storage or retrieval system, without written permission from the publishers.

For permission to photocopy or use material electronically from this work, please access www.copyright.com (http://www.copyright.com/) or contact the Copyright Clearance Center, Inc. (CCC), 222 Rosewood Drive, Danvers, MA 01923, 978-750-8400. CCC is a not-for-profit organization that provides licenses and registration for a variety of users. For organizations that have been granted a photocopy license by the CCC, a separate system of payment has been arranged.

Trademark Notice: Product or corporate names may be trademarks or registered trademarks, and are used only for identification and explanation without intent to infringe.

British Library Cataloguing in Publication Data

Data available on application

Library of Congress Cataloging-in-Publication Data

**Visit the Taylor & Francis Web site at
http://www.taylorandfrancis.com**

**and the CRC Press Web site at
http://www.crcpress.com**

Contents

List of contributors

A. Balen MD FRCOG
Department of Reproductive Medicine
Leeds General Infirmary
Leeds LS2 9NS
UK

F. Blake
Addenbrooke's Hospital
Hills Road
Cambridge CB2 2QQ
UK

T.J. Child MA MRCOG
Nuffield Department of Obstetrics and
  Gynaecology
University of Oxford
John Radcliffe Hospital
Oxford OX3 9DU
UK

L.B. Davis MD
Department of Obstetrics and Gynecology
Brigham and Women's Hospital
75 Francis Street
Boston, MA 02115
USA

R. Erkkola MD PhD
Department of Obstetrics and Gynecology
University Central Hospital
20520 Turku
Finland

S. Hope MA BMBCh FRCGP DRCOG
Park Lane Surgery
Woodstock
Oxfordshire OX20 1UD
UK

M.D. Hornstein MD
Department of Obstetrics and Gynecology
Brigham and Women's Hospital
75 Francis Street
Boston, MA 02115
USA

E.A. MacGregor MFFP
The City of London Migraine Clinic
22 Charterhouse Square
London EC1M 6DX
UK

I.Z. MacKenzie MA MD FRCOG DSc
Nuffield Department of Obstetrics and
  Gynaecology
John Radcliffe Hospital
Oxford OX3 9DU
UK

J. Moore
Nuffield Department of Obstetrics and
  Gynaecology
John Radcliffe Hospital
Oxford OX3 9DU
UK

J. Morrison
Nuffield Department of Obstetrics and
  Gynaecology
John Radcliffe Hospital
Oxford OX3 9DU
UK

M.K. Oehler

Department of Obstetrics and Gynaecology
Monash Medical Centre
Moorabbin Campus
865 Centre Road
East Bentleigh, VIC 3165
Australia

D.E. Parkin MD FRCOG

Gynaecological Oncology Unit
Aberdeen Royal Infirmary
Foresterhill
Aberdeen AB25 2ZN
Scotland
UK

A. Perheentupa MD PhD

Departments of Obstetrics and Gynecology and
  Physiology
University of Turku
Kiinamyllynkatu 10
20520 Turku
Finland

I.R. Pirwany MB BS MRCOG MD

McGill Reproductive Center
687 Pine Avenue West
Montreal, Quebec
Canada H3A 1A1

Address for correspondence:

Medicine Hat Regional Hospital
Medicine Hat, Alberta
Canada T1B 2A8

V. Ravnikar MD

Department of Obstetrics and Gynecology
St Barnabas Medical Center
94 Old Short Hills Road
Livingston, NJ 07039
USA

K. Reddy FRCS MRCOG

Department of Obstetrics and Gynaecology
St Paul's Wing
Cheltenham General Hospital
Sandford Road
Cheltenham GL53 7AN
UK

M. Rees DPhil FRCOG

Nuffield Department of Obstetrics and
  Gynaecology
University of Oxford
John Radcliffe Hospital
Oxford OX3 9DU
UK

T.C. Rowe FRCSC, FRCOG, MB BS

Department of Obstetrics and Gynecology
University of British Columbia
805 West 12th Avenue
Vancouver, BC
Canada V5Z 1M9

D. Tucker MRCOG

Nuffield Department of Obstetrics and
  Gynaecology
University of Oxford, Women's Centre
John Radcliffe Hospital
Oxford OX3 9DU
UK

Preface

Disorders of menstruation are among the most common problems encountered in women's health and their treatment presents a variety of complex challenges. This is not surprising since in Western societies women will each experience about 400 menstruations between the menarche and the menopause over a period of about 40 years. It has been estimated that the prevalence of menstrual disorders is 53 in 1000 in the general US population. Thirty-seven percent of women in the USA and 20 percent of women in the UK have had a hysterectomy by the age of 60. Women will seek advice from either family doctors or gynaecologists.

The range of problems women may complain of is wide encompassing excessive menstrual bleeding, pelvic pain, mood changes, migraine and irregular cycles. Symptoms can be indicative of different pathologies; for example irregular cycles may be a sign of either early ovarian failure or polycystic ovary syndrome.

Written by international experts from Europe and North America, The Abnormal Menstrual Cycle provides a comprehensive review of our current knowledge of the causes of these conditions, their investigation, and the treatment options available. Medical and surgical treatments are examined as well as the limited evidence regarding alternative and complementary therapies as women often feel that they are safer and 'more natural'. The final chapter is on the perimenopause and assesses the controversies regarding management following publication of the Women's Health Initiative with specific reference to hormone replacement.

A practical reference, the book highlights the role of the family doctor, the initial assessment and the importance of effective liaison between primary care physicians and hospital specialists. Each chapter begins with investigation and concludes with treatment, management options, and practice points.

Margaret Rees
April 2005

Consultation for an abnormal menstrual cycle

1

S. Hope

IS IT NORMAL TO HAVE PERIODS?

Modern woman is a victim of her own success. One of her priorities was to have safe, effective contraception. A natural consequence of this is that we now have regular menstrual periods or withdrawal bleeds. If you summate the number of days a 21st century woman bleeds for throughout her lifetime it is between 4 and 6 years. Effective contraception had a major impact on the 20th century and within three generations of women there has been a complete role reversal. Our great grandmothers got married and had up to 17 children and spent most of their adult life pregnant and breast feeding. Most late 20th and 21st century women want one or two children and therefore the vast majority of their adult life is dominated by cyclical menstruation. Women now perceive periods as being 'natural' whereas one could argue they are highly unnatural. Women often ask for advice but do not necessarily want treatment, as they feel inducing amenorrhea by various methods would be 'interfering with nature'. However, one could argue that amenorrhea is the 'natural' state of an adult primate.

THE SIZE OF THE PROBLEM

Women are brought up to believe that they have a menstrual cycle that lasts 28 days and that they bleed for between 4 and 7 days. Women do come and seek advice if they are outside these strict parameters. Often young girls who have just started the menarche are very worried by highly irregular cycles and also women in their mid- to late forties are again worried by irregularity of cycles. It is obvious living in a community with other women one's own age, either at school or work, that different women experience different amounts of pain and disability from their menstrual cycle. This is another reason why women seek advice from their family doctor or primary-care nurse, often with opportunism when they are having a cervical smear.

In many cases, the most challenging part of the consultation for a general practitioner is to obtain an accurate history. Discussions about periods are common; for example, 5% of women between the ages of 30 and 49 consult their general practitioner in the UK for excessive menstrual blood loss in one year[1].

Menorrhagia has the gynecological definition of heavy cyclical menstrual bleeding occurring over several consecutive cycles (blood loss > 80 ml per menstruation)[2]. However, blood loss is not routinely measured either in general practice or in gynecological out-patient clinics. It is therefore impossible for a general practitioner to apply objective evidence-based

1

medicine in this field as a primary diagnosis cannot be made with certainty in most cases. One population study accurately measuring women's menstrual loss showed that 30% of women think they have menorrhagia, compared with 10% who actually do[3]. The number of pads or tampons used does not correlate with blood loss, and the validity of a menstrual blood loss pictorial chart is debated. Measurement of menstrual blood lost using the alkaline hematin method with collected sanitary pads is accurate, but is only used in the research setting. To help in the primary-care setting a pictorial blood loss assessment chart (PBAC) was developed. However, the results of studies correlating PBAC scores and menstrual blood loss are conflicting, and it has not been widely adopted[4]. The definition of menorrhagia is utterly useless in clinical practice until someone comes up with a simple, cheap acceptable way of measuring menstrual blood loss accurately.

There is no actual difference in blood loss between patients who have periods of different length because the vast majority of blood loss happens in the first 3 days of a period. Accepting the complaint a woman gives of 'heavy periods' may commit that woman to very expensive drug treatments for a number of years or even major surgery; a sobering thought when 40–60% of women may not have menorrhagia at all but only perceived menorrhagia[5,6]. This may reach the extreme of actually removing the uterus simply because the woman finds periods unacceptable. In the UK one in five women under the age of 60 has had a hysterectomy, at least 50% of which are found to be normal at histological examination[7]. A woman with menorrhagia may not be anemic, although menorrhagia is the commonest cause of anemia in menstruating women[2,8].

SECRET AGENDAS

Physicians need to be aware of possible secret agendas that cause a woman to discuss abnormalities of her periods. Such agendas can take various forms. Consider the teenager who is really hoping that her general practitioner will offer an oral contraceptive as a means of 'normalizing' her periods because she is too shy or frightened to ask for contraception but needs it desperately. Or, the teenager who discusses her abnormal menstrual cycle in the hope of being examined because she is actually concealing a 6-month pregnancy, and who is too terrified to admit it to herself or to anyone else. Similarly, some cases of sexual abuse may be too difficult to raise openly but women come in complaining bitterly of gynecological problems in the hope that the doctor will either raise this issue, or notice something at examination, and thus enable these women to discuss the issues that are destroying their lives.

Other women may actually be worried that they have some real or imagined venereal disease and wish for a gynecological examination to reassure them in the misplaced belief that a doctor will detect any sexually transmitted disease by a simple examination. Older women in their mid- to late forties may be worried about issues surrounding the menopause, and loss of fertility and femininity, and may be grieving if infertility has occurred. Some women desire a hysterectomy as an ultimate means of contraception when they have failed to persuade their partner to volunteer for sterilization and who simply cannot contemplate another pregnancy. Others, who are prevented by their religious beliefs from using any contraception, may consciously or subconsciously wish for a hysterectomy, as will women with lesbian orientation whose monthly menstruation is a constant reminder of their femininity.

ABNORMAL PAIN

Some women have a change in the pain of their periods, which brings them to the doctor's surgery. This implies a disease process is going on. Specific chapters in this book are devoted to dysmenorrhea and endometriosis. Secondary dysmenorrhea is associated with pelvic pathology such as endometriosis, adenomyosis, pelvic inflammatory disease, submucous leiomyomas and endometrial polyps[9]. Others have always had painful periods, but for some reason, just reach the end of their tether and want relief.

Abnormal pain can be associated with menstruation but other pelvic and musculoskeletal causes must be excluded. Again, the woman might have a secret agenda that she is unable to explain. For example, a regretted termination 8 years ago may be weighing on her mind every time she has a period and she may attribute the extra pain perceived to that termination and have issues regarding future fertility. Similar problems occur with people who have been treated for sexually transmitted diseases in the past or abnormal smears with colposcopy. The complex interaction between irritable bowel syndrome and pain perceived as gynecological pain is discussed at length in a special chapter of this book.

It is always worth remembering that rare things can occur and women can have more than one complaint at one time. For example, to my shame, I treated a lady for 10 years for iron-deficient anemia as did the gynecologist for menorrhagia. It was only after the menopause when she still had iron-deficient anemia that I investigated her further and found that she had celiac disease.

WHAT IS ABNORMAL?

Delayed menarche: primary amenorrhea

The menarche occurs between the ages of 10 and 16 in most girls in developed countries[10]. Some children in the UK are now getting their periods at 8 years of age. 'Early' menarchy is a more common reason for consultation than delayed menarche, as mothers can remember getting their periods at the age of 12, and are shocked when their daughters start menstruating when still at primary school. Because the first cycles tend to be without ovulation there is a wide variation of cycle length and menstrual pain and loss. Intense exercise from ballet dancers, marathon runners and gymnasts is associated with a delayed menarche and indeed women who take up such exercises can become amenorrheic. Any girl who has not had her first period by the age of 16 should be investigated (full history, family history, examination for secondary sexual characteristics, follicle stimulating hormone (FSH), luteinizing hormone (LH), estrogen, testosterone, prolactin, thyroid function test (TFT), ?chromosomes).

Secondary amenorrhea or oligomenorrhea

Women who have had periods which then become very infrequent or non-existent should be investigated. The patient might have polycystic ovary syndrome[11,12] (see Chapter 7).

Irregular periods

As already mentioned periods become irregular with both the long and short cycles at either end of reproductive life, around the time of the menarche or in the perimenopause. These cycles are usually anovulatory. Usually a young girl with irregular periods just needs a discussion of what can be expected for the future, although it may be that she is actually requesting contraception. For a woman in the perimenopause irregularity of periods is extremely common and indeed she may be wishing for a discussion about contraception or abortion too. If periods become heavy and irregular or there is intermittent or postcoital bleeding, further investigation is advised.

Prolonged menstruation

Women on average menstruate 6 days per cycle. For the management of menorrhagia, medical and surgical see Chapters 5 and 10[13,14]. Most blood loss occurs during the first 3 days of menstruation. Periods may be prolonged by using the progesterone-only pill or depot injection or by using a copper intrauterine device (IUCD). Women may experience continual slight spotting after insertion of a levonorgestrel intrauterine contraceptive system (LNG-IUS, Mirena®), but the levonorgestrel IUS can be a very helpful solution[15,16].

There have been published guidelines for menorrhagia in primary and secondary care by the Royal College of Obstetricians and Gynecologists (RCOG)[17,18], but uptake of the recommendations in primary care has not been uniform throughout the UK and substantial differences in management still exist between practices when investigating and prescribing for menorrhagia[19,20].

Days of spotting before a period can be a sign of an endometrial or cervical polyp or a sexually transmitted disease (STD), or even a malignancy and examination should therefore be performed.

Variations in smell of vaginal discharge or color of vaginal blood

If a woman complains of an unpleasant smell she should be investigated, either for the presence of a foreign body (e.g. a forgotten tampon) or for the existence of all the various STDs. A full sexual history should be taken and appropriate swabs sent for culture.

Women often get thrush in reaction to using very alkaline preparations such as bubble baths, bath salts or heavily perfumed soaps; discussing such issues goes a long way towards prevention. Recurrent thrush is a classic sign of diabetes mellitus, and the general practitioner can do a finger-prick blood glucose in the consultation, and progress to a full fasting blood sugar and HbA1C if appropriate.

Some women worry about the change in the color of their menstrual blood and occasionally women mention passing black pieces of blood which may indicate that an endometrial cyst has discharged (see Chapter 2 on endometriosis).

Period and pelvic pain

Period pain can vary from cycle to cycle and different women in different times of their life experience different types of period pain often depending on the type of contraception they may or may not be using[21]. It is worth getting the woman to make a proper diary of her period pain to record the intensity and position and any relation to bleeding; this will provide a better understanding of her problems and how they affect her life. It will also make it clear to the woman and her doctor whether the pain is related to cycles or whether it has an entirely different etiology and falls into the areas of pelvic pain[22,23] or irritable bowel syndrome[24].

Examination

Most women fear a gynecological examination because they do not want their intimacy violated. This is especially true of women who have been sexually abused in the past and those who are virgins. Care and sensitivity must be the core part of the consultation. Some women refuse to be examined. Quite often a woman does not wish to be examined at the initial consultation and agrees to come back at a later date for an examination. This should be noted in her records. Some women do not need to be examined and have come purely for reassurance or contraceptive advice or information about other gynecological issues.

The following is a possible template for the clinical evaluation of the complaint of menorrhagia and a checklist for examination:

(1) Does the woman look pale (think of anemia)? Check hemoglobin and fecal occult blood if appropriate.
(2) Does she look as though she has other systemic disease, e.g. thyroid, etc.?
(3) Does she need to have her blood pressure checked?
(4) Have you talked about smoking?
(5) Is she up to date on contraception?
(6) Does she need to have a cervical smear?

(7) Does she require abdominal bimanual examination and visualization of the cervix?

Investigations

All investigations are dealt with in more detail in the chapters on specific problems. A hemoglobin estimation is mandatory[17,18], with total iron binding capacity and iron stores. If there is doubt as to whether the blood loss is coming from the uterus or the gut, a fecal occult blood test may be helpful. Hormone profiles for excessive menstrual bleeding and irregular cycles may be helpful.

Further referral

Further referral needs to be considered depending on the outcome of examinations and investigations as described in subsequent chapters and as appropriate to the system the individual family doctor is familiar with, as different areas of the world have different investigations. However, it would be advisable to refer in the following cases:

(1) If there is a pelvic mass on clinical examination;
(2) If 3 months of medical treatment have failed to improve symptoms;
(3) Unresolved anemia;
(4) Evidence-based patient choice.

The Royal College of Obstetricians and Gynaecologists recommends considering referral for symptoms that suggest conditions other than menorrhagia and/or if there are risk factors for endometrial cancer[17], such as polycystic ovary syndrome, gross obesity, older nulliparous women, and use of tamoxifen or unopposed estrogen.

If the woman has menorrhagia and is iron deficient, she should be treated with iron and a medical treatment for the menorrhagia[6,25], and have a repeat hemoglobin in 2 months. A transvaginal ultrasound could also be considered appropriate[26,27].

Follow-up

Planned follow-up appointments for these women are useful to feedback the results of investigations, such as hemoglobin, and also to look at charts and diaries regarding cycle length and pain in relation to bleeding. These details should be entered in the notes in case the patient fails to re-attend.

If the woman had a normal physical examination and blood tests, she would be followed up in 3 months, or sooner if she was experiencing problems with the medication[28,29]. If she had a normal physical examination but was found to be anemic she should be treated with iron and medical treatment for the menorrhagia, and have a repeat hemoglobin in 2 months. See also Appendix, p.8.

REFERENCES

1. Vessey MP, Villard-MacKintosh L, McPherson K, et al. The epidemiology of hysterectomy: findings in a large cohort study. Br J Obstet Gynaecol 1992; 99: 402–7

2. Hallberg L, Hogdahl AM, Nilsson L, Rybo G. Menstrual blood loss – a population study. Variation at different ages and attempts to define normality. Acta Obstet Gynecol Scand 1966; 45: 320–51

3. MORI. Women's Health in 1990. London: Market and Opinion Research International, 1990

4. Reid PC, Coker A, Coltart R. Assessment of menstrual blood loss using a pictorial chart: a validation study. BJOG 2000; 107: 320–2

5. Haines PJ, Hodgson H, Anderson AB, Tendle AC. Measurement of menstrual blood loss in patients complaining of menorrhagia. Br J Obstet Gynaecol 1977; 84: 763–8

6. Duckitt K, McCully K. Menorrhagia. Clinical Evidence: Women's Health. Search Date Feb 2003. BMJ Pub Group Ltd. 2151–69. www.clinicalevidence.com

7. Vessey MP, Villard-Mackintosh L, McPherson K, et al. The epidemiology of hysterectomy findings in a large cohort study. Br J Obstet Gynaecol 1992; 99: 402–7

8. Oehler MK, Rees MC. Menorrhagia: an update. Acta Obstet Gynecol Scand 2003; 82: 405–22

9. Proctor M, Farquhar C. Dysmenorrhoea: Women's Health. Search Date Feb 2003. BMJ www.clinicalevidence.com

10. Rees M. Menarche when and why? Lancet 1993; 342: 1375–6

11. Tackling polycystic ovary syndrome. Drug Ther Bull 2001; 39: 1–5

12. Kovacs GT, ed. Polycystic Ovary Syndrome. Cambridge: Cambridge University Press, 2000

13. Coulter A, Kelland J, Long A, et al. The management of menorrhagia. Effective Health Care Bulletin, no 9. Halifax: Stott Bros, 1995

14. Which operation for menorrhagia? Drug Ther Bull 2000; 38: 77–80

15. Lethaby AE, Cooke I, Rees M. Progesterone/progestogen releasing intra-uterine systems for heavy menstrual bleeding (Cochrane Review). In The Cochrane Library, Issue 1. Chichester, UK: John Wiley & Sons Ltd, 2004

16. Lahteenmaki P, Haukkamaa M, Puolakka J, et al. Open randomised study of use of levonor-gestrel releasing intrauterine system as an alternative to hysterectomy. BMJ 1998; 316: 1122–6

17. The Royal College of Obstetricians and Gynaecologists. The Initial Management of Menorrhagia. Evidence-based Guidelines 1. London: RCOG, 1998

18. The Royal College of Obstetricians and Gynaecologists. The Management of Menorrhagia in Secondary Care. Evidence-based Guidelines 5. London: RCOG, 1999

19. Grant C, Gallier L, Fahey T, et al. Management of menorrhagia in primary care – impact on referral and hysterectomy: data from the Somerset Morbidity Project. J Epidemiol Community Health 2000; 54: 709–13

20. Turner E, Bowie P, McMullen KW, Kellock C. First-line management of menorrhagia: find-ings from a survey of general practitioners in Forth Valley. Br J Fam Plann 2000; 26: 227–8

21. The Royal College of Obstetricians and Gynaecologists. The Investigation and Management of Endometriosis. RCOG Guideline No. 24. July 2000. Available at www.rcog.org.uk

22. Moore J. Chronic pelvic pain and endo-metriosis. In Rees M, Hope S, eds. Specialist Training in Gynaecology. Mosby Ltd, 2005

23. Moore J, Kennedy S. Causes of chronic pelvic pain. Baillière's Clin Obstet Gynaecol 2000; 14: 1–14

24. Camilleri M. Management of irritable bowel syndrome. Gastroenterology 2001; 120: 652–68

25. Zhang WY, Li Wan Po A. Efficacy of minor analgesics in primary dysmenorrhoea: a systematic review. Br J Obstet Gynaecol 1998; 105: 780–9

26. Vercellini P, Cortesi I, Oldani S, et al. The role of transvaginal ultrasonography and outpatient diagnostic hysteroscopy in the evaluation of patients with menorrhagia. Hum Reprod 1997; 12: 1768–71

27. Smith-Bindman R, Kerlikowske K, Feldstein VA, et al. Endovaginal ultrasound to exclude endometrial cancer and other endometrial abnormalities. JAMA 1998; 280: 1510–17

28. Hope S. Menorrhagia. BMJ 2000; 321: 935

29. Prentice A. Medical management of menorrha-gia. BMJ 1999; 319: 1343–5

30. Just in time: menorrhagia. BMJ learning module. Margaret Rees, Sally Hope, Martin Oehler. BMJlearning. www.bmjlearning.com

Appendix

Algorithm for management of menorrhagia. Reproduced from reference 30 with kind permission of the BMJ

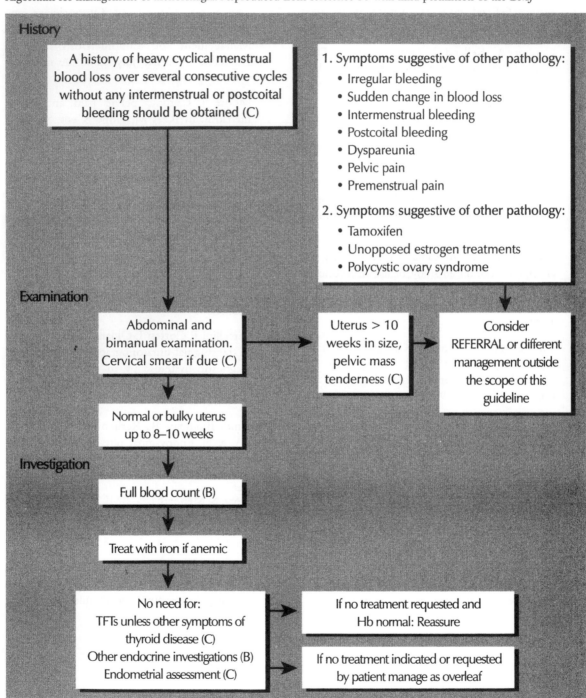

History

A history of heavy cyclical menstrual blood loss over several consecutive cycles without any intermenstrual or postcoital bleeding should be obtained (C)

1. Symptoms suggestive of other pathology:
   - Irregular bleeding
   - Sudden change in blood loss
   - Intermenstrual bleeding
   - Postcoital bleeding
   - Dyspareunia
   - Pelvic pain
   - Premenstrual pain

2. Symptoms suggestive of other pathology:
   - Tamoxifen
   - Unopposed estrogen treatments
   - Polycystic ovary syndrome

Examination

Abdominal and bimanual examination. Cervical smear if due (C)

Uterus > 10 weeks in size, pelvic mass tenderness (C)

Consider REFERRAL or different management outside the scope of this guideline

Normal or bulky uterus up to 8–10 weeks

Investigation

Full blood count (B)

Treat with iron if anemic

No need for:
TFTs unless other symptoms of thyroid disease (C)
Other endocrine investigations (B)
Endometrial assessment (C)

If no treatment requested and Hb normal: Reassure

If no treatment indicated or requested by patient manage as overleaf

Painful menstruation: endometriosis

2

L.B. Davis and M.D. Hornstein

ETIOLOGY

Endometriosis is defined as the presence of endometrial glands and stroma outside the uterine cavity. It is typically confined to the pelvis, particularly the ovaries, posterior cul-de-sac, anterior uterovesical peritoneum, uterosacral ligaments, fallopian tubes, uterus, and rectovaginal septum; however, it has been reported to occur in more remote locations including the lung, pleura, extremities, pelvic lymph nodes, and surgical scars.

There are several theories regarding the etiology of endometriosis including Sampson's theory of retrograde menstruation, celomic metaplasia, and lymphatic and vascular metastasis. Furthermore, genetic predisposition and the importance of immune function and hormonal influences have also been noted.

Retrograde menstruation

First reported by Sampson in 1921, the retrograde menstruation theory states that fragments of endometrial tissue are carried through the fallopian tubes with subsequent implantation on peritoneal structures. There are a number of observations that support this theory. First, retrograde regurgitation of desquamated endometrium at the time of menstruation has been directly observed by laparoscopy and laparotomy[1]. Second, some fragments of desquamated endometrium have proven to be viable and able to implant and grow on peritoneal structures. Third, women at higher risk of retrograde flow seem to have higher rates of endometriosis and *vice versa*. For example, women with müllerian anomalies in whom antegrade menstrual flow is blocked have higher rates of endometriosis[2]. Endometriosis has also been shown to be more common in women with cycle lengths less than 27 days and menstrual flow greater than 7 days[3]. This is in contrast to women who have had multiple pregnancies or prolonged use of oral contraceptives, and therefore probable decreased retrograde flow, who experience lower rates of endometriosis. The retrograde menstruation theory is generally the most favored among authorities, but does have its shortcomings. Specifically, endometriosis differs in many fundamental ways from eutopic endometrium, including clonality of origin, enzymatic activity, and protein expression, and therefore lacks the characteristics that would be expected of an autotransplant[4]. Furthermore, Sampson's theory does not account for the fact that endometriosis does not occur in all women with retrograde menstruation.

Celomic metaplasia

The celomic metaplasia theory states that the epithelial lining of the ovary and mesothelial lining of the peritoneal structures are capable of differentiating into müllerian elements (i.e. endometrium). Contributing factors to this process have been difficult to identify but probably include inflammation and/or sub-clinical infection. This theory could account for the rare case reports of endometriosis in men.

Lymphatic and vascular dissemination

Support for the lymphatic and vascular metastasis theories comes primarily from the fact that endometrial tissue has been identified in pelvic lymphatic and blood vessels. This theory would account for the reports of endometriosis in ectopic sites remote from the pelvic cavity.

Genetic predisposition

There are multiple sources of evidence suggesting a genetic basis for endometriosis. First, significant familial clustering particularly in the maternal line has been observed. For example, first-degree relatives of a woman with endometriosis have a seven-fold increased risk of developing endometriosis compared with the general population[5,6]. Furthermore, according to the Australian National Health and Medical Research Council Twin Register, there is increased concordance of endometriosis among monozygotic twins compared with dizygotic twins (0.52 vs. 0.19, respectively)[7]. Additionally, there is a similar age of onset in affected non-twin sisters, which supports a genetic basis as opposed to a common exposure (i.e. if both sisters were exposed to a causative agent with a fixed incubation time, one would expect onset of symptoms in the same year, not at the same age)[8].

Immune function

Endometriosis is associated with alterations in both cell-mediated and humoral immunity. Small fragments of regurgitated endometrial tissue may not be eradicated in women with diminished immune function. Impaired natural killer cell activity may play a role in the development of endometriosis by limiting adequate removal of endometrial debris[9]. Macrophages have been shown to exist in increased concentrations in the peritoneal fluid of women with endometriosis[10], yet act to enhance endometrial cell proliferation by secreting growth factors and cytokines[11].

Several growth factors and cytokines including tumor necrosis factor-α (TNF-α) and vascular endothelial growth factor (VEGF) are found in higher concentrations in the peritoneal fluid of women with endometriosis, and may promote the growth and development of endometriotic tissue by inducing proliferation and angiogenesis[12]. Matrix metalloproteinases, a family of endopeptidases that play a role in the degradation and turnover of extracellular matrix proteins, are also found in higher concentrations in the peritoneal fluid of patients with endometriosis[13], and may play an important role in the pathogenesis of the disease.

Interestingly, women with endometriosis have been shown to have higher rates of rheumatoid arthritis, systemic lupus erythematosus, Sjögren's syndrome, hypothyroidism, multiple sclerosis, allergies, and asthma compared with women without endometriosis[14].

This association also supports the role of the immune system in the etiology of endometriosis.

Hormonal factors

Endometriotic tissue is dependent on estrogen for growth and development. Progesterone antagonizes the mitogenic effects of estrogen; however, this effect is less pronounced in endometriotic implants than in endometrium. Aromatase is the rate-limiting enzyme that is responsible for the conversion of C19 steroids to estrogen in many human tissues. The enzyme 17β-hydroxysteroid dehydrogenase type 2 catalyzes the conversion of the potent estrogen, estradiol, to a biologically less potent estrogen, estrone[15]. These enzymatic pathways of estrogen metabolism have important implications for the pathophysiology, and hence, the medical treatment of endometriosis.

PRESENTATION

The prevalence of endometriosis has been difficult to establish owing to the fact that definitive diagnosis requires surgical intervention, but is estimated at 2.5–15% of reproductive-aged women[16]. Endometriosis can develop between 10 and 60 years of age. The average age of diagnosis is 27 years[17]; however, women typically report symptomatology many years prior to the diagnosis. Endometriosis is more common in women of Asian origin than in Caucasian women[18]. While some patients with endometriosis are asymptomatic, the most common presentations are pain, infertility, and pelvic mass.

Pain

Patients with endometriosis characteristically complain of acquired, progressive, severe pain occurring just before or during menstruation. The pain is usually bilateral, may range from mild to severe, is often described as dull and aching, may radiate to the low back and legs, and may be associated with rectal pressure, nausea, and diarrhea. Dyspareunia, dysuria, and painful defecation may also be presenting symptoms, as well as premenstrual staining, hypermenorrhea, and hematuria. Interestingly, the severity of pain does not consistently correlate with the severity of endometriosis[19]. Patients with stage I or stage II disease often have more pain than those with advanced disease[20]. Some authors suggest that it is the adhesions associated with endometriosis that cause pelvic pain[21], but others maintain that pain is mediated by prostaglandin release from miniature menstruation and bleeding[22].

Infertility

Endometriosis can cause subfertility and infertility, but rarely precludes conception in an absolute way. The association between advanced endometriosis and infertility is well established, but in patients with minimal to moderate disease, the data are less convincing. The primary mechanism for infertility in severe endometriosis, is probably adhesive disease that results in a mechanical barrier between the ovary and the uterus. In the absence of adhesions, other mechanisms are less well defined. Some authors suggest that endometriotic implants are associated with diffuse pelvic inflammation, increased peritoneal fluid volume, and increased numbers of activated macrophages, all of which may play a role in a more hostile environment to egg and sperm interaction[12]. The stability of the microenvironment of the eutopic endometrium leading to disruption of the implantation process has also been questioned. Of course, dyspareunia leading to decreased coital frequency may also play a role.

Pelvic mass

An otherwise asymptomatic patient with endometriosis may present with an incidental finding of a pelvic mass either on pelvic examination or imaging. An area of endometriosis that becomes sufficiently large to be classified as a tumor, typically in the ovary, is defined as an endometrioma. These are commonly called chocolate cysts in reference to the filling of the cyst with old blood that resembles chocolate syrup or tar. The management of a patient with an asymptomatic pelvic mass should be focused on excluding malignancy. While malignant transformation in endometriotic implants is uncommon, it is a well-documented phenomenon[23]. Women with endometriosis-associated cancers are typically premenopausal, have a high incidence of endometrioid and clear cell histologies, and have early-stage disease[24].

INVESTIGATION

Physical examination

Ideally, physical examination should be performed while the patient is experiencing symptoms, preferably during menstruation. In some cases, the pelvic examination may be completely unremarkable as the sensitivity, specificity, and predictive values of the examination in the diagnosis of endometriosis are low. The pathognomonic sign of endometriosis is uterosacral nodularity[25]. Other common findings include a fixed retroverted uterus with tenderness of the uterosacral ligaments and posterior cul-de-sac. Tender masses, nodules, and fibrosis may also be palpated. Clinicians may find that the cervix is laterally displaced due to unequal shortening of the uterosacral ligaments (Propst's sign)[26].

Laboratory studies

There have been multiple attempts to identify a serum marker that would function as a screening test for endometriosis. To date, however, none have been shown to have adequate sensitivity and specificity to serve as a reliable screening tool. CA-125 is often elevated in advanced endometriosis; however, the sensitivity of the assay is too low to be clinically useful in mild to moderate disease. There are conflicting reports on whether or not following serial serum CA-125 levels may help predict the response to medical and surgical treatment[27,28]. Other markers that have been evaluated include CA-72, CA-15–3, TAG-72, CA-19–9, PP14, TATI, CRP, and anti-endometrial antibodies[29]. Research in this area is ongoing.

Imaging

Ultrasound examination is the most common imaging modality for evaluation of suspected endometriosis. Ultrasound is particularly helpful in women with endometriotic cysts, but its role is limited in the diagnosis of peritoneal implants and adhesive disease. Endometriomas typically appear as cystic structures with diffuse low-level internal echoes and echogenic wall foci. Septations, thickened walls, and wall nodularity may also be observed. Ultrasound was found to have up to 84% sensitivity and 90% specificity for the detection of endometriomas, confirmed by surgery and histopathology[30]. Other types of pelvic masses including dermoid cysts, hemorrhagic cysts, and cystic neoplasms may resemble endometriomas, and should be considered in the differential diagnosis[29].

Magnetic resonance imaging (MRI) is also helpful in the identification of endometriomas. In addition, it may occasionally visualize solid endometriotic implants and adhesions. Endometrial implants typically express an intensity signal similar to normal endometrium – hypointense on T1- and hyperintense on T2-weighted images. The addition of gadolinium contrast has not been shown to improve sensitivity or specificity over MRI alone[31]. MRI has been reported as a valuable tool in the identification of deep infiltrating lesions of the rectovaginal septum and uterosacral ligaments[32]. While direct comparison of ultrasound and MRI in the same population has not been made, there does seem to be an adjunctive role for this modality in a small high-risk subset of the population[29].

Surgery

The gold standard for the diagnosis of endometriosis is generally considered to be laparoscopic assessment. Endometriosis has a myriad of visual presentations upon laparoscopic examination. The classic appearance is the so-called powder-burn lesion, which is a small, punctate, brown or purple discoloration of the peritoneal surface. The dark coloration is attributed to hemosiderin deposits from entrapped endometriotic debris. Atypical lesions may appear red, white, clear, nodular, as a peritoneal window, or may be invisible to the surgeon altogether. Red lesions are highly vascularized and proliferative and tend to represent early disease. In contrast, white lesions contain fibrous tissue, are poorly vascularized, and probably represent healed or latent disease[33]. Endometriomas tend to appear as dark, brown, smooth-walled cysts often in the presence of adhesive disease. Careful inspection of the ovaries is highly reliable in the identification of endometriomas; however, enlarged ovaries in infertile patients may contain occult small deep endometriomas, which can be detected by ovarian puncture and aspiration[34]. Deep endometriotic lesions, defined as infiltration more than 5 mm beneath the peritoneal surface, may be difficult to evaluate laparoscopically, but meticulous palpation with a blunt probe may help identify these lesions. Because endometriotic implants are so diverse in appearance, the expertise of the surgeon may significantly influence diagnostic accuracy.

The most widely used method for staging is the revised American Fertility Society classification of endometriosis, despite the fact that intraobserver and interobserver variability is high[35]. The staging system for endometriosis was initially established to assess in a standardized way a patient's prognosis in terms of fertility outcome. However, in the era of assisted reproductive technologies (ART), formal staging becomes less relevant as patients who do not conceive spontaneously after surgery still have a reasonable chance of success with the aid of ART. Furthermore, since there is little correlation between pain symptoms and severity of disease, formal staging is of limited use in this patient population as well.

MEDICAL MANAGEMENT

Therapeutic intervention should be targeted at resolving the patient's specific problem. For endometriosis there are two therapeutic goals of treatment: pain relief and improved fertility. Medical remedies have a role in the management of pain symptoms, but have not been demonstrated to improve fertility when compared to expectant management. Thus medical management is presented here as a modality to reduce pain. The role of medical therapy in conjunction with surgery has also been examined. In general, postoperative hormonal therapy improves duration of pain relief after surgery if administered for at least 6 month's duration.

Antiprostaglandins

Non-steroidal anti-inflammatory drugs (NSAIDs) are the first-line treatment for pain relief in women with endometriosis. Ibuprofen 600 mg every 6 h up to 2400 mg per day, or naproxen (Naprosyn®) 550 mg every 12 h up to 1100 mg per day are excellent choices for most patients (Table 1). Mefenamic acid (Ponstel®) is an anti-inflammatory agent indicated for the treatment of primary dysmenorrhea. The recommended dosage is 500 mg as an initial dose followed by 250 mg every 6 h. It should be initiated at the start of menses and should not be necessary for more than 2–3 days per month. Caution should be used with NSAIDs in patients with underlying gastrointestinal or renal disease. Tramadol (Ultram®) may be considered

as a second-line drug. The recommended dosage is 50–100 mg (for moderate and severe pain, respectively) every 4–6 h as needed, not to exceed 400 mg per day.

Progestogens

The established mechanism of action of progestogens appears to be initial decidualization followed by eventual atrophy of endometrial tissue. Newer evidence also suggests suppression of matrix metallo-proteinases, enzymes that promote implantation and growth of ectopic endometrium[36]. There are multiple types of progestogens including medroxyprogesterone (administered both orally and in depot form), norethindrone, and levonorgestrel. Medroxyprogesterone 30 mg orally per day has been shown to be as effective as danazol in the treatment of endometriosis[37]. The depot form is of limited use in the infertility patient because of the varying length of time for resumption of ovulation after discontinuation of the drug. Side-effects of these agents include breakthrough bleeding, weight gain, fluid retention, nausea, breast tenderness, and osteopenia. Depression should be considered a contraindication to the use of progestogens for the treatment of endo-metriosis.

Gestrinone

Gestrinone is a mixed progestin/antiprogestin that has been shown to have roughly equivalent efficacy to danazol and gonadotropin releasing hormone (GnRH) agonists in terms of pain relief[38]. Dosage ranges from 2.5 to 10 mg weekly, typically divided into twice-weekly dosing. The side-effects are similar to those of danazol.

Table 1 Medical management

	Mechanism of action	Common dosing regimen	Side-effects
NSAIDs	decreased prostaglandin production	ibuprofen 600 mg p.o. q. 6 h	nausea, heartburn, GI ulceration, bleeding, renal toxicity, rash
Progestogens	endometrial atrophy	medroxyprogesterone acetate 30 mg p.o. q.d.	breakthrough bleeding, weight gain, fluid retention, nausea, breast tenderness, depression
OCs	endometrial pseudo-decidualization	1 low-dose tab p.o. q.d.	minor: breakthrough bleeding, fluid retention, melasma, nausea, headache, mood changes; major: thromboembolism, cerebrovascular disease, myocardial infarction
GnRH agonists	hypoestrogenic, hypoandrogenic state → endometrial atrophy and amenorrhea	leuprolide acetate depot 3.75 mg i.m. q. mo	hot flushes, bone loss, vaginal dryness, vaginal bleeding, decreased libido, insomnia, fatigue, depression, amenorrhea, headache, breast tenderness, decreased skin elasticity
Danazol	hypoestrogenic, hyperandrogenic state → endometrial atrophy and amenorrhea	danazol 600 mg p.o. t.i.d.	weight gain, edema, decreased breast size, acne, oily skin, hirsutism, voice deepening, headache, hot flushes, changes in libido, muscle cramps, fetal androgenization

NSAIDs, non-steroidal anti-inflammatory drugs; OCs, oral contraceptive pills; GnRH agonists, gonadotropin releasing hormone agonists; GI, gastrointestinal

It has been used extensively in Europe, but is not currently approved for use in the United States.

Combined estrogen–progesterone

Oral contraceptive pills (OCs) are currently the most commonly prescribed treatment for endometriosis-associated pain. OCs produce a 'pseudo' decidualized endometrium, a condition that may apply to ectopic as well as eutopic endometrium. The mechanism of action is not clearly defined, but may involve suppression of cell proliferation and enhancement of programed cell death or apoptosis. In a randomized, controlled trial comparing cyclic low-dose OCs with a GnRH agonist, OCs were found to be equally efficacious in relieving non-specific pelvic pain, but less effective in the treatment of dysmenorrhea[39]. It is likely that all low-dose monophasic pills are of equal efficacy. Continuous non-cycling OCs may offer improved pain relief over cyclic therapy. The usual dose is one pill per day for 3–6 months. Minor side-effects include breakthrough bleeding, fluid retention, melasma, nausea, headache, and mood changes. Potential serious side-effects include thromboembolism, cerebrovascular disease, and myocardial infarction. OCs are contraindicated in women with thromboembolic disorders, cerebrovascular or coronary artery disease, breast cancer or any cancer suspected to be estrogen-dependent, jaundice, hepatic adenomas, undiagnosed abnormal genital bleeding, or known or suspected pregnancy. Non-contraceptive health benefits should be considered which include improved cycle regularity, diminished acne, diminished blood loss and iron-deficiency anemia, decreased incidence of functional ovarian cysts and acute pelvic inflammatory disease, and decreased incidences of benign breast diseases as well as endometrial and ovarian cancers.

Gonadotropin releasing hormone agonists

GnRH agonists (e.g. nafarelin, leuprorelin, buserelin, goserelin, histrelin, and triptorelin) bind to the pituitary GnRH receptors and, after initial stimulation of follicle stimulating hormone (FSH) and luteinizing hormone (LH) secretion, ultimately result in down-regulation of pituitary gonadotropin secretion. Diminished levels of FSH and LH reduce secretion of estrogen from the ovary and result in endometrial atrophy and amenorrhea. Newer evidence also suggests additional mechanisms of action including suppression of matrix metalloproteinases. These medications can be administered intramuscularly, subcutaneously, or intranasally. One common dosing regimen includes leuprolide acetate 3.75 mg i.m. every 4 weeks or 11.25 mg i.m. every 12 weeks. In a placebo-controlled trial, more than 80% of women who failed treatment of presumed

endometriosis with OCPs experienced pain relief in 3 months with a GnRH agonist[40]. Pain associated with endometriosis is generally well controlled during and immediately after treatment with GnRH agonists; however, pain returns in up to 75% of treated women. Side-effects are related to hypoestrogenism and include hot flushes, bone loss, vaginal dryness, transient vaginal bleeding, decreased libido, insomnia, irritability, fatigue, depression, headache, breast tenderness, and decreased skin elasticity.

While endometriosis itself does not increase the risk of osteopenia or osteoporosis, iatrogenic hypoestrogenism via the use of GnRH agonists puts a patient at significant risk of this long-term sequela. This observation initially led the Federal Drug Administration (FDA) to limit the use of these medications to 6 months duration. Numerous well-designed studies have documented a 0.5–1% decrease in bone density for each month of GnRH agonist use. While many studies suggest that bone loss will not be fully recovered by 6 or 12 months after treatment, complete recovery by 24 months may be possible[41]. The addition of hormonal add-back therapy, in the form of progestins with or without estrogen, significantly reduces the hypoestrogenic side-effects of GnRH agonists, including that of osteopenia/osteoporosis, without stimulating growth of endometriotic implants[42]. Hormonal add-back is primarily accomplished by the supplementation of a progestin. Norethindrone acetate 5 mg in conjunction with leuprolide acetate depot has been shown to protect against bone loss while still allowing for effective suppression of pelvic pain[43]. Addition of an estrogen to the progestin may also be employed. This use of estrogen add-back may be explained by a proposed hierarchy of tissue responsiveness to levels of circulating estradiol. Barbieri proposed a hormonal threshold (e.g. an estradiol level of 30–50 pg/ml) below which endometriosis is suppressed whereas bone density may be maintained[44]. Add-back therapy does not diminish the efficacy of GnRH agonists even when started during the first month of treatment; therefore, an add-back-free interval at the beginning of treatment is not necessary[45]. Other regimens to diminish bone loss in women using GnRH agonists include human parathyroid hormone and the bisphosphonates[46,47]. The addition of the bisphosphonate, sodium etidronate, to low-dose norethindrone has been shown to preserve bone density fully in women receiving prolonged GnRH agonist therapy[47]. All women using a GnRH agonist should consume adequate amounts of calcium and vitamin D, and perform regular weight-bearing exercise.

Danazol

Danazol, the first drug to be approved by the FDA for the treatment of endometriosis, is now rarely used due to high rates of masculinizing side-effects. Danazol is a steroid derivative of 17α-ethinyltestosterone, which acts in part to eliminate the mid-cycle surge of LH and FSH. It is metabolized to at least 60 different by-products, which may account for its multitude of effects. The resultant high-androgen, low-estrogen state inhibits endometrial growth and promotes amenorrhea[48]. Pain relief is obtained in approximately 90% of patients; however, symptoms may recur within one year after discontinuation of the drug. The usual dose is two 200 mg tablets 3 times daily for 6 months. Doses less than 800 mg per day may be associated with fewer side-effects but have been shown to be less effective[49]. Androgenizing side-effects include weight gain, edema, decreased breast size, acne, oily skin, hirsutism, voice deepening, headache, hot flushes, change in libido, and muscle cramps[50]. Voice deepening may be irreversible so danazol should not be given to patients for whom voice quality is particularly important. Barrier methods of contraception or other effective forms of birth control are required due to the possibility of androgenization of a female fetus should pregnancy occur. Danazol is contraindicated in women with liver disease, severe hypertension, congestive heart failure, or impaired renal function. It should also be avoided in women with hypercholesterolemia as danazol can exacerbate this condition.

OTHER MEDICATIONS ON THE HORIZON

Aromatase inhibitors

Endometriotic cells aberrantly express aromatase[51], the enzyme that converts androstenedione and testosterone to estrone and estradiol. Estrogens in turn stimulate cyclo-oxygenase activity, which increases prostaglandin formation, and because prostaglandins stimulate aromatase activity, an autocrine positive feedback loop is completed. In normal endometrial cells, aromatase expression is inhibited by the binding of a transcription factor COUP-TF to the promoter. However, in endometriotic cells an aberrantly expressed factor, SF-1, displaces COUP-TF to bind to this same promoter and activate aromatase expression and subsequently increase estrogen biosynthesis (Figure 1)[52].

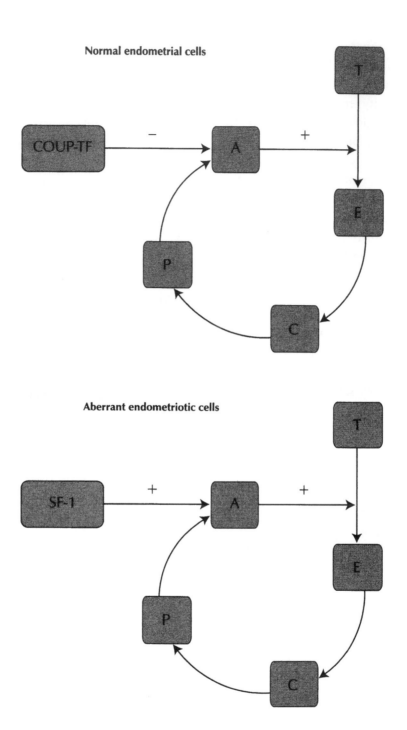

Figure 1 The role of aromatase in normal and aberrant endometrial cells. T, testosterone and adrostenedione; E, estrone and estradiol; C, cyclo-oxygenase; P, prostaglandins; A, aromatase; COUP-TF, chicken ovalburmin upstream promoter transcription factor; SF-1, steroidogenic factor

Table 2 Other medications on the horizon

	Mechanism of action	Common dosing regimen	Side-effects
Aromatase inhibitors	hypoestrogenic state → endometrial atrophy and amenorrhea	anastrozole 1 mg p.o. q.d. letrozole 2.5 mg p.o. q.d.	GI disturbance, hot flushes, bone loss, vaginal dryness, headache
Pentoxifylline	anti-inflammatory	trental 400 mg p.o. t.i.d.	nausea, vomiting, dyspepsia, dizziness, headache
Gestrinone	mixed progestin/ antiprogestin	gestrinone 2.5 mg p.o. b.i.w.	weight gain, edema, decreased breast size, acne, oily skin, hirsutism, voice deepening, headache, hot flushes
Mifepristone	antiprogestin	mifepristone 50 mg p.o. q.d.	hot flushes, fatigue, nausea, transient liver transaminase changes, abortifacient
SPRMs	progesterone agonist– antagonist	not defined	unknown
SERMs	estrogen agonist– antagonist	raloxifene 60 mg p.o. q.d.	hot flushes, leg cramps, thromboembolism, fetal toxicity

SPRMs, selective progesterone receptor modulators; SERMs, selective estrogen receptor modulators; GI, gastrointestinal

Aromatase inhibitors are an exciting new area of research in the medical treatment of endometriosis (Table 2). This class of drug has already been tested in the rodent model with good success. There has also been a case report of a postmenopausal woman with severe persistent endometriosis, despite hysterectomy and bilateral oophorectomy, who achieved complete resolution of her symptoms[53]. Additionally, the aromatase inhibitor, anastrozole (Arimidex®), has been studied in conjunction with a GnRH agonist in 80 women with severe endometriosis, and found to significantly increase the pain-free interval after conservative laparoscopic surgery compared to a GnRH agonist alone[54]. As in other medical treatments that act to decrease estrogen formation, long-term effects such as osteoporosis must be considered.

Pentoxifylline

Pentoxifylline (Trental®) is an immuno-modulating agent that acts to diminish the production of inflammatory mediators and the response of these mediators on their target cells. Indicated for the treatment of intermittent claudication, it has been suggested as a novel approach for the treatment of endometriosis-related subfertility. It should be noted that thus far there are no adequate, well-controlled studies of this drug in pregnant women should pregnancy be achieved.

Mifepristone

Mifepristone (also known as RU-486) is an antiprogesterone and antiglucocorticoid that inhibits ovulation and disrupts endometrial integrity. Thus far, one small, uncontrolled trial suggests possible improvement in pelvic pain[55]. Typical dosage is 50–100 mg daily. Side-effects include hot flushes, fatigue, nausea, and transient liver transaminase changes. No effect upon bone mineral density has been reported.

Selective progesterone receptor modulators (SPRMs)

SPRMs are agonist–antagonists of progesterone depending on tissue type, and hold promise as a possible treatment for endometriosis if they are able to inhibit endometrial growth without the progesterone-like side-effects.

Selective estrogen receptor modulators (SERMs)

SERMs are agonist–antagonists of estrogen depending on tissue type, and also may be of therapeutic value in the treatment of endometriosis. Raloxifene, for example, inhibits endometrial growth while promoting bone density; however, vasomotor side-effects can be limiting. Investigation continues for a SERM with an ideal agonist–antagonist profile.

Other

Other promising medications including TNF-α inhibitors, angiogenesis inhibitors, and matrix metalloproteinase inhibitors have been studied in animal models; however, human trials have yet to be conducted.

SURGICAL MANAGEMENT

As is the case in medical management, the decision to proceed with surgical treatment should be based on the patient's particular symptomatology, e.g. pain, infertility, or mass. For patients with pain unresponsive to conservative treatment, surgical intervention at all stages of endometriosis may be beneficial. While evaluation of pelvic pain is complex and may be imprecise, surgical success in relieving pain has been reported in uncontrolled trials to be greater than 70%[56].

The more advanced the endometriosis, the greater the likelihood that surgical intervention will be required. For women who wish to maintain or restore fertility, 'conservative' surgery is indicated. This is in contradistinction to 'radical' surgery, which typically involves hysterectomy and bilateral salpingo-oophorectomy. Surgical removal of both ovaries is the definitive treatment for endometriosis and should be considered for women over the age of 35 who have completed their childbearing[57].

In general, a pregnancy rate of approximately 65% can be reached in the first 1–2 years following surgery without the aid of ART[58]. If conception has not occurred within 2 years of surgery, the likelihood of a spontaneous pregnancy is low. For women with moderate or severe endometriosis who want to maintain or restore fertility, surgery is the treatment of choice. For minimal or mild endometriosis (e.g. minimal anatomic distortion), the decision to proceed with surgery used to be less straightforward until the Canadian Collaborative Group on Endometriosis performed a multicenter, prospective, randomized, controlled, double-blind study that revealed significantly higher pregnancy rates in laparoscopic treatment compared with expectant management after 9 months (37.5% vs. 22.5%, $p = 0.002$)[59]. It should be noted that in this study the number requiring treatment was 7.7, meaning that approximately 7.7 women would have to undergo laparoscopy to obtain one additional pregnancy at 9 months. This result, coupled with considerations of cost, surgical risk, and the availability of alternative approaches to infertility, makes the decision to perform surgery for minimal or mild endometriosis an individual one, based on patient preference and physician discretion.

The goals of surgical treatment are to restore normal anatomy, eliminate endometrial implants, and delay recurrence of the disease. For patients with a persistent adnexal mass greater than 4 cm, surgery, usually via laparoscopy, is also indicated. For the treatment of endometriomas, procedures involving wide incision and drainage, cyst stripping or ablation, have similar efficacy in improving pain immediately after surgery, reportedly as high as 61–100%[60–62]. Excision of endometriomas, however, may be associated with increased adhesion formation without improvement in pain or residual endometriosis at follow-up laparoscopy[61]. Minimal sutures (if any) should be used to restore the anatomy of the ovary after cystectomy to diminish the risk of adhesion formation.

Adhesions should be excised rather than simply lysed because of the possibility of occult endometriosis within adhesive tissue. Elimination of endometriosis may be performed by sharp resection, laser ablation, or electrosurgical desiccation. Sharp resection, while effective, increases the risk of bleeding and also of subsequent adhesion formation. Laser ablation, also effective, may have limited precision (e.g. KTP532, argon; Nd:YAG) or limited coagulating ability (e.g. CO_2) depending on the type of laser selected. Electrosurgical desiccation, while relatively simple to perform, increases the risk of inadequate treatment as depth of tissue destruction cannot be determined by the operator.

The surgical approach to endometriosis may be accomplished either by laparoscopy or laparotomy. Due to advancements in laparoscopic equipment and technique, laparoscopy is now the more common modality. In general, laparoscopy allows for better visualization, less tissue trauma, possibly less adhesion formation, and faster recovery time. However, it tends to be more expensive, time consuming, and does not allow for three-dimensional viewing or palpation of structures. Laparotomy is generally preferred for extensive enterolysis, bowel resection, or other difficult situations too complex for the laparoscopic approach. When deciding between the two techniques it is most important to choose the one that will allow the best surgical result with the lowest risk of injury or complication.

HORMONE REPLACEMENT THERAPY AFTER ENDOMETRIOSIS

There is no absolute contraindication to hormone replacement therapy (HRT) in women with endometriosis. It has been established that among women with endometriosis who have had a bilateral oophorectomy, the risk of recurrence with HRT is low; approximately 1% per year[63]. In general, HRT may be started in the immediate postoperative period with negligible risk of recurrent endometriosis or pain. However, the risk of recurrence seems to increase with peritoneal involvement greater than 3 cm, making HRT less straightforward in these patients[63]. The decision to proceed with HRT is exceedingly complex, especially in light of the results of the Women's Health Initiative[64], and should be made on an individual basis depending on the patient's symptomatology, risk factors, and acceptance of risk. It may be reasonable to introduce a progestin such as medroxyprogesterone acetate in high doses, around 20–30 mg per day, in the initial postoperative period to reduce the risk of hot flushes.

PRACTICE POINTS

- Endometriosis is defined as the presence of endometrial glands and stroma outside the uterine cavity
- There are several theories regarding the etiology of endometriosis including Sampson's theory of retrograde menstruation, celomic metaplasia, and lymphatic and vascular metastasis
- Endometriotic tissue is dependent on estrogen for growth and development. This fact has important implications for the medical treatment of endometriosis
- The most common presentations of endometriosis are pain, infertility, and pelvic mass. Some patients are asymptomatic
- The severity of pain does not consistently correlate with the severity of endometriosis
- Endometriosis can cause subfertility and infertility, but rarely precludes conception in an absolute way
- An area of endometriosis that becomes sufficiently large to be classified as a tumor, typically in the ovary, is defined as an endometrioma
- While malignant transformation in endometriotic implants is uncommon, it is a well-documented phenomenon
- There are no serum markers that have been shown to have adequate sensitivity and specificity to serve as a reliable screening tool for endometriosis
- Ultrasound is the most common imaging modality for evaluation of suspected endometriosis. It is particularly helpful in women with endometriotic cysts, but its role is limited in the diagnosis of peritoneal implants and adhesive disease
- The gold standard for the diagnosis of endometriosis is generally considered to be laparoscopic assessment. Endometriosis has a myriad of visual presentations and the expertise of the surgeon may significantly influence diagnostic accuracy
- The two therapeutic goals of treatment are pain relief and improved fertility
- Medical remedies have a role in the management of pain symptoms, but have not been demonstrated to improve fertility when compared to expectant management
- The goals of surgical treatment are to restore normal anatomy, eliminate endometrial implants, and delay recurrence of disease
- There is no absolute contraindication to HRT in women with endometriosis. The decision to proceed with HRT is complex and should be made on an individual basis depending on the patient's symptomatology, risk factors, and acceptance of risk

REFERENCES

1. Liu DT, Hitchcock A. Endometriosis: its association with retrograde menstruation, dysmenorrhoea, and tubal pathology. Br J Obstet Gynaecol 1986; 93: 859–62

2. Olive DL, Henderson DY. Endometriosis and müllerian anomalies. Obstet Gynecol 1987; 69: 412–15

3. Cramer DW. Epidemiology of endometriosis. In Wilson EA, ed. Endometriosis. New York: Alan R Liss, 1987

4. Redwine DB. Was Sampson wrong? Fertil Steril 2002; 78: 686–93

5. Moen MH, Magnus P. The familial risk of endometriosis. Acta Obstet Gynecol Scand 1993; 72: 560–4

6. Simpson JL, Elias S, Malinak LR, Buttram VC Jr. Heritable aspects of endometriosis. I. Genetic studies. Am J Obstet Gynecol 1980; 137: 327–31

7. Treloar SA, O'Connor DT, O'Connor VM, Martin NG. Genetic influences on endometriosis in an Australian twin sample. Fertil Steril 1999; 71: 701–10

8. Kennedy SH, Hadfield RM, Mardon H, Barlow D. Age of onset of pain symptoms in non-twin sisters concordant for endometriosis. Hum Reprod 1996; 11: 403–5

9. Ho HN, Chao KH, Chen HF, et al. Peritoneal natural killer cytotoxicity and CD25+ CD3+ lymphocyte subpopulation are decreased in women with stage III-IV endometriosis. Hum Reprod 1995; 10: 2671–5

10. Haney AF, Muscato JJ, Weinberg JB. Peritoneal fluid cell populations in infertility patients. Fertil Steril 1981; 35: 696–8

11. Lebovic DI, Mueller MD, Taylor RN. Immunobiology of endometriosis. Fertil Steril 2001; 75: 1–10

12. Seli E, Arici A. Endometriosis: interaction of immune and endocrine systems. Semin Reprod Med 2003; 21: 135–44

13. Szamatowicz J, Laudanski P, Tomaszewska I. Matrix metalloproteinase-9 and tissue inhibitor of matrix metalloproteinase-1: a possible role in the pathogenesis of endometriosis. Hum Reprod 2002; 17: 284–8

14. Sinaii N, Cleary SD, Ballweg ML, et al. High rates of autoimmune and endocrine disorders, fibromyalgia, chronic fatigue syndrome and atopic diseases among women with endometriosis: a survey analysis. Hum Reprod 2002; 17: 2715–24

15. Gurates B, Bulun SE. Endometriosis: the ultimate hormonal disease. Semin Reprod Med 2003; 21: 125–34

16. Guzick DS. Clinical epidemiology of endometriosis and infertility. Obstet Gynecol Clin North Am 1989; 16: 43–59

17. Kuohung W, Jones GL, Vitonis AF, et al. Characteristics of patients with endometriosis in the United States and the United Kingdom. Fertil Steril 2002; 78: 767–72

18. Arumugam K, Templeton AA. Endometriosis and race. Aust NZ J Obstet Gynaecol 1992; 32: 164–5

19. Vercellini P, Trespidi L, De Giorgi O, et al. Endometriosis and pelvic pain: relation to disease stage and localization. Fertil Steril 1996; 65: 299–304

20. Fukaya T, Hoshiai H, Yajima A. Is pelvic endometriosis always associated with chronic pain? A retrospective study of 618 cases diagnosed by laparoscopy. Am J Obstet Gynecol 1993; 169: 719–22

21. Porpora MG, Koninckx PR, Piazze J, et al. Correlation between endometriosis and pelvic pain. J Am Assoc Gynecol Laparosc 1999; 6: 429–34

22. Koike H, Egawa H, Ohtsuka T, et al. Correlation between dysmenorrheic severity and prostaglandin production in women with endometriosis. Prostaglandins Leukot Essent Fatty Acids 1992; 46: 133–7

23. Heaps JM, Nieberg RK, Berek JS. Malignant neoplasms arising in endometriosis. Obstet Gynecol 1990; 75: 1023–8

24. Modesitt SC, Tortolero-Luna G, Robinson JB, et al. Ovarian and extraovarian endometriosis-associated cancer. Obstet Gynecol 2002; 100: 788–95

25. Matorras R, Rodriguez F, Pijoan JI, et al. Are there any clinical signs and symptoms that are related to endometriosis in infertile women? Am J Obstet Gynecol 1996; 174: 620–3

26. Propst AM, Storti K, Barbieri RL. Lateral cervical displacement is associated with endometriosis. Fertil Steril 1998; 70: 568–70

27. Parazzini F, Fedele L, Busacca M, et al. Postsurgical medical treatment of advanced endometriosis: results of a randomized clinical trial. Am J Obstet Gynecol 1994; 171: 1205–7

28. Chen FP, Soong YK, Lee N, Lo SK. The use of serum CA-125 as a marker for endometriosis in patients with dysmenorrhea for monitoring therapy and for recurrence of endometriosis. Acta Obstet Gynecol Scand 1998; 77: 665–70

29. Spaczynski RZ, Duleba AJ. Diagnosis of endometriosis. Semin Reprod Med 2003; 21: 193–208

30. Mais V, Guerriero S, Ajossa S, et al. The efficiency of transvaginal ultrasonography in the diagnosis of endometrioma. Fertil Steril 1993; 60: 776–80

31. Ascher SM, Agrawal R, Bis KG, et al. Endometriosis: appearance and detection with conventional and contrast-enhanced fat-suppressed spin-echo techniques. J Magn Reson Imaging 1995; 5: 251–7

32. Kinkel K, Chapron C, Balleyguier C, et al. Magnetic resonance imaging characteristics of deep endometriosis. Hum Reprod 1999; 14: 1080–6

33. Nisolle M, Donnez J. Peritoneal endometriosis, ovarian endometriosis, and adenomyotic nodules of the rectovaginal septum are three different entities. Fertil Steril 1997; 68: 585–96

34. Candiani GB, Vercellini P, Fedele L. Laparoscopic ovarian puncture for correct staging of endometriosis. Fertil Steril 1990; 53: 994–7

35. Hornstein MD, Gleason RE, Orav J, et al. The reproducibility of the revised American Fertility Society classification of endometriosis. Fertil Steril 1993; 59: 1015–21

36. Bruner KL, Eisenberg E, Gorstein F, Osteen KG. Progesterone and transforming growth factor-beta coordinately regulate suppression of endometrial matrix metalloproteinases in a model of experimental endometriosis. Steroids 1999; 64: 648–53

37. Hull ME, Moghissi KS, Magyar DF, Hayes MF. Comparison of different treatment modalities of endometriosis in infertile women. Fertil Steril 1987; 47: 40–4

38. Fedele L, Bianchi S, Viezzoli T, et al. Gestrinone versus danazol in the treatment of endometriosis. Fertil Steril 1989; 51: 781–5

39. Vercellini P, Trespidi L, Colombo A, et al. A gonadotropin-releasing hormone agonist versus a low-dose oral contraceptive for pelvic pain associated with endometriosis. Fertil Steril 1993; 60: 75–9

40. Ling FW. Randomized controlled trial of depot leuprolide in patients with chronic pelvic pain and clinically suspected endometriosis. Pelvic Pain Study Group. Obstet Gynecol 1999; 93: 51–8

41. Paoletti AM, Serra GG, Cagnacci A, et al. Spontaneous reversibility of bone loss induced by gonadotropin-releasing hormone analog treatment. Fertil Steril 1996; 65: 707–10

42. Gargiulo AR, Hornstein MD. The role of GnRH agonists plus add-back therapy in the treatment of endometriosis. Semin Reprod Endocrinol 1997; 15: 273–84

43. Hornstein MD, Surrey ES, Weisberg GW, Casino LA. Leuprolide acetate depot and hormonal add-back in endometriosis: a 12-month study. Lupron Add-Back Study Group. Obstet Gynecol 1998; 91: 16–24

44. Barbieri RL. Gonadotropin-releasing hormone agonists: treatment of endometriosis. Clin Obstet Gynecol 1993; 36: 636–41

45. Moghissi KS, Schlaff WD, Olive DL, et al. Goserelin acetate (Zoladex) with or without hormone replacement therapy for the treatment of endometriosis. Fertil Steril 1998; 69: 1056–62

46. Finkelstein JS, Arnold AL. Increases in bone mineral density after discontinuation of daily human parathyroid hormone and gonadotropin-releasing hormone analog administration in women with endometriosis. J Clin Endocrinol Metab 1999; 84: 1214–19

47. Surrey ES, Voigt B, Fournet N, Judd HL. Prolonged gonadotropin-releasing hormone agonist treatment of symptomatic endometriosis: the role of cyclic sodium etidronate and low-dose norethindrone 'add-back' therapy. Fertil Steril 1995; 63: 747–55

48. Barbieri RL, Hornstein MD. Medical therapy for endometriosis. In Liss AR, ed. Endometriosis. New York: Alan R. Liss, Inc., 1987: 111

49. Dmowski WP, Kapetanakis E, Scommegna A. Variable effects of danazol on endometriosis at 4 low-dose levels. Obstet Gynecol 1982; 59: 408–15

50. Barbieri RL, Evans S, Kistner RW. Danazol in the treatment of endometriosis: analysis of 100 cases with a 4-year follow-up. Fertil Steril 1982; 37: 737–46

51. Bulun SE, Zeitoun K, Takayama K, et al. Estrogen production in endometriosis and use of aromatase inhibitors to treat endometriosis. Endocr Relat Cancer 1999; 6: 293–301

52. Zeitoun KM, Bulun SE. Aromatase: a key molecule in the pathophysiology of endometriosis and a therapeutic target. Fertil Steril 1999; 72: 961–9

53. Takayama K, Zeitoun K, Gunby RT, et al. Treatment of severe postmenopausal endometriosis with an aromatase inhibitor. Fertil Steril 1998; 69: 709–13

54. Soysal S, Soysal ME, Ozer S, et al. The effects of post-surgical administration of goserelin plus anastrozole compared to goserelin alone in patients with severe endometriosis: a prospective randomized trial. Hum Reprod 2004; 19: 160–7

55. Kettel LM, Murphy AA, Mortola JF, et al. Endocrine responses to long-term administration of the antiprogesterone RU486 in patients with pelvic endometriosis. Fertil Steril 1991; 56: 402–7

56. Redwine DB. Treatment of endometriosis-associated pain. Infertil Reprod Med Clin Am 1994; 3: 697–720

57. Barbieri RL. Endometriosis 1990. Current treatment approaches. Drugs 1990; 39: 502–10

58. Adamson GD, Pasta DJ. Surgical treatment of endometriosis-associated infertility: meta-analysis compared with survival analysis. Am J Obstet Gynecol 1994; 171: 1488–505

59. Marcoux S, Maheux R, Bérubé S. Laparoscopic surgery in infertile women with minimal or mild endometriosis. Canadian Collaborative Group on Endometriosis. N Engl J Med 1997; 337: 217–22

60. Reich H, McGlynn F. Treatment of ovarian endometriomas using laparoscopic surgical techniques. J Reprod Med 1986; 31: 577–84

61. Fayez JA, Vogel MF. Comparison of different treatment methods of endometriomas by laparoscopy. Obstet Gynecol 1991; 78: 660–5

62. Kojima E, Morita M, Otaka K, Yano Y. Nd:YAG laser laparoscopy for ovarian endometriomas. J Reprod Med 1990; 35: 592–6

63. Matorras R, Elorriaga MA, Pijoan JI, et al. Recurrence of endometriosis in women with bilateral adnexectomy (with or without total hysterectomy) who received hormone replacement therapy. Fertil Steril 2002; 77: 303–8

64. Manson JE, Hsia J, Johnson KC, et al. Estrogen plus progestin and the risk of coronary heart disease. N Engl J Med 2003; 349: 523–34

Painful menstruation: primary dysmenorrhea

3

A. Perheentupa and R. Erkkola

INTRODUCTION

The term dysmenorrhea is derived from the Greek (*dys*, difficult; *men*, month) and in medical terms means painful menstruation. Primary dysmenorrhea is defined as lower abdominal pain during menstrual bleeding in the absence of pelvic pathology. Dysmenorrhea is a very common complaint particularly among adolescent girls. It is so frequent that many girls and women fail to report it in medical interviews, even when it regularly interferes with their daily activities. Primary dysmenorrhea can be disabling and causes high rates of school and work absenteeism. Although our understanding of the etiology and physiology of primary dysmenorrhea has increased and the available treatments have improved, a great proportion of affected young girls unfortunately never seek medical advice, and thus their problem remains untreated.

Prostaglandins (PGs) have several important roles in female reproductive physiology. With regard to uterine function they stimulate uterine contractions, the intensity and frequency of which change throughout the menstrual cycle; more contractions occur during menstruation itself especially in women with dysmenorrhea compared with women without pain. In women with primary dys-

menorrhea prostaglandin release is increased. During contractions uterine blood flow is reduced leading to ischemia which may contribute to menstrual pain. The role of PGs is crucial in primary dysmenorrhea and the inhibition of their production is the cornerstone of its medical treatment. Therefore, a short overview of PG biosynthesis and factors involved in the process is included in this chapter.

Non-steroidal anti-inflammatory drugs (NSAIDs) have retained their role as the primary medical treatment. If pain relief with NSAIDs is not sufficient and contraception is also an issue, a trial treatment with combined oral contraceptive pill (COC) should be offered. Those who do not respond to either of these treatments should undergo laparoscopy in order to exclude secondary causes of dysmenorrhea.

Primary dysmenorrhea presents an unorthodox challenge. Whereas efficient modes of management exist, awareness of the problem and the availability of successful treatments need to be increased through means of education. The socioeconomic impact of the high prevalence of dysmenorrhea which may lead to recurrent absenteeism should not be underestimated. Those involved in adolescent health care have an important role in counseling girls about menstruation-associated symptoms and evaluating the need for treatment of dysmenorrhea.

ETIOLOGY

Primary dysmenorrhea is defined as lower abdominal pain during menses in the absence of identifiable pelvic pathology. The pain may be accompanied by gastrointestinal and neurological symptoms, e.g. nausea, vomiting, diarrhea, dizziness and headache. Primary dysmenorrhea is typically associated with ovulatory cycles. Its primary cause remains incompletely understood, but evidently, potent PGs and, possibly, leukotrienes (LTs) are involved in generating the symptoms (Figure 1).

Hyperactivity of the uterus in women with primary dysmenorrhea was first suggested in 1932[1]. Administration of $PGF_{2\alpha}$ causes uterine contractions and vasoconstriction resulting in pain similar to that of dysmenorrhea. While the contractility is increased, there is no unusual uterine sensitivity to $PGF_{2\alpha}$ in dysmenorrheic women, they simply seem to have increased endometrial production of the PGs[2]. The most excessive release of the PGs occurs during the first 2 days of menstrual bleeding; this is closely associated with the severity of symptoms. $PGF_{2\alpha}$ activity in menstrual blood was reported to be doubled in dysmenorrheic compared with asymptomatic women[3,4]. An even greater difference was observed in the endometrial $PGF_{2\alpha}$ levels during the first day of the menstrual cycle – the dysmenorrheic levels were four-fold[5]. In dysmenorrheic women intrauterine pressure may increase to 200 mmHg during the contractions[6]. However, it is the elevated resting pressure and increased frequency of contractions that are most clearly associated with the ischemic pain[7]. Reflecting this, Doppler ultrasonography shows elevated flow impedance at all levels of uterine arteries in dysmenorrheic women[8].

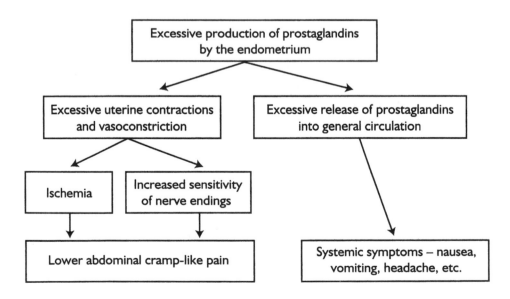

Figure 1 Schematic presentation of the etiology of primary dysmenorrhea

There is increasing evidence of the involvement of LTs in the etiology of dysmenorrhea. LTs are potent vasoconstrictors and also mediators of inflammation that may cause uterine contractions. In addition to PGs, excess levels of LTs have been observed in women suffering from primary dysmenorrhea[9]. Endometrial LT concentrations were highest in women with dysmenorrhea[10]. Furthermore, a close correlation was observed between menstrual blood levels of LTC_4 and LTD_4 and the severity of dysmenorrhea[11]. Moreover, increased urinary output of LTE_4 has been demonstrated in adolescent girls with dysmenorrhea[12]. It seems likely that LTs in concert with PGs generate the symptoms of primary dysmenorrhea. However, other factors may well exist.

Biosynthesis of prostaglandins and leukotrienes

PGs are produced in practically all cells of the human body. The biosynthesis of PG is mainly regulated by the liberation of arachidonic acid from the membrane-bound phospholipids, primarily by phospholipase A_2. Phospholipase A_2 requires calcium and calmodulin to be activated. PGG_2 and PGH_2 are formed from arachidonic acid in reactions induced by the two cyclo-oxygenase enzymes, COX-1 and COX-2. First the cyclo-oxygenase activity forms a cyclic endoperoxide PGG_2 and, subsequently, PGH_2 is formed as a result of the peroxidase activity of the COX enzymes. PGH_2 can be metabolized further by different enzyme pathways to a range of biologically active products. Downstream enzymes determine the final products made by cells expressing COX-1 and COX-2. PGs D_2, E_2, I_2 and thromboxane A_2 are synthesized from PGH_2 by specific PGD,

PGE, PGI and thromboxane synthases, respectively. Some of these synthases may be inducible in certain situation, e.g. pregnancy or labor. PGF_2 is synthesized through three different pathways from PGE_2, PGD_2 and PGH_2 by PGE 9-ketoreductase, PGD 11-ketoreductase and PGH 9-, 11-endoperoxide reductase, respectively (Figure 2; for review see reference 13).

Since the 1990s it has been clear that COX-1 and COX-2 are responsible for the production of PGH_2, which is the first step in the synthesis of the PGs. Although COX-1 and 2 are products of two different genes, they share approximately 60% amino acid homology, and have similar molecular mass (70 kDa) and identical length. They both catalyze the formation of PGH_2 from arachidonic acid. Although COX-1 and COX-2 have nearly identical kinetic properties, COX-1 shows negative alloterism at low arachidonic acid levels suggesting that COX-2 may more readily bind to available arachidonic acid. The COX-1 gene has several features of a house-keeping gene. In contrast, the COX-2 gene is a primary response gene with a number of regulatory sites.

Accordingly, COX-1 appears to be responsible for a steady physiological production of PGs. Small physiological amounts of PGE_2 are constantly produced to protect the gastric mucosa, and prostacyclin from the endothelial cells inhibits platelet aggregation. COX-2 induces the increased PG production that occurs during disease and inflammation. Thus, theoretically, COX-2 should be the primary therapeutic target (e.g. anti-inflammatories), while COX-1 inhibition is undesirable as it results in side-effects. Unfortunately, the roles of COX-1 and COX-2 are probably not quite so clear cut in all organs. Contrary to

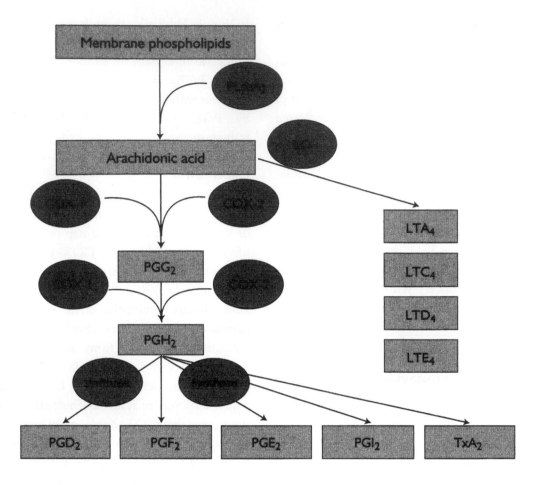

Figure 2 Biosynthesis of prostaglandins and leukotrienes. PLseA2, phospholipase A_2; LO, lipoxygenase; COX, cyclo-oxygenase; PG, prostaglandin; TxA_2, thromboxane; LT, leukotriene

earlier belief, COX-2 seems to be constitutively expressed in some tissues such as the kidney. COX-2 inhibitors should still not be used in patients with active gastrointestinal ulceration or bleeding. COX-2 inhibition may in some patients cause sodium and potassium retention.

Glucocorticoids inhibit the liberation of arachidonic acid by inducing the synthesis of lipocortin that inhibits the activity of phospholipase. Also, glucocorticoids decrease the amount of COX-2 thus alleviating inflammation.

A third COX enzyme, COX-3, appears to be formed as a splice variant of COX-1. In humans, COX-3 appears to be expressed most abundantly in the cerebral cortex and heart. Its inhibition could represent a primary central mechanism by which the drugs decrease pain and possibly fever. Paracetamol, with its well-established analgesic and antipyretic effects but little anti-inflammatory action, may act through an inhibitory effect on COX-3 activity[14]. However, the physiological significance of

COX-3 in human remains to be properly proven[13].

LTs are synthesized (together with other eicosanoids) from membrane phospholipids (arachidonic acid) through the lipoxygenase enzyme pathway. The LTs are mainly produced by myeloid-derived cells in the lungs and the uterus[15]. Receptors for LTs are located in the plasma membranes of smooth muscle cells and other types of cells. Most of the biological effects of LTs are mediated through LT receptor type 1, a glycosylated G-protein-coupled receptor. LT antagonists are competitors of LTD_4 for binding to the LT_1 receptor. In the uterus, the LTs stimulate contractions in smooth muscle[16]. Patients with primary dysmenorrhea have excessive amounts of LTs in the endometrium and myometrial smooth muscle[16]. In these women, excessive uterine concentrations of LTC_4 and LTD_4 have been demonstrated[10,11] (for review see reference 17).

Presentation and prevalence

Primary dysmenorrhea typically presents in adolescence, usually 2–3 years after the menarche. Symptoms seldom start during the first 6 months after menarche, probably because initial cycles are anovulatory. Although dysmenorrhea is the most common gynecological complaint of adolescent girls, it may only be revealed when the medical history is taken. The intensity of the pain ranges from a dull ache to tightening sensation, contractions, and sometimes to intolerable colic-like pain. Sharp intermittent waves of cramps in the suprapubic area are typical. But also, the pain may radiate to the inguinal region, lower back and/or to the back of the legs. Systemic symptoms are common and may include nausea, vomiting, diarrhea, fatigue, fever, irritability, myalgia, dizziness and headache. The pain usually begins within hours before or after the start of menstruation and its intensity follows the amount of menstrual flow, being worse during the first day or two. Several risk factors for severe episodes of dysmenorrhea have been suspected: early age at menarche, long menstrual periods, obesity and smoking[18]. However, other studies have not confirmed all of them. Family antecedents (grandmother, mother, sister with dysmenorrhea) have been observed in 39% of the adolescent patients[19]. Women with dysmenorrhea may have an increased risk of other syndromes associated with pain, e.g. migraine[20], fibromyalgia[21], and irritable bowel syndrome[22].

Critical evaluation of the publications on the frequency of dysmenorrhea is compromised by the subjective nature of the symptoms that are difficult if not impossible to standardize. This partly explains the large variation of findings across different studies. Although, generally, symptoms are thought to decrease with age and particularly as a result of parturition, no consensus exists about these effects. A limited number of studies exist on the prevalence of dysmenorrhea. Andersch and Milsom[23] found that 72% of unselected 19-year-old Swedish women reported dysmenorrhea, with nearly 40% regularly using medication for the pain. Of these women, 18% had consequently limited their daily activities and felt no alleviation of the symptoms by analgesics, and 8% stayed absent from work or school at every period. The majority of women suffer from dysmenorrhea during the first three postmenarchal years. According to a study in the United States, 60% of menstruating young women suffered from dysmenorrhea and 14% regularly missed school. Only 29% of those who experienced severe dysmenorrhea had consulted a health-care professional with their problem[24]. In another study, 73% of high-school girls reported menstrual pains, but a mere 16% had discussed the problem with their doctor or nurse. Only 26% of the girls who missed school or work because of dysmenorrhea had discussed the subject with a health-care professional[25]. Of those who did not seek advice, 68% thought their cramps were not severe enough to warrant medical advice, 20% felt sceptical about the alleviation provided by medical treatment, 5% were afraid of the gynecological examination, and 3% did not know where to go for advice[25]. Despite the above, a vast majority of adolescent girls use a variety of non-pharmacological methods (e.g. rest, topical heat, etc.) to treat the symptoms of dysmenorrhea, albeit with limited success[26]. Furthermore, up to 70% admitted using non-prescription drugs at one time or another to treat cramps, but most were unaware of the adequate doses required for pain alleviation[27].

Some estimate that dysmenorrhea is the single most important reason for lost working hours and school absence. However, the data are scant and no studies have prospectively examined the cost or the impact of dysmenorrhea on quality of life.

INVESTIGATIONS

The diagnosis of primary dysmenorrhea is one of exclusion. If symptoms are typical of primary dysmenorrhea, a therapeutic trial may be embarked on before considering any examination and investigation especially in adolescents. Due to the high incidence of Chlamydia and human papilloma virus infections and the severity of their possible complications, cervical smear and Chlamydia test are indicated in sexually active adolescents who complain of menstrual symptoms. Other laboratory tests are seldom required. If clinical evaluation raises suspicion of secondary causes of dysmenorrhea, such as endometriosis or pelvic inflammatory disease, then laparoscopy should be considered. Likewise, if symptoms of primary dysmenorrhea are not alleviated either with prostaglandin inhibitors or treatment with COC, 3 months each, in this order, or the combination of the two, secondary causes of dysmenorrhea need to be considered and pelvic pathology excluded. Secondary dysmenorrhea should also be suspected: if symptoms start after the age of 25 years; if they begin with the very first few menstrual cycles; and if those initially typical of primary dysmenorrhea worsen in duration (starting premenstrually) and intensity.

In individual cases, e.g. with suspicion of pelvic anomalies, pelvic imaging using transvaginal ultrasound or magnetic resonance imaging may be warranted.

MANAGEMENT

Even the severe symptoms of dysmenorrhea can be effectively alleviated with sufficient pharmacological management. The patient should be advised about the importance of starting the NSAID as soon as any symptoms or menstrual bleeding appear and of continuing regular intake until the pain has subsided (Table 1). In addition to the well-established drugs, NSAIDs, and COC, several other forms of treatment are available. A number of drugs that have been shown to decrease the uterine contractility, and thus the symptoms, will also be discussed shortly.

Table 1 Pharmacological treatment of primary dysmenorrhea. Medication should be started as soon as any symptoms or menstrual bleeding are evident and continued until symptoms subside

Pharmaceutical agent	Usual dose
NSAIDs	
Naproxen sodium	550 mg initially, then 275 mg every 8 h
Ibuprofen	400–600 mg every 6 h as required
Ketoprofen	50–100 mg every 8 h as required
Diclofenac	50 mg every 8–12 h as required
Mefenamic acid	500 mg initially, then 250 mg every 6 h

NSAIDS, non-steroidal anti-inflammatory drugs

Non-steroidal anti-inflammatory drugs

NSAIDs have anti-inflammatory, antipyretic and analgesic properties and have been used widely in the treatment of pain for years. NSAIDs are inhibitors of the cyclo-oxygenase enzyme pathway and, consequently, reduce the production of PGs. NSAIDs inhibit both COX-1 and COX-2. Some NSAIDs more readily inhibit COX-1 than COX-2. Lower PG levels result in uterine contractions of lower intensity and alleviated experience of discomfort and pain. Several studies have shown the efficacy of NSAIDs in providing relief from the pain of primary dysmenorrhea. NSAIDs have conventionally been the treatment of choice for primary dysmenorrhea reducing the interference of daily activities[28]. In addition, NSAIDs reduce menstrual flow (see Chapter 5). Propionic acid derivatives (naproxen, ibuprofen, ketoprofen and diclofenac) and the fenamates (mefenamic acid, meclofenamate and flufenamic acid) have all been used with success in relieving the pain associated with primary dysmenorrhea[29,30]. No single NSAID has been shown to display significant advantages over others in the treatment of dysmenorrhea[31,32]. However, ibuprofen may be preferred because of its favorable efficacy and safety profile[31]. There are data supporting the use of an initial loading dose (double the regular dose) for the optimal response to NSAIDs treatment[33]. NSAIDs should then be continued with the regular dose until symptoms subside. The patient should be advised to take NSAIDs with food in order to minimize the gastrointestinal side-effects. About 80% (64–100%) of dysmenorrheic women obtain symptom relief with NSAIDs therapy[34] (Table 1).

As a point of interest, traditional healers have used plants with significant COX inhibitory activity to treat menstrual pain[35].

COX-2 inhibitors

The cyclo-oxygenase pathway is the main route for oxidative metabolism of arachidonic acid to the PGs. Two COX enzymes exist, and are very similar in structure. They do, however, differ significantly in their regulation and expression. COX-1 is involved in homeostasis (integrity of the gastric mucosa, renal tract and platelet aggregation) and it is expressed constitutively. COX-2 in turn is more involved in pathways of inflammation and pain. NSAIDs non-specifically inhibit both of the COX enzymes. Many of the adverse effects observed with conventional NSAIDs, particularly disruption of platelet function, and gastrointestinal ulceration and bleeding are consequences of the inhibition of the COX-1 enzyme. NSAIDs largely exert their therapeutic effects by inhibiting COX-2 and their gastrointestinal adverse effects by inhibiting COX-1. Even short-term use of conventional NSAIDs is associated with gastrointestinal symptoms in some patients.

Specific inhibitors of the COX-2 were developed in the 1990s. They provide analgesia with fewer gastrointestinal side-effects.

COX-2 inhibitors provide an efficient therapeutic alternative to conventional NSAIDs in treating primary dysmenorrhea. Since in the doses used these agents have little or no effects on COX-1, it can be concluded that the efficacy of NSAIDs in the treatment of pain accounts for the inhibition of COX-2. The COX-2 inhibitors, rofecoxib and valdecoxib, have recently been withdrawn from the market due to increased risk of cardiovascular events.

The combined oral contraceptive pill

COCs are the second-line therapy for most women unless contraception is also required. In such cases they are the obvious treatment of choice. However, commonly used clinically, solid evidence supporting their efficacy in primary dysmenorrhea is limited. The COCs are thought to reduce the endometrial production of PGs and LTs by limiting endometrial thickness and therefore reducing the amount of endometrial tissue available to produce these mediators. Furthermore, COCs inhibit ovulation. Several small studies have evaluated the effect of COCs. Lower $PGF_{2\alpha}$ levels of menstrual fluid have been reported in two women with dysmenorrhea treated with COC in comparison with six women with untreated dysmenorrhea or eumenorrhea[36]. In another study, the concentrations of both PG and LT were found to be lower in the menstrual fluid of women taking COCs[9]. In a study by Creatsas et al.[37] serum levels of $PGF_{2\alpha}$ and PGE_2 were measured in ten adolescent women

with dysmenorrhea before and after a cycle of COC (50 µg ethinylestradiol and 2.5 mg lynestrenol). Slightly lower PG levels were observed on the first day of bleeding following the COC treatment; furthermore, the patients reported alleviation in the symptoms of dysmenorrhea. Similar studies have found highly variable serum levels of $PGF_{2\alpha}$ and vasopressin and no differences in the levels of first day of bleeding[38]. As the increased intrauterine pressure appears to be significant in causing the symptoms of dysmenorrhea, the findings of decreased intrauterine pressure and alleviated pain following treatment with modern COCs appear perhaps most convincing[39,40]. The conclusion from these studies is that COCs may alleviate pain through reduction of the production of the PGs and LTs and consequently uterine contractions. Several larger studies have confirmed this beneficial effect of COC on symptoms of dysmenorrhea with both monophasic and triphasic formulations[41,42]. COCs are estimated to be effective in about 70% of patients[43].

In addition to the relief of primary dysmenorrhea, COCs offer effective protection from unwanted pregnancies and abortions, which remain a high concern among the adolescents having often unplanned sex. There seem to be surprising unwarranted fears associated with the use of COCs, risk of cancer being the main concern. Most patients are unaware of the health benefits of COCs, yet, particularly in women suffering from severe dysmenorrhea, the health benefits of COCs clearly outweigh their risks[43]. COCs are effective in treatment of acne, irregular menstrual periods, iron deficiency, and in the prevention of pelvic inflammatory disease. The use of COCs also protects against ovarian and endometrial cancer, and probably has beneficial effects on bone mineral density, and against colorectal carcinoma, uterine leiomyomas and toxic shock syndrome.

COCs containing a potent progestogen (e.g. desogestrel or levonorgestrel) may offer better efficacy for pain relief and may be preferred for girls with severe symptoms[44]. Women using COCs and suffering symptoms of dysmenorrhea during the pill-free interval, should be considered for an uninterrupted cycle regimen with menstrual bleeding every 3–6 months. Such extended regimens appear to be well tolerated and efficacious in alleviating menstrual symptoms[45,46]. The combined hormonal contraception in the form of a patch or a vaginal ring may reduce the side-effects and improve patient compliance. The recently introduced COC containing a new progestin, drospirenone, which has some anti-mineralo-corticoid effects, may present fewer side-effects than its predecessors[47]. Poor compliance however, is seldom a real problem as those dysmenorrheic women who get pain alleviation from the COC are far more likely to continue therapy than non-responders.

Other hormonal methods

NSAIDs and COCs comprise the usual treatment of primary dysmenorrhea. COCs prevent menstrual pain through a different mechanism than NSAIDs, and there is no reason why these two treatments should not be combined. However, it is logical to avoid the combination of COX-2 inhibitors and COCs as their co-use may increase the risk of cardiovascular problems. Patients with special needs, poor tolerance of or compliance with these treatments may require other approaches (e.g. mentally handi-capped women, who may have problems with menstrual hygiene).

Although primarily designed for parous women, the levonorgestrel-releasing intra-uterine system (LNG-IUS, Mirena®, Schering AG, Berlin) may be an effective treatment for nulliparous adolescent women who have trouble in remembering to take daily oral medication or who would rather have minimal menstrual bleedings. In older women (25–47 years old), the frequency of menstrual pain decreased from 60% to 29% after 36 months' use of LNG-IUS[50]. In cases where the effects of this treatment seem desirable, but insertion is difficult, the LNG-IUS can be inserted during a brief general anesthestic. The LNG-IUS dramatically reduces the amount of menstrual bleeding through strong suppression of endometrial growth. Amenorrhea results typically in about 50% of women following LNG-IUS insertion[48]. The LNG-IUS may even be effective in alleviating the pain associated with endometriosis[49]. Other alternatives include the progestogen implants, or the long-acting medroxyprogesterone acetate (DMPA) injection. The levonorgestrel-releasing implants disrupt follicular growth and ovulation with the ensuing endometrial changes. On the other hand, the desogestrel-releasing implants suppress ovulation[50]. Both implants are effective in providing relief of dysmenorrhea. Amenorrhea develops in about 30–40% of desogestrel and 20–30% of levonorgestrel users by 12 months of treatment[51]. DMPA injections are required every 3 months for effective contraception[52]. Amenorrhea is experienced by a majority of women using DMPA injections, and this consequently alleviates symptoms of both menorrhagia and dysmenorrhea.

Some of the new progestogen-only contraceptive pills (e.g. 75 μg desogestrel) effectively inhibit ovulation and thus probably relieve symptoms of dysmenorrhea.

Other methods

Several other therapies for alleviation of dysmenorrhea have been tried. Benefits may be gained through dietary changes[53], cessation of smoking[54] and increase in the amount of physical exercise[55]. Small observational studies have reported improvement of dysmenorrhea following interventions by herbal preparations[56], topical heat[57] and transcutaneous nerve stimulation[58].

A number of other pharmaceutical agents exist that alleviate the symptoms of dysmenorrhea. Vasopressin, better known as a vasoconstrictor, causes contractions of the (non-pregnant) uterus. Dysmenorrheic women have elevated levels of circulating vasopressin[59]. An orally active vasopressin VIa receptor antagonist has been shown to be effective in preventing dysmenorrhea in young women[60].

Beta-adrenergic agonists have a utero-relaxing quality, which could be used to alleviate the uterine discomfort of dysmenorrhea. Vaginal administration of such an agonist could diminish typical side-effects associated with oral administration[61]. Ca^{2+} channel blockers are better tolerated and could be effective in decreasing uterine contractility[62]. Transdermal glyceryl trinitrate has also been evaluated[63]. Recently, vitamin E was reported to be effective in the treatment of adolescent dysmenorrhea[64]. In this study, the severity of pain was significantly reduced even in the placebo group. A randomized control study found supplementation with omega-3 polyunsaturated fatty acids

beneficial in the management of dysmenorrhea in adolescents[65]. The mode of action is presumed to involve altered PG synthesis.

CONCLUSIONS

In conclusion, dysmenorrhea leads to significant morbidity in adolescent girls, a large part of which is undertreated if not untreated. This is very unfortunate, as effective treatment options are presently available. It remains an important task to educate and counsel these young patients both on the problem itself and on the alleviating treatments that are available. This is a challenge for all pediatricians, gynecologists and generalists who treat these adolescents. In order to ensure basic knowledge of common menstrual problems, it would seem logical to include this topic in the regular school curriculum of all pupils. Suspicion, proper diagnosis and treatment thereafter of secondary dysmenorrhea should be a high priority, as early treatment not only reduces human suffering but may also benefit long-term reproductive health.

PRACTICE POINTS

- Primary dysmenorrhea is defined as painful menstruation in the absence of pelvic pathology
- Primary dysmenorrhea is very common; it may, however, first be revealed through careful medical history
- The diagnosis of primary dysmenorrhea is based on characteristic medical history and requires exclusion of other causes
- The endometrium secretes prostaglandins in excess in women with primary dysmenorrhea

- Primary dysmenorrhea is typically associated with ovulatory cycles and increased uterine contractility
- The COX-2 enzyme is responsible for inducing the elevated prostaglandin levels in disease and inflammation
- NSAIDs are the first line of pharmacological treatment
- If COX inhibition does not effectively alleviate the symptoms or if contraception is required, combined oral contraceptive pills should be used
- Uninterrupted use of an oral contraceptive is an effective and well-tolerated treatment option

- Patients with special needs may benefit most from optional treatment, e.g. levonorgestrel-releasing intrauterine system
- Treatment of secondary dysmenorrhea should be a high priority as it may benefit the long-term reproductive health
- The doctors and nurses involved in adolescent health care should inform their patient of the symptoms of primary dysmenorrhea, available treatments and practical points regarding management
- It would seem logical to include menstrual problems as one topic in the general curriculum of all pupils to ensure basic knowledge of these common complaints

REFERENCES

1. Novak E, Reynolds SRM. The cause of primary dysmenorrhea with special reference to hormonal factors. JAMA 1932; 99: 1466–72

2. Lumsden MA, Kelly RW, Baird DT. Is prostaglandin F_2 alpha involved in the increased myometrial contractility of primary dysmenorrhea? Prostaglandins 1983; 25: 683–92

3. Chan WY, Hill JC. Determination of menstrual prostaglandin levels in non-dysmenorrheic and dysmenorrheic subjects. Prostaglandins 1978; 15: 365–75

4. Rees MC, Anderson AB, Demers LM, et al. Prostaglandins in menstrual fluid in menorrhagia and dysmenorrhoea. Br J Obstet Gynaecol 1984; 91: 673–80

5. Lundstrom V, Green K. Endogenous levels of prostaglandin F_2alpha and its main metabolites in plasma and endometrium of normal and dysmenorrheic women. Am J Obstet Gynecol 1978; 130: 640–6

6. Pulkkinen MO. Alterations in intrauterine pressure, menstrual fluid prostaglandin F levels, and pain in dysmenorrheic women treated with nimesulide. J Clin Pharmacol 1987; 27: 65–9

7. Csapo AI, Pulkkinen MO, Henzl MR. The effect of naproxen-sodium on the intrauterine pressure and menstrual pain of dysmenorrheic patients. Prostaglandins 1977; 13: 193–9

8. Pirhonen J, Pulkkinen M. The effect of nimesulide and naproxen on the uterine and ovarian arterial blood flow velocity. A Doppler study. Acta Obstet Gynecol Scand 1995; 74: 549–53

9. Bieglmayer C, Hofer G, Kainz C, et al. Concentrations of various arachidonic acid metabolites in menstrual fluid are associated with menstrual pain and are influenced by hormonal contraceptives. Gynecol Endocrinol 1995; 9: 307–12

10. Rees MC, DiMarzo V, Tippins JR, et al. Leukotriene release by endometrium and

myometrium throughout the menstrual cycle in dysmenorrhoea and menorrhagia. J Endocrinol 1987; 113: 291–5

11. Nigam S, Benedetto C, Zonca M, et al. Increased concentrations of eicosanoids and platelet-activating factor in menstrual blood from women with primary dysmenorrhea. Eicosanoids 1991; 4: 137–41

12. Harel Z, Lilly C, Riggs S, et al. Urinary leukotriene (LT) E(4) in adolescents with dys- menorrhea: a pilot study. J Adolesc Health 2000; 27: 151–4

13. Warner TD, Mitchell JA. Cyclooxygenases: new forms, new inhibitors, and lessons from the clinic. FASEB J 2004; 18: 790–804

14. Chandrasekharan NV, Dai H, Roos LT, et al. COX-3, a cyclooxygenase-1 variant inhibited by acetaminophen and other analgesic/ antipyretic drugs: cloning, structure, and expression. Proc Natl Acad Sci USA 2002; 99: 13926–31

15. Ritchie DM, Hahn DW, McGuire JL. Smooth muscle contraction as a model to study the mediator role of endogenous lipoxygenase products of arachidonic acid. Life Sci 1984; 34: 509–13

16. Chegini N, Rao CV. The presence of leukotriene C4- and prostacyclin-binding sites in nonpregnant human uterine tissue. J Clin Endocrinol Metab 1988; 66: 76–87

17. Abu JI, Konje JC. Leukotrienes in gynae- cology: the hypothetical value of anti- leukotriene therapy in dysmenorrhoea and endometriosis. Hum Reprod Update 2000; 6: 200–5

18. Harlow SD, Park M. A longitudinal study of risk factors for the occurrence, duration and severity of menstrual cramps in a cohort of college women. Br J Obstet Gynaecol 1996; 103: 1134–42

19. Sultan C, Jeandel C, Paris F, Trimeche S. Adolescent dysmenorrhea. Endocr Dev 2004; 7: 140–7

20. Bousser MG, Massiou H. Migraine in the reproductive cycle. In Olesen J, Felt-Hansen PT, Welch KMA, eds. The Headaches. New York: Raven Press, 1993: 413–19

21. Yunus MB, Masi AT, Aldag JC. A controlled study of primary fibromyalgia syndrome: clinical features and association with other functional syndromes. J Rheumatol Suppl 1989; 19: 62–71

22. Jamieson DJ, Steege JF. The prevalence of dysmenorrhea, dyspareunia, pelvic pain, and irritable bowel syndrome in primary care practices. Obstet Gynecol 1996; 87: 55–8

23. Andersch B, Milsom I. An epidemiologic study of young women with dysmenorrhea. Am J Obstet Gynecol 1982; 144: 655–60

24. Klein JR, Litt IF. Epidemiology of adolescent dysmenorrhea. Pediatrics 1981; 68: 661–4

25. Johnson J. Level of knowledge among adolescent girls regarding effective treatment for dysmenorrhea. J Adolesc Health Care 1988; 9: 398–402

26. Campbell MA, McGrath PJ. Non-pharmaco- logic strategies used by adolescents for the management of menstrual discomfort. Clin J Pain 1999; 15: 313–20

27. Campbell MA, McGrath PJ. Use of medication by adolescents for the management of menstrual discomfort. Arch Pediatr Adolesc Med 1997; 151: 905–13

28. Mehlisch DR, Fulmer RI. A crossover comparison of bromfenac sodium, naproxen sodium, and placebo for relief of pain from primary dysmenorrhea. J Womens Health 1997; 6: 83–92

29. Chan WY, Dawood MY, Fuchs F. Relief of dysmenorrhea with the prostaglandin synthetase inhibitor ibuprofen: effect on

prostaglandin levels in menstrual fluid. Am J Obstet Gynecol 1979; 135: 102–8

30. Milsom I, Andersch B. Effect of ibuprofen, naproxen sodium and paracetamol on intrauterine pressure and menstrual pain in dysmenorrhoea. Br J Obstet Gynaecol 1984; 91: 1129–35

31. Zhang WY, Li Wan Po A. Efficacy of minor analgesics in primary dysmenorrhoea: a systematic review. Br J Obstet Gynaecol 1998; 105: 780–9

32. Roy S. A double-blind comparison of a propionic acid derivative (ibuprofen) and a fenamate (mefenamic acid) in the treatment of dysmenorrhea. Obstet Gynecol 1983; 61: 628–32

33. DuRant RH, Jay MS, Shoffitt T, et al. Factors influencing adolescents' responses to regimens of naproxen for dysmenorrhea. Am J Dis Child 1985; 139: 489–93

34. Smith RP. Cyclic pelvic pain and dysmenorrhea. Obstet Gynecol Clin North Am 1993; 20: 753–64

35. Lindsey K, Jager AK, Raidoo DM, van Staden J. Screening of plants used by Southern African traditional healers in the treatment of dysmenorrhea for prostaglandin-synthesis inhibitors and uterine relaxing activity. J Ethnopharmacol 1999; 64: 9–14

36. Chan WY, Dawood MY. Prostaglandin levels in menstrual fluid of nondysmenorrheic and of dysmenorrheic subjects with and without oral contraceptive or ibuprofen therapy. Adv Prostaglandin Thromboxane Res 1980; 8: 1443–7

37. Creatsas G, Deligeoroglou E, Zachari A, et al. Prostaglandins: PGF2 alpha, PGE2, 6-keto-PGF1 alpha and TXB2 serum levels in dysmenorrheic adolescents before, during and after treatment with oral contraceptives. Eur J Obstet Gynecol Reprod Biol 1990; 36: 292–8

38. Hauksson A, Akerlund M, Forsling ML, Kindahl H. Plasma concentrations of vasopressin and a prostaglandin F2 alpha metabolite in women with primary dysmenorrhoea before and during treatment with a combined oral contraceptive. J Endocrinol 1987; 115: 355–61

39. Ekstrom P, Juchnicka E, Laudanski T, Akerlund M. Effect of an oral contraceptive in primary dysmenorrhea – changes in uterine activity and reactivity to agonists. Contraception 1989; 40: 39–47

40. Ekstrom P, Akerlund M, Forsling M, et al. Stimulation of vasopressin release in women with primary dysmenorrhoea and after oral contraceptive treatment – effect on uterine contractility. Br J Obstet Gynaecol 1992; 99: 680–4

41. Robinson JC, Plichta S, Weisman CS, et al. Dysmenorrhea and use of oral contraceptives in adolescent women attending a family planning clinic. Am J Obstet Gynecol 1992; 166: 578–83

42. Weber-Diehl F, Unger R, Lachnit U. Triphasic combination of ethinyl estradiol and gestodene. Long-term clinical trial. Contraception 1992; 46: 19–27

43. Fraser IS, Kovacs GT. The efficacy of non-contraceptive uses for hormonal contraceptives. Med J Aust 2003; 178: 621–3

44. Milsom I, Andersch B. Effect of various oral contraceptive combinations on dysmenorrhea. Gynecol Obstet Invest 1984; 17: 284–92

45. Wiegratz I, Hommel HH, Zimmermann T, Kuhl H. Attitude of German women and gynecologists towards long-cycle treatment with oral contraceptives. Contraception 2004; 69: 37–42

46. Braunstein JB, Hausfeld J, Hausfeld J, London A. Economics of reducing menstruation with trimonthly-cycle oral contraceptive therapy: comparison with standard-cycle regimens. Obstet Gynecol 2003; 102: 699–708

47. Sillem M, Schneidereit R, Heithecker R, Mueck AO. Use of an oral contraceptive containing drospirenone in an extended regimen. Eur J Contracept Reprod Health Care 2003; 8: 162–9

48. Baldaszti E, Wimmer-Puchinger B, Loschke K. Acceptability of the long-term contraceptive levonorgestrel-releasing intrauterine system (Mirena): a 3-year follow-up study. Contraception 2003; 67: 87–91

49. Fedele L, Bianchi S, Zanconato G, et al. Use of a levonorgestrel-releasing intrauterine device in the treatment of rectovaginal endometriosis. Fertil Steril 2001; 75: 485–8

50. Meirik O, Fraser IS, d'Arcangues C. Implantable contraceptives for women. Hum Reprod Update 2003; 9: 49–59

51. Varma R, Mascarenhas L. Endometrial effects of etonogestrel (Implanon) contraceptive implant. Curr Opin Obstet Gynecol 2001; 13: 335–41

52. Westhoff C. Depot-medroxyprogesterone acetate injection (Depo-Provera): a highly effective contraceptive option with proven long-term safety. Contraception 2003; 68: 75–87

53. Deutch B. Menstrual pain in Danish women correlated with low n-3 polyunsaturated fatty acid intake. Eur J Clin Nutr 1995; 49: 508–16

54. Hornby PP, Wilcox AJ, Weinber CR. Cigarette smoking and disturbance of menstrual function. Epidemiology 1998; 9: 193–8

55. Golomb LM, Solidum AA, Warren MP. Primary dysmenorrhea and physical activity. Med Sci Sports Exerc 1998; 30: 906–9

56. Kotani N, Oyama T, Sakai I, et al. Analgesic effect of a herbal medicine for treatment of primary dysmenorrhea – a double-blind study. Am J Chin Med 1997; 25: 205–12

57. Akin MD, Weingand KW, Hengehold DA, et al. Continuous low-level topical heat in the treatment of dysmenorrhea. Obstet Gynecol 2001; 97: 343–9

58. Kaplan B, Rabinerson D, Lurie S, et al. Clinical evaluation of a new model of a transcutaneous electrical nerve stimulation device for the management of primary dysmenorrhea. Gynecol Obstet Invest 1997; 44: 255–9

59. Åkerlund M, Stromberg P, Forsling ML. Primary dysmenorrhoea and vasopressin. Br J Obstet Gynaecol 1979; 86: 484–7

60. Brouard R, Bossmar T, Fournie-Lloret D, et al. Effect of SR49059, an orally active V1a vasopressin receptor antagonist, in the prevention of dysmenorrhoea. Br J Obstet Gynaecol 2000; 107: 614–19

61. Bulletti C, de Ziegler D, de Moustier B, et al. Uterine contractility: vaginal administration of the beta-adrenergic agonist, terbutaline. Evidence of direct vagina-to-uterus transport. Ann N Y Acad Sci 2001; 943: 163–71

62. Bakheet DM, El Tahir KE, Al-Sayed MI, et al. Studies on the spasmolytic and uterine relaxant actions of n -ethyl and n -benzyl-1,2-diphenyl ethanolamines: elucidation of the mechanisms of action. Pharmacol Res 1999; 39: 463–70

63. Moya RA, Moisa CF, Morales F, et al. Transdermal glyceryl trinitrate in the management of primary dysmenorrhea. Int J Gynaecol Obstet 2000; 69: 113–18

64. Ziaei S, Faghihzadeh S, Sohrabvand F, et al. A randomised placebo-controlled trial to determine the effect of vitamin E in treatment of primary dysmenorrhoea. Br J Obstet Gynaecol 2001; 108: 1181–3

65. Harel Z, Biro FM, Kottenhahn RK, et al. Supplementation with omega-3 polyunsaturated fatty acids in the management of dysmenorrhea in adolescents. Am J Obstet Gynecol 1996; 174: 1335–8

Chronic pelvic pain without endometriosis

4

J. Moore

INTRODUCTION

Chronic pelvic pain (CPP) is a common condition affecting approximately one in six of the adult female population in the UK[1]. It presents in primary care as commonly as asthma and migraine[2]. For many women it is a debilitating and depressing condition that can lead to breakdown of relationships, social isolation and loss of earnings. Some women with CPP feel they do not get the help and support they need from their doctors[3]. There is a lot that is unknown or poorly understood about CPP, its etiology and how best to treat it, and this may leave the doctor feeling inadequate and uncomfortable. But even if an accurate diagnosis cannot be made, there is huge value to the patient in listening to her story, accepting the reality of her pain and attempting to treat the pain on an empirical basis if nothing else. The stories women tell of the support they receive from their general practitioners bear testament to this.

CPP has been defined in a number of ways. Some definitions require a degree of functional impairment such as time off work, while others define the condition by the presence or exclusion of specific pathology. In this chapter, however, a purely symptom-based definition is presented:

Chronic pelvic pain may be defined as pain felt in the lower abdomen or pelvis, of at least 6-months' duration, occurring continuously or intermittently, not associated exclusively with menstruation or sexual intercourse, and not associated with pregnancy or malignancy

Known possible causes of the symptom of CCP are explored and the features that might point towards a particular diagnosis are described. Suggestions for investigations and treatments are also discussed.

ETIOLOGY

The nature of chronic pain

As with other chronic pain syndromes, CPP should be viewed as a symptom with a number of contributory factors rather than a condition with a single etiology. Pain is defined as an unpleasant sensory or emotional experience associated with actual or potential tissue damage or described in those terms[4]. The sufferer's experience of the pain will inevitably be affected by such factors as other diseases or conditions, the patient's mental health, beliefs about the pain, social circumstances and so forth. Also, the balance between them does not matter but it is important to try to address all components of the pain. The balance between these factors may change over the course of the illness.

Two important points should be made about the nature of chronic pelvic pain. First, pain may arise from somatic or visceral structures and the two types of pain tend to have different characteristics.

- Somatic pain arises from the body wall and is usually highly localized
- Visceral pain tends to be more diffuse and to be associated with systemic symptoms such as nausea and vomiting

Second, the mechanism of chronic pain is very different to that of acute pain. In acute pain, nerve signals reach the central nervous system (CNS) in response to actual or potential tissue damage. Pain is experienced and behavior is likely to change in response to the pain. The central nervous system is of course crucial to the experience of acute pain, both in modifying perception and interpreting the pain. The hallmark of acute pain is that as the stimulus resolves, the pain resolves.

Chronic pain is very different. The nervous system is plastic and changes may occur at a number of different levels:

- Local inflammation or perhaps signals from the CNS may recruit additional nociceptors or nerve fibers that are usually silent. This may lead to modification of sensation at the site of the original injury such that previously painless or imperceptible sensations become painful. This is known as primary hyperalgesia
- Within the CNS, inputs from one dermatome will send signals that spread several segments up and down the spinal cord which may result in altered nerve

function or heightened sensation in surrounding areas as well. This is known as secondary hyperalgesia

- Because sensory signals from somatic and visceral structures connect to the same spinal segments, inputs from the viscera may alter the perception of sensation from somatic structures such as the abdominal wall. This viscerosomatic mapping accounts for referred pain in which pain from an organ may be perceived as arising from the abdominal wall, but it may also lead to altered sensation or even function in the 'referred area'
- Inputs from higher centers within the cortex are known to modify pain transmission within the CNS

It can be seen that the perception of chronic pain is complex and dynamic and can be modified at a number of levels. Abnormal sensation can become independent of the original insult and may persist long after tissue healing.

It has been suggested that the development of chronic pain can be seen as a time line beginning before birth and having perhaps three phases:

- Several factors may make an individual vulnerable to a chronic pain syndrome such as genetic factors, child abuse or intrauterine exposure to unknown factors
- During adolescence or early adult life further events may trigger the development of pain such as a severe infection, surgery or the onset of a condition such as endometriosis
- During the course of the illness, factors may contribute to the maintenance of the chronic pain syndrome such as the patient's

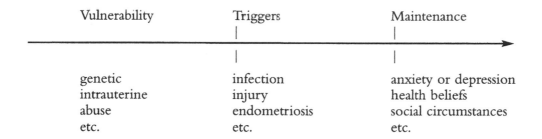

Figure 1 Time-line to conceptualize the development of chronic pelvic pain

beliefs about the pain, work circumstances or the attitude of carers

This idea is summarized in Figure 1.

Contributory factors

CPP may arise from any structure in or related to the pelvis, including the abdominal and pelvic walls. Table 1 summarizes the common contributory factors in women in their reproductive years but it is acknowledged that our understanding of this subject is still developing[5]. In one individual there may be more than one source of pain.

Gynecological causes

Endometriosis can occur throughout reproductive life including teenage years. It may be asymptomatic, but women with endometriosis are more likely to complain of pain than women with a laparoscopically normal pelvis. For a more detailed discussion of pain associated with endometriosis see Chapter 2.

The hallmark of the pain of endometriosis is its striking variation with the menstrual cycle. (Many pains will vary a little across the menstrual cycle due to the effect of hormonal fluctuation on nerve function.) Pain is often dull and aching or cramping in nature and felt in the lower abdomen but it may be anywhere. There may be a peak at the time of ovulation but pain characteristically increases towards the period. In addition to CPP, the cardinal symptoms associated with endometriosis are dysmenorrhea

Table 1 Possible contributory factors in the genesis of chronic pelvic pain

Gynecological causes
    endometriosis or adenomyosis
    pelvic inflammatory disease
    adhesions
Bowel-related pain
    irritable bowel syndrome
    constipation
Bladder-related pain
    interstitial cystitis
    urethral syndrome
Musculoskeletal pain
    mechanical pelvic pain
    muscle pain and trigger points
Neurological factors
    nerve entrapment
    neuropathic pain
    moderation by the peripheral and central nervous
      system
Psychosocial factors
    psychogenic pain
    physical and sexual abuse
    depression

(pain with menstruation) and dyspareunia (pain with sexual intercourse). Sufferers frequently experience other symptoms particularly just before or during menstruation such as fatigue and malaise, nausea and sometimes excruciating pain on defecation.

Adenomyosis is a form of endometriosis in which endometrioid tissue is found within the myometrium. Like endometriosis, it causes pain in a cyclical pattern often associated with deep dyspareunia, menorrhagia and menstrual irregularities. The uterus may be bulky but adenomyosis is otherwise undetectable at laparoscopy.

The term chronic pelvic inflammatory disease (PID) is used to mean either damage from a past upper genital tract infection or sometimes, episodic pain considered to be due to recurrent infection. In most cases the original infection is sexually transmitted. Pelvic infection is common, particularly with chlamydia, and persisting pelvic damage such as adhesions may be identified at diagnostic laparoscopy. However, such damage may be an incidental finding and not the cause of pain. Another possible explanation for pain following PID is that the presence of the infection may alter nerve function in such a way as to sensitize the pelvis so that physiological activity is subsequently perceived as painful.

Although it is important that sexually transmitted infections (STIs) are identified and treated, it is equally important that a woman is not incorrectly labeled as having chronic PID. Other more relevant factors may be missed and great damage may be done to her personal relationships by insensitive discussion. The presence of an STI at the cervix does not prove that pelvic pain is due to PID[6].

Pelvic adhesions are common and frequently asymptomatic. They may be caused by previous surgery or infection or by endometriosis. Although difficult to demonstrate, it seems likely that some peritoneal adhesions can cause pelvic pain, particularly pain associated with stretching movements or organ distension. Division of adhesions may result in pain relief although the only randomized evidence of benefit applies to dense or highly vascular adhesions divided at laparotomy[7].

In addition to peritoneal adhesions, two distinct forms of adhesive disease are recognized:

- The ovarian remnant syndrome describes CPP associated with a fragment of ovary left behind following oophorectomy
- The trapped ovary syndrome refers to CPP associated with the conservation of one or both ovaries at hysterectomy

In both conditions, the ovarian tissue continues to function and dense adhesions form around it. The pain is typically cyclical in nature, and may be associated with dyspareunia or a postcoital ache. Suppressing or removing the remnant may relieve symptoms.

Bowel-related pain

Although conditions such as inflammatory bowel disease may present with pelvic pain, there are usually other symptoms present such as bloody diarrhea or excessive weight loss. Constipation is very common among women and although rarely the primary source of pain, may make an important and treatable contribution to the overall pain burden.

Irritable bowel syndrome (IBS) is very common, affecting 10–20% of the general population and 50% of patients with pain symptoms attend a gynecology clinic[8]. Although essentially a diagnosis of exclusion, it can be diagnosed with confidence from the history alone in the absence of other abnormal symptoms such as weight loss and rectal bleeding[9]. Symptoms of IBS may vary with the menstrual cycle[10]. The agreed features, known as the Rome II criteria, are shown in Table 2. The etiology of IBS is unknown but in one-third of cases an infective episode is identified at the onset of symptoms. It is proposed that the presence of infection sets up an abnormal responsiveness within the bowel; so called visceral hypersensitivity occurs[11], whereby previously imperceptible movements or sensations are now considered painful.

Bladder-related pain

The principal urological causes of pelvic pain are interstitial cystitis and urethral syndrome. These conditions are characterized by irritative

Table 2 Diagnostic features of irritable bowel syndrome (IBS)[9]

Rome II criteria
At least 12 weeks or more, which need not be consecutive, in the previous 12 months of abdominal pain or discomfort that has two of three features:
   relief with defecation
   onset associated with a change in the frequency of the stool
   onset associated with a change in form (appearance) of stool

Other features associated with IBS
Abdominal distension
Passage of mucus
Sensation of incomplete evacuation

---

bladder symptoms such as urgency, frequency and nocturia associated with lower abdominal pain. They may be versions of the same condition. Irritative bladder symptoms are known to be common in the community affecting approximately 25% of women of reproductive age[1] but the prevalence of interstitial cystitis is unknown. If pelvic pain is due to interstitial cystitis then the pain would be expected to vary with the severity of urinary symptoms and be affected by emptying the bladder (see Table 3).

In the presence of symptoms, the diagnosis is made by finding characteristic appearances at cystoscopy and hydrodistension associated with a chronically contracted bladder. These fairly restrictive criteria were developed for the purposes of research and have become clinical criteria for diagnosis by default. It may be that a looser definition based on symptoms might help to identify the condition earlier in its pathogenesis allowing the possibility of more effective treatment. As with other conditions associated with chronic pelvic pain, the etiology of interstitial cystitis is poorly understood but involvement of the peripheral and central nervous systems in the pathophysiology of the chronic pain has been proposed[12].

Musculoskeletal pain

The hallmark of musculoskeletal pain is its variation with movement and posture. Mechanical pelvic pain describes pain due to abnormalities of the joints and ligaments of the pelvis or lower back. Damage may occur as a result of trauma, pregnancy or congenital abnormality but only come to light years later. The symphysis pubis or the sacroiliac joints may be unstable. Pain in the sacroiliac joints may be

Table 3 Signs and symptoms suggestive of particular diagnoses

Diagnosis	Nature of pain	Associated features	Examination findings
Endometriosis	marked variation with menstrual cycle	dyspareunia, dysmenorrhea, painful defecation family history	Focal tenderness, thickening of uterosacral ligaments, nodularity
Adenomyosis	marked variation with menstrual cycle	menstrual irregularities and menorrhagia	tender, globular uterus
Pelvic inflammatory disease	little variation in pain	vaginal discharge, irregular bleeding, recent change of partner	cervical excitation, cervical contact bleeding
Adhesions	?variation with movement or organ distension	previous surgery or infection	scars
Irritable bowel syndrome	related to opening bowels	constipation or diarrhea, mucus, bloating	nothing abnormal per vaginam, but abdomen generally tender
Urological pain	associated with passing urine	nocturia, frequency	tenderness under bladder base
Musculoskeletal pain	association with movement or posture	history of injury or strain, possibly old	pain elicited by specific movement. Examine the back
Nerve entrapment	associated with movement	often shooting or burning	scars; tenderness highly localized
Psychogenic pain	?? history difficult to grasp	??sadness, multiple previous symptoms	??examination traumatic

referred to the iliac fossae. It has been suggested that women in chronic pain may adopt an abnormal 'pelvic pain posture' in response to their pain, which, combined with a sedentary lifestyle, may result in additional pain arising from the pelvis[13].

Muscles themselves or associated fascia may be a source of pain, perhaps due to chronic muscle imbalance resulting from a distorted pelvis. Myofascial trigger points may be present, perhaps created by viscero-somatic mapping from painful organs within the pelvis. These may be present in the abdominal wall and possibly also the pelvic floor. This is one of many under-researched areas.

Nerve-related pain

Nerve entrapment may occur in scar tissue or fascia in the abdominal wall or in tight foramina in the pelvis or spine. Pain may be shooting in nature, associated with particular movements, or experienced as an ache locally or in the distribution of the nerve. Abnormal touch sensation may be detected in areas supplied by the nerve.

Neuropathic pain is the term given to pain that arises from a damaged nerve itself. Damage may occur as a result of surgery or injury or as part of a fibrotic process such as endometriosis. Pain is characteristically burning in nature or may have a knife-like quality.

Psychosocial factors

Research in other chronic pain syndromes suggests that a predisposition to the development of chronic pain and disability may be associated with certain personality traits such as a tendency to 'catastrophize', use of negative coping strategies, feeling no control over the pain, and a belief that pain represents ongoing tissue damage.

Psychogenic pain Almost all pain will have some physical and some psychological components. For some women a past experience or present emotion can be too terrible or difficult to bear conscious processing. It has become unspeakable and is expressed through the experience of pain. Unless the fear or concern is uncovered it will be difficult to resolve the pain. Often the traumatic experience is linked to a specific but terrifying worry such as the fear that she has been damaged by a difficult childbirth, or the fear that a sexual assault has led to infection or loss of fertility.

Physical and sexual abuse Sadly, many women have been or are being abused. However, a history of abuse is not necessarily relevant to pelvic pain. The link between pain and physical or sexual abuse is complex but recent studies have found an increased prevalence of major sexual abuse (meaning unwanted direct genital contact or penetrative sex at any age) in women with CPP compared to women with another pain complaint[14–17].

PRESENTATION

Women may present because they want an explanation for their pain. Even if their life is not disrupted by the pain they want to know why the pain is there[18]. And yet many women with chronic pelvic pain have no explanation for their pain, either because they do not seek advice or because no diagnosis has been made. In primary care, 29% of CPP sufferers remain without a diagnosis 2 years after presentation to their general practitioner[19] and in the community 50% of sufferers do not have an explanation for their pain[20]. Even if a diagnosis cannot be made, the reality of the pain must be accepted and attempts made to treat the pain empirically.

Living with chronic pain can be a debilitating and depressing experience during which many aspects of the woman's life may fall apart, including her job and her relationships. It is important to try to intervene early before patterns of chronic pain behavior both in the patient and those around her become established.

History

CPP is a symptom and not a diagnosis. Its association with other symptoms and events is the key to diagnosis. Allowing the patient to tell her story may allow her to make connections or associations in her own mind that may reveal clues as to the origin of the pain. Fears or beliefs

Table 4 Questions to consider

Careful description of the duration, nature, site and
  radiation of the pain

Is there more than one pain?

(It may be helpful to note a pain score for each pain at best
  and worst)

Factors that provoke or relieve the pain, particularly
  movement or posture

Variation of the pain over time, especially with the
  menstrual cycle

Gynecological symptoms including irregular bleeding and
  vaginal discharge

Is there dyspareunia, and what effect is it having?

Is there dysmenorrhea, and does the CPP feel any
  different?

Bladder and bowel symptoms (ask directly for symptoms of
  IBS)

Drugs that have been helpful, e.g. COC or NSAIDs

Are there any symptoms suggestive of depression or sleep
  disorder?

Is there any significant past medical or family history?

What was happening at the time the pain began?

Is there any experience that the pain reminds her of?

In what way does the pain affect day-to-day life?

What does the woman believe the pain is due to?

What does she want to achieve by coming for help? Why
  now?

CPP, chronic pelvic pain; IBS, irritable bowel syndrome; COC,
combined oral contraceptive pill; NSAIDs non-steroidal anti-
inflammatory drugs

about the origin of the pain may be uncovered (see Table 4).

The nature of the pain, its localization, its radiation, its duration are all important points. Asking whether the pain reminds her of something may be helpful. It may remind her of another kind of pain such as dysmenorrhea or it may be an event, a trauma perhaps. The precise circumstances surrounding the onset of the pain or her reasons for presenting at this time may give an important clue to the origin of the pain.

Dysmenorrhea and dyspareunia are important additional symptoms. Any abnormality in the bleeding pattern should be noted. The variation of the pain with the menstrual cycle, with movement, or with activity should be recorded. Enquiries should be made about bowel or bladder problems or vaginal discharge and the way in which the pain varies with these symptoms. It is also important to ask directly about other contributory problems such as depression or sleep disturbance.

It is useful to be able to record the severity of the pain both to get an idea of the scale of the problem and so that progress with treatment can be recorded. Using a score out of 10 can be useful, perhaps at different points in the pain cycle. It is important to try to record the degree to which pain is currently disrupting the patient's life. This could be time off work, disruption of domestic roles, avoidance of sex or use of pain killers. The woman's previous experience of investigations and treatment and her feelings about surgery or hormones may be important in planning future management.

Particularly in the context of primary care, the patient may have several 'attempts' at presenting with her pain. She may come with a related complaint and if she receives what she feels is the response she is looking for she may come back to ask for help with her pelvic pain. This has been referred to as the 'calling card' consultation. She may choose to give the doctor only part of the story at the first consultation, not knowing whether it is safe to reveal her own knowledge of the origins of the pain. Respectful listening, even if the story does not make sense or does not fit into a recognizable diagnostic pattern, may allow her to come back and trust her doctor with the whole story and thereby start the process of moving forward.

This process takes time and it may be appropriate to ask the patient to come back at a later date. If time is short, or the pattern of the pain is unclear, consider asking her to keep a pain diary for a few months.

'It is the theory that should be discounted when the patient's symptoms refuse to fit, not the patient's account of the reality of their experience.'[21]

Examination

During the examination it is useful if the pain can be recreated. This not only helps to make a more accurate assessment but gives the patient confidence that *you do know* the type of pain she is talking about and that you believe that this pain is real (Table 5).

In the abdomen, the presence of scars and any associated tenderness or numbness should be noted. This may suggest nerve entrapment in

Table 5 Points to consider in the examination

Can the pain be recreated?
Is there any associated numbness or altered sensation?
Is the tenderness highly localized or diffuse?
Does it get worse if the patient tenses the recti?

Vaginal examination:
Does her behavior strike you as unusual or different in any way?
Is there any particularly tender spot?
Can you recreate the pain?
Is there any tenderness under the bladder base?
Is the uterus normal size and shape?
Is it unusually tender?
Are there any adnexal masses or tenderness?
Is there any nodularity in the uterosacral ligaments or rectovaginal space?

the scar. Areas of abnormal sensation on the abdominal wall where light touch is perceived as painful or unpleasant (allodynia) may indicate neurological dysfunction associated with either nerve entrapment or referred pain. Asking the patient to point to the pain may indicate highly localized (suggesting somatic pain) as opposed to diffuse pain (more suggestive of visceral pain). This has been called 'the single finger sign'. Pressure over the precise point indicated may recreate the pain. Tensing the recti by the patient raising her shoulders off the bed whilst continuing the pressure on the point usually enhances the tenderness significantly if it is arising from the abdominal wall. Some authorities view these points as entrapments of perforating nerves. Others consider them to be trigger points in the abdominal musculature. A useful diagnostic test is to inject local anesthetic at the site at the level of the rectus sheath. This should bring complete relief if the pain is arising from the abdominal wall.

Case history (a composite of many cases)

Aged 34 she had been under the care of gynecologists for many years with severe endometriosis. She had had several laparoscopies to treat the disease that were generally successful for a year or two. This time her pain had come back but she could not face another laparoscopy. She opted to try gonadotropin releasing hormone (GnRH) analogs with hormone replacement therapy (HRT) for a while until she was clearer in her mind whether she ever wanted to have children. At review she was very much better but still troubled by an unpleasant shooting pain in the right iliac fossa that she thought was linked to movement. She was able to put her finger precisely on the tender spot. This tenderness got worse when she was asked to raise her shoulders off the bed whilst the doctor maintained pressure on the tender area. Complete pain relief, by injection of 10 ml of bupivicaine into the tender spot, was maintained several days after the injection. The sensitive spot may have been a nerve entrapment related to previous surgery or a trigger point in the abdominal wall.

The vaginal examination is not only a physical examination but also an important moment in the doctor–patient relationship – 'a psychodynamic event'. It is an opportunity to demonstrate respect and sympathy. In her vulnerability, a patient may reveal fears or secrets that are crucial to the understanding of her pain. The doctor should be prepared for this and not embark on the examination unless there is time to respond[22].

Case history 2 (a composite of many cases)

She presented aged 19 with chronic pelvic pain and dyspareunia of 3-years' duration. She looked much older than her years and was dressed in leathers. Her attitude appeared rather offhand. She found the pain difficult to describe and did not volunteer much information, but she thought it varied a bit with the menstrual cycle. She hated having periods. During the vaginal examination she seemed surprisingly vulnerable in contrast to her earlier hardness. The examination caused her pain and when asked if it reminded her of anything she started to talk about her experiences working in a massage parlor as a young teenager. When she returned for follow-up some months later, having been on the combined pill continuously, she looked completely different and appeared relaxed and at ease with herself. She had made a number of changes in her circumstances and rarely had pain.

In addition to assessing uterine size and tenderness and feeling for adnexal masses and cervical excitation, features should be sought such as vaginal nodules or thickening of the uterosacral ligaments (palpable laterally in the posterior fornix). Such areas might suggest endometriosis. Tenderness anteriorly under the bladder base may suggest interstitial cystitis. The exact site of the tenderness should be identified with the patient.

In the presence of an up-to-date smear history, a cervical smear is not required. Swabs for infection may be necessary (although referral to a genitourinary medicine clinic for this to be performed may be preferable – see below). A speculum examination is therefore not usually needed. Urinalysis should be performed in the presence of bladder symptoms to rule out infection and microscopic hematuria.

INVESTIGATIONS

Decisions about further investigation and treatment should be made in partnership with the patient. Knowing what the patient wants to achieve will define the extent of investigations required and will influence treatment options. For women in their reproductive years, CPP is rarely a presentation of life-threatening or progressive disease in the absence of other significant symptoms such as rectal bleeding. So called 'red flag' symptoms need to be investigated as appropriate (see Table 6). Investigations should be aimed at excluding serious pathology if appropriate and finding a

Table 6 Red flag symptoms

Bleeding per rectum
New bowel symptoms over 50
New pain after the menopause
Pelvic mass
Suicidal ideation
Excessive weight loss
Irregular vaginal bleeding over 40
Postcoital bleeding

satisfactory explanation for the patient's symptoms including her own concerns or theories (see Table 7).

Screening for STIs may be required and is best performed in a genitourinary medicine (GUM) clinic. It would be particularly relevant in women under 25, when there has been a recent change of partner and in the presence of vaginal discharge. If the patient has particular concerns about STIs, screening may also be helpful. Not only is the sensitivity of the investigation improved at the GUM clinic but also contact tracing can readily be arranged. However, if referral does not seem appropriate endocervical swabs for chlamydia and routine culture can be taken at the initial examination, when indicated.

Table 7 Investigations to consider

Pain diary
Screening for STDs
Pelvic ultrasound scan
Therapeutic trial of COC or GnRH analog
Diagnostic laparoscopy +/- cystoscopy
Conscious pain mapping?
Referral to another discipline

STDs, sexually transmitted diseases; COC, combined oral contraceptive pill; GnRH, gonadotropin releasing hormone

An ultrasound scan of the pelvis (usually transvaginal) can reliably exclude an ovarian cyst or endometrioma. Hydrosalpinges or tubo-ovarian abscesses may be identified. An ultrasound scan may be particularly helpful when vaginal examination reveals an abnormality. A magnetic resonance imaging (MRI) scan may be helpful in the diagnosis of adenomyosis[23].

Diagnostic laparoscopy is the conventional investigation for the diagnosis of CPP. Endometriosis and adhesions may be identified and possibly also treated at one operation. However, the role of diagnostic laparoscopy has been questioned. In approximately one-third of cases (depending on the population studied) no pathology will be identified[24]. Where pathology is identified, its relevance to the pain is not always clear. Many of the possible causes of pain listed above cannot be seen at laparoscopy. Women find it very disheartening to go through a laparoscopy and no cause to be identified. In the absence of pathology at laparoscopy, they feel that doctors are more likely to label them as having 'no organic pathology' meaning 'they think it's all in my head'[18,25].

The risks of diagnostic laparoscopy are significant. One in 500 will suffer a significant injury such as perforation of bowel or blood vessel[26,27]. The patient needs to know the limitations of the test in order to decide whether her symptoms justify the risk and inconvenience incurred. Arguably diagnostic laparoscopy should be reserved for patients thought likely to need surgical treatment such as those with abnormal findings at vaginal examination or ultrasound scan.

Laparoscopic conscious pain mapping describes the use of a fine laparoscope while the patient is sedated but conscious. This allows the surgeon to touch abnormal areas and ask the patient about the pain[28]. Although theoretically appealing, questions remain as to its acceptability and whether it improves outcomes. Its use has not become widespread in the UK.

In women with urinary symptoms, consideration should be given to performing a cystoscopy with hydrodistension at the time of the diagnostic laparoscopy to look for interstitial cystitis. If hematuria is identified in urinalysis a cystoscopy should be performed to rule out malignancy.

Referral to other professionals such as physiotherapists, osteopaths or specialist counselors may be helpful in assessing and treating various components of the pain. Many patients may be managed in primary care but when pain is not adequately controlled, or the explanation for the pain is not satisfactory, referral should ideally be directed to a team with an interest in pelvic pain. A multidisciplinary approach is likely to be most effective[29,30].

MEDICAL TREATMENT

Management of CPP should be directed at identifying the components of pain and treating these specifically where possible. The treatment of endometriosis is described in Chapter 2. The treatment of IBS is described more fully elsewhere but involves the use of antispasmodics, laxatives if appropriate and dietary modification[31]. Interstitial cystitis is probably best managed by a team with an interest in the condition. Treatment may include anticholinergics, analgesics and bladder instillations. Dietary modification may help. Treating contributory factors such as depression, poor sleep and constipation may help to reduce the overall pain burden and should not be overlooked.

Treating the pain

Even if the precise cause or causes of the pain cannot be identified, the pain should be treated empirically. Anti-inflammatory drugs can be very helpful. Patients should be advised to take them regularly on the days of the cycle in which they are in pain. Paracetamol or codeine-based analgesics can be used in addition. Other measures such as development of a regular exercise program, dietary changes or psychological techniques may have a place. Transcutaneous electrical nerve stimulation (TENS) may also be helpful. Where possible, the patient's own coping strategies should be harnessed to manage the pain.

Tricyclic antidepressants such as amitriptyline are particularly useful for neuropathic pain. It may take several weeks for the drug to reach its full effect. The anticholinergic side-effects, which usually diminish in the first couple of weeks, should be explained to the patient. There is a sedative effect and this can be harnessed to improve sleep pattern. Amitriptyline may also help to lift the spirits. As one patient put it, 'It's not that the pain isn't there, it's just that it doesn't dominate everything anymore'. However, if depression is thought to be a major component, ideally it should be discussed openly and consideration given to using a more modern formulation such as an SSRI (selective serotonin re-uptake inhibitor). Carbamazepine or gabapentin may also have a role in treating neuropathic pain particularly when pain is shooting in nature.

Suggestions for the management of pain on an empirical basis are given in Table 8.

Table 8 Empirical treatments for pain

Non-steroidal anti-inflammatory drugs preferably used on a regular basis
    e.g. diclofenac 50 mg t.d.s. or 100 mg per rectum 16 hourly.
    +/– paracetamol or stronger analgesic, e.g. codydramol
Tricyclic antidepressant
    e.g. amitriptyline 25 mg nocte, increasing by 25 mg every 2 weeks until symptoms controlled to maximum of 150 mg
    (usually 75–125 mg)
Complementary therapy, e.g. acupuncture, herbal medicine
Dietary changes
Conservative measures, e.g. regular exercise, relaxation, stress management, TENS
Support, e.g. self-help groups, 'an open door'

TENs, transcutaneous electrical nerve stimulation

Therapeutic trials

It is reasonable to suggest that pain which is strikingly cyclical in nature, particularly when associated with dyspareunia and dysmenorrhea, may be due to 'an endometriosis-like condition'. If the pelvis is clinically normal and fertility is not desired, a trial of the combined oral contraceptive pill is worthwhile[32]. This is commonly undertaken in primary care. Continuous progesterone aiming to induce amenorrhea may control cyclical pain for the duration of treatment[29] (see Table 9). Patients should be warned about side-effects.

A trial of a GnRH analog may be used as a first-line treatment for cyclical pain even if the laparoscopy has been negative. If successful the pain is clearly hormone dependent. Although pain due to endometriosis or adenomyosis will improve with this regime, other conditions may also improve. For example, a 'trapped ovary' will be less painful when 'shut down' by GnRH analogs. There is some evidence that IBS[33] and even interstitial cystitis may be improved with GnRH analogs. Success with GnRH analogs should therefore be interpreted with care.

Patients should be carefully warned about the side-effects, which include hot flushes (experienced by 98% of users), and other symptoms associated with the menopause. Patients should be aware of the so-called flare effect in which symptoms get worse before getting better. If successful, treatment may be continued with the addition of HRT to prevent osteoporosis and hypoestrogenic side-effects. Tibolone is licensed for this use but continuous combined preparations may also be used. With this regime bone mass is maintained and usage is safe for many months[34].

Such a trial may be helpful in making a decision about surgery in women who have unexplained CPP. If the GnRH analogs do not control the pain, hysterectomy and bilateral oophorectomy are unlikely to be successful. The treatment is also particularly useful for patients who are not yet ready to have a hysterectomy but who feel their pain is forcing them towards

Table 9 Medical treatments for chronic pelvic pain

Empirical analgesia
Combined oral contraceptive
Continuous progestogen
GnRH analogs
Mirena® coil

GnRH, gonadotropin releasing hormone

this. The treatment may offer very good quality of life and allow these women time to reach a decision about a permanent solution to their pain.

Although it does not in general inhibit ovulation, the Mirena® coil is also being used empirically in the treatment of strikingly cyclical pelvic pain particularly where menorrhagia is also present.

Non-medical strategies

For some patients psychosocial factors contribute significantly to the overall problem often co-existing with physical causes. It may be necessary to address physical factors first and achieve some improvement and perhaps an element of trust before tackling other components. Some practitioners have the skills and time to deal with psychosocial problems but in both primary and secondary care referral to a specialist may be desirable.

Self-help groups offer an excellent source of support and information. Directing a patient towards a relevant organization or web site and requesting her to come back to discuss matters further, may prove time saving.

Dietary modification may also be helpful. Up to a third of patients with IBS will gain considerable relief from changing their diet. Interstitial cystitis sufferers may also be able to identify specific food or drinks that make their symptoms worse. Patients should try excluding items for at least 2 weeks at a time. There may be more than one provoking food.

Physiotherapy can play a major component in pain management. It can be used to improve stamina and muscle function and may also be important in retraining muscles and dispersing trigger points. Physiotherapy can also be used to

teach relaxation techniques and stress management.

In many areas multidisciplinary pain management services exist and can be very helpful particularly when the cause of the pain is unknown or untreatable. Pain management teams will generally not investigate the cause of the pain any further and should therefore probably be involved only when a patient has already seen a specialist with a particular interest in pelvic pain. The aim of the treatment is to improve the patient's function, not to make a diagnosis.

CPP sufferers are likely to need ongoing support whatever the cause of their pain. This does not necessarily mean that patients should continue to be seen on a regular basis in either primary or secondary care but they should know where to turn for help. Periodic exacerbations are to be expected.

SURGICAL TREATMENT

As emphasized throughout this chapter, CPP is a symptom and not a diagnosis. Treatment should ideally be directed at a specific pathology (Table 10). Surgical intervention for pain of unknown origin seems more than likely to fail.

Table 10 Surgical treatments for chronic pelvic pain

Laparoscopic management of endometriosis
Laparoscopic adhesiolysis
Total abdominal hysterectomy and bilateral salpingo-
  oophorectomy
Laparoscopic uterosacral nerve ablation?
Presacral neurectomy?
Implanted nerve stimulator?

Laparoscopy is the surgical management of choice for endometriosis and is discussed in Chapter 2. Adhesions can be divided laparoscopically, and anecdotal evidence suggests that it may be of value in some patients. However, the only randomized evidence of benefit comes from a trial involving laparotomy not laparoscopy in which only the division of dense or vascular adhesions was shown to produce pain relief[7].

Total abdominal hysterectomy with or without oophorectomy is commonly performed as a treatment for CPP. The decision to perform a hysterectomy is obviously highly dependent on the woman's age and her fertility aspirations. The presence of menstrual chaos may contribute to the woman's desire to have a hysterectomy. If hysterectomy is to be performed for pain, the ovaries should probably be removed as well. If the pain is due to a hormone-dependent condition, the pain may well continue or recur if the uterus is removed but the ovaries remain, allowing the hormones to continue unabated. An ovary left behind following hysterectomy may well become encased in scar tissue (residual ovary syndrome) and become a source of pain in itself. The removal of an ovary post hysterectomy can be technically challenging. If the woman considering hysterectomy is too young to contemplate bilateral oophorectomy it may be better to use a medical treatment for a few years and then perform the hysterectomy at a later date removing the ovaries at the same time.

Prior to hysterectomy, attempts should be made to establish that the pain can be controlled by removing the ovarian hormones. GnRH analogs can be used to induce a 'medical oophorectomy'. If the pain is completely resolved with this treatment it is likely to be resolved permanently by oophorectomy. Persistent pain in the presence of adequate ovarian suppression should lead to reconsideration of the diagnosis and management plan.

Few of the other conditions discussed above are amenable to specific surgical intervention, at least not until end-stage disease (e.g. cystectomy in end-stage interstitial cystitis). A number of other empirical surgical treatments for chronic pelvic pain have been described. A major flaw in their use is the assumption that pelvic pain is generated wholly in the end organ, usually the uterus.

The use of laparoscopic uterosacral nerve ablation (LUNA) has been advocated as a treatment for pelvic pain. Whilst theoretically appealing due to the rich nerve supply that travels through the uterosacral ligaments, evidence of benefit is poor[35]. A large multi-center trial is underway to assess its place in the management of pelvic pain[36].

Some have advocated presacral neurectomy (PSN) as an empirical treatment for CPP. In a systematic review, no evidence of benefit was found for the treatment of secondary dysmenorrhea[35]. However, a recent randomized controlled trial involving 141 women with CPP associated with endometriosis demonstrated reduced pain scores in patients undergoing PSN in addition to conservative laparoscopy for endometriosis[37]. Complications with this treatment may be significant including bladder and bowel dysfunction.

The surgical implantation of a nerve stimulator within the spinal cord is designed to harness the plasticity of the CNS in the treatment of chronic pain. Some success has been achieved but evidence so far is largely anecdotal.

CONCLUSION

Living with chronic pelvic pain is a debilitating and depressing condition. Although the understanding of pelvic pain is developing rapidly there is still a great deal unknown regarding its etiology and most effective treatments.

Acceptance and validation of the patient's experience is important and may be of great benefit to the patient even if her symptoms do not fit with accepted medical understanding of the condition. Investigation should be directed at excluding serious pathology and addressing the patient's need for an explanation or the exclusion of a specific concern.

Pelvic pain may arise from any structure in or related to the pelvis. Often more than one factor is contributing to the overall pain burden. Teasing out these factors and treating at least some of them may make a huge difference. New insights into the response of the CNS to pain may help to understand the nature of some kinds of pelvic pain and to explain the large overlap in symptoms of conditions such as irritable bowel syndrome, interstitial cystitis and endometriosis.

Even if the specific cause or causes cannot be identified, empirical treatments can be used to treat the pain with good effect. Where pain is strikingly cyclical in nature a therapeutic trial of GnRH analogs may be better first-line management than diagnostic laparoscopy.

Case history 3 (a composite of many cases)

She presented aged 50 having experienced many years of pain. The account of her pain was overwhelming and punctuated by tears. She was open in her opinion that everything was hopeless and she could not be helped. Goals were set at the first visit with the acceptance that achieving a pain-free state was probably unrealistic. She wanted to be able to hold down a job and resume her sex life. Over several visits, she was able to identify at least two pains. First, she addressed pain that seemed to be related to her abnormal bowel habit and was helped by changing her diet. Second, she had a different pain that was associated with movement and thought to come from a distorted pelvis. This pain was helped by specific exercises; a regular exercise program was then established. She was already taking antidepressants and gradually established a regular part-time working pattern. Finally, she was able to examine her feelings about the violence she had suffered at the end of a pregnancy many years ago and her fears about a recent miscarriage that had marked the start of the dyspareunia.

PRACTICE POINTS

- Listen to the patient: allow her to tell her story
- Make sure the patient knows that you acknowledge the reality of her pain
- Allow or create enough time
- Establish what she wants to achieve or what she fears
- Involve the patient in decision-making
- Consider asking her to keep a pain diary
- Look for contributory factors, rather than a single cause
- Exclude serious pathology, even if a positive diagnosis cannot be made
- Do something about the pain itself
- Offer access to information and support

REFERENCES

1. Zondervan KT, Yudkin PL, Vessey MP, et al. The community prevalence of chronic pelvic pain in women and associated illness behaviour. Br J Gen Pract 2001; 51: 541–7

2. Zondervan KT, Yudkin PL, Vessey MP, et al. Prevalence and incidence of chronic pelvic pain in primary care: evidence from a national general practice database. Br J Obstet Gynaecol 1999; 106: 1149–55

3. Grace VM. Problems women patients experience in the medical encounter for chronic pelvic pain: a New Zealand study. Health Care Women Int 1995; 16: 509–19

4. IASP. Classification of chronic pelvic pain. Pain 1986; Suppl 3: S217

5. Howard FM. Chronic pelvic pain. Obstet Gynecol 2003; 101: 594–611

6. Royal College of Obstetricians and Gynecologists. Management of Acute Pelvic Inflammatory Disease. Clinical Green Top Guidelines, 32. London: RCOG, 2003

7. Peters AAW, Trimbos-Kemper GCM, Admiraal C, et al. A randomized clinical trial of the benefits of adhesiolysis in patients with intraperitoneal adhesions and chronic pelvic pain. Br J Obstet Gynaecol 1992; 99: 59–62

8. Prior A, Wilson K, Whorwell PJ, Faragher EB. Irritable bowel syndrome in the gynaecological clinic. Survey of 798 new referrals. Dig Dis Sci 1989; 34: 1820–4

9. Talley NJ. Definition, diagnosis and epidemiology. Baillieres Best Pract Res Clin Gastroenterol 1999; 13: 371–84

10. Moore J, Barlow DH, Jewell D, et al. Do gastrointestinal symptoms vary with the menstrual cycle? Br J Obstet Gynaecol 1998; 105: 1322–5

11. Collins SM, Barbara G, Vallance B. Stress, inflammation and the irritable bowel syndrome. Can J Gastroenterol 1999; 13 (Suppl A): 47A–49A

12. Wesselmann U, Czakanski PP. Pelvic pain: a chronic visceral pain syndrome. Curr Pain Headache Rep 2001; 5: 13–19

13. King PM, Myers CA, Ling FW, et al. Musculoskeletal factors in chronic pelvic pain. J Psychosom Obstet Gynaecol 1991; 12: 87–98

14. Collett BJ, Cordle CJ, Stewart CR, Jagger C. A comparative study of women with chronic pelvic pain, chronic nonpelvic pain and those with no history of pain attending general practitioners. Br J Obstet Gynaecol 1998; 105: 87–92

15. Walling MK, Reiter RC, O'Hara MW, et al. Abuse history and chronic pain in women: I. Prevalences of sexual abuse and physical abuse. Obstet Gynecol 1994; 84: 193–9

16. Lampe A, Solder E, Ennemoser A, et al. Chronic pelvic pain and previous sexual abuse. Obstet Gynecol 2000; 96: 929–33

17. Lampe A, Doering S, Rumpold G, et al. Chronic pain syndromes and their relation to childhood abuse and stressful life events. J Psychsom Res 2003; 54: 361–7

18. Moore J, Ziebland S, Kennedy S. 'People sometimes react funny if they're not told enough': women's views about the risks of diagnostic laparoscopy. Health Expect 2002; 5: 302–9

19. Zondervan KT, Yudkin PL, Vessey MP, et al. Patterns of diagnosis and referral in women consulting for chronic pelvic pain in UK primary care. Br J Obstet Gynaecol 1999; 106: 1156 61

20. Zondervan K, Yudkin PL, Vessey MP, et al. Chronic pelvic pain in the community – symptoms, investigations and diagnoses. Am J Obstet Gynecol 2001; 184: 1149–55

21. Heath I. Following the story: continuity of care in general practice. In Greenhalgh T, Hurwitz B, eds. Narrative Based Medicine. London: BMJ Books, 1998: 83–92

22. Smith A. The skills of psychosexual medicine. In Skrine RL, Mountford H, eds. Psychosexual Medicine: An Introduction. London: Hodder Arnold, 2001; 62–75

23. Cody RF Jr, Ascher SM. Diagnostic value of radiological tests in chronic pelvic pain. Baillières Best Pract Res Clin Obstet Gynaecol 2000; 14: 433–66

24. Howard FM. The role of laparoscopy as a diagnostic tool in chronic pelvic pain. Baillieres Best Pract Res Clin Obstet Gynaecol 2000; 14: 467–94

25. Grace VM. Mind/body dualism in medicine: the case of chronic pelvic pain without organic pathology: a critical review of the literature. Int J Health Serv 1998; 28: 127–51

26. Chapron C, Querleu D, Bruhat MA, et al. Surgical complications of diagnostic and operative gynaecological laparoscopy: a series of 29 966 cases. Hum Reprod 1998; 13: 867–72

27. Jansen FW, Kapiteyn K, Trimbos-Kemper T, et al. Complications of laparoscopy: a prospective multicentre observational study. Br J Obstet Gynaecol 1997; 104: 595–600

28. Palter SF. Microlaparoscopy under local anaesthetia and conscious pain mapping for the diagnosis and management of pelvic pain. Curr Opin Obstet Gynecol 1999; 11: 387–93

29. Stones RW, Mountfield J. Interventions for treating chronic pelvic pain in women. In The Cochrane Library. Issue 4. Chichester UK: John Wiley and Sons Ltd, 2003

30. Peters AAW, van Dorst E, Jellis B, et al. A randomized clinical trial to compare two different approaches in women with chronic pelvic pain. Obstet Gynecol 1991; 77: 740–4

31. Camilleri M. Management of the irritable bowel syndrome. Gastroenterology 2001; 120: 652–68

32. Gambone JC, Mittman BS, Munro MG, et al. Consensus statement for the management of chronic pelvic pain and endometriosis: proceedings of an expert-panel consensus process. Fertil Steril 2002; 78: 961–72

33. Mathias JR, Clench MH, Reeves-Darby VG, et al. Effect of leuprolide acetate in patients with moderate to severe functional bowel disease. Double-blind, placebo-controlled study. Dig Dis Sci 1994; 39: 1155–62

34. Hornstein MD, Surrey ES, Weisberg GW, Casino LA. Leuprolide acetate depot with hormonal add-back in endometriosis: a 12-month study. Lupron Add-Back Study Group. Obstet Gynecol 1998; 91: 16–24

35. Proctor ML, Farquhar CM, Sinclair OJ, Johnson NP. Surgical interruption of pelvic nerve pathways for primary and secondary dysmenorrhoea (Cochrane review). In The Cochrane Library, Issue 4. Chichester UK: John Wiley and Sons Ltd, 2003

36. Latthe PM. LUNA Trial Collaboration. A randomised controlled trial to assess the efficacy of Laparoscopic Uterosacral Nerve Ablation (LUNA) in the treatment of chronic pelvic pain. BMC Womens Health 2003; 3: 6

37. Zullo F, Palomba S, Zupi E. Effectiveness of presacral neurectomy in women with severe dysmenorrhea caused by endometriosis who were treated with laparoscopic conservative surgery: a 1-year prospective randomized double-blind controlled trial. Am J Obstet Gynecol 2003; 189: 5–10

Self-help organizations and useful web sites

Endometriosis Society
Suite 50, Westminster Palace Gardens,
1–7 Artillery Row, London SW1P 1RL
Tel: +44 (0) 207 222 2781 (admin);
+44 (0) 207 222 2776 (Helpline 7–10pm)
www.endo.org.uk

Women's Health *Good source of information about chronic PID and other conditions*
52 Featherstone St, London EC1Y 8RT
Tel: +44 (0) 207 251 6333 (admin);
+44 (0) 207 251 6580 (enquiry line)
Womenshealth@pop3.poptel.4

IBS Network
Ms PJ Nunn, Northern General Hospital,
Sheffield S5 7AU
Tel: +44 (0) 114 261 1531
www.uel.ac.uk/c.p.dancey/ibs.html

Women's Nutrition Advisory Service
PO Box 268, Lewis, Sussex BN7 2QN
Tel: +44 (0) 1273 487 366

Female Action Against Abuse of Women and Girls *(for victims and workers)*
PO Box 124, Bognor Regis, W Sussex
PO21 5JT
Tel: +44 (0) 1243 860 003

The Cystitis and Overactive Bladder Foundation
76 High Street, Stony Startford,
Buckinghamshire MK11 1AH
Tel: +44 (0) 1908 569169
www.cobfoundation.org

The British DSP Support Group *(Symphisis pubis dysfunction)*
Mont Hamel House, Office 2, Chapel Place,
Ramsgate, Kent CT11 9RY
Tel: +44 (0) 1843 587 356
www.dsp.future.easyspace.com

Miscarriage Association
Clayton Hospital, Northgate, Wakefield WF1 3JS
Tel: +44 (0) 1924 200799

Other suggested web sites:
www.pelvicpain.org
(International Pelvic Pain Society)

www.psiesys.com
(British-based site focusing on endometriosis)

www.obgyn.net
(American-based wide-ranging site for doctors and patients)

Excessive menstrual bleeding 5

M.K. Oehler and M. Rees

INTRODUCTION

Excessive menstrual bleeding is a significant cause of morbidity during the reproductive years. Approximately 30% of women complain of menorrhagia and it is the main presenting problem of women consulting a gynecologist[1]. In addition, excessive menstrual bleeding accounts for about two-thirds of all hysterectomies and a large proportion of endoscopic endometrial destructive surgery, therefore using substantial health-care resources[2].

Menorrhagia can be defined subjectively as 'a complaint of excessive menstrual bleeding occurring over several consecutive cycles'[3]. Objectively it is 'a total menstrual blood loss greater or equal to 80 ml per period'[4]. This degree of blood loss can cause disturbances of the woman's social, occupational or sexual life, and give rise to concern about possible underlying serious disease (in particular cancer), as well as medical risks such as chronic iron-deficiency anemia.

ETIOLOGY

The volume of menstrual blood loss is controlled by local uterine vascular tone and hemostasis. Menorrhagia may be due to systemic or pelvic pathology, or iatrogenic causes. However, this widespread view perpetrated by many gynecological textbooks is based on clinical impression without essential objective menstrual blood loss measurement in many cases. With regard to pelvic pathology, uterine fibroids (leiomyomas), endometriosis (adenomyosis), pelvic inflammatory disease, and endometrial polyps are thought to be causes of menorrhagia. Again there is a paucity of data with objective menstrual blood loss measurement. In 50% of cases of objective menorrhagia no pathology is found at hysterectomy[5] (Table 1).

Leiomyomas are a very common finding in women with menorrhagia. It is estimated that 20–50% of women of childbearing age have leiomyomas[6]. Fibroids that involve the uterine cavity are believed to cause menorrhagia by inhibition of local hemostasis and/or expansion of the surface area of the endometrium[6]. Furthermore, recent work demonstrates dysregulation of a number of growth factors in the myomatous uterus. As many of these factors regulate the process of angiogenesis or have other effects on vascular structures, it is hypothesized that dysregulated angiogenesis with the formation of abnormal vessels might be the reason why women with fibroid uteri experience menorrhagia. Angiogenic factors

Table 1 Causes of menorrhagia

Uterine
Fibroids
Endometrial polyps
Endometriosis
Pelvic inflammatory disease

Systemic
Coagulation disorders
 Von Willebrand's disease
 Idiopathic thrombocytopenic purpura
 Factor V, VII, X, and XI deficiency
Hypothyroidism

Iatrogenic
Progestogen-only contraceptives
Intrauterine devices
Anticoagulants

that may prove to be important in this process include the vascular endothelial growth factor (VEGF) and adrenomedullin[7].

Uterine adenomyosis, defined by the presence of ectopic endometrial glands and stroma in the uterine myometrium, has been reported to be accompanied by fibroids in up to 80% of cases[8] and is also believed to be a cause of menorrhagia.

Occasionally excessive menstrual bleeding can result from bleeding diatheses. According to various studies these disorders can have a prevalence of up to 17% in menorrhagia cases[9,10]. Von Willebrand's disease (vWD), an autosomal disorder located on chromosome 12, is the most common of these coagulopathies and may be underdiagnosed in many women with unexplained menorrhagia. About 80% of women with vWD develop menorrhagia, and a relatively significant proportion (about 8–18%) of vWD patients undergo surgical interventions such as hysterectomies for control of their

excessive menstrual bleeding[11]. Other more rare disorders that impair blood platelets and clotting factors (e.g. idiopathic thrombocytopenic purpura, deficiencies of factors V, VII, X, and XI) can also account for some cases of menorrhagia. As most coagulopathies have a genetic basis they should be suspected especially in adolescent girls who experience excessive bleeding.

Many iatrogenic causes of menorrhagia exist, the most common being oral, implantable, or injectible progestogen-only contraceptives. Copper-containing and inert intrauterine contraceptive devices (IUCDs), especially those with a large surface area, are also known to result frequently in increased menstrual bleeding. The mechanism of menorrhagia with IUCDs is believed to be related to a combination of local inflammatory reaction and foreign body-induced fibrinolytic activity. Although the true significance of anticoagulants on menorrhagia is unknown, warfarin therapy has objectively been shown to increase menstrual blood loss[12]. However, use of thrombolytic therapy (e.g. with tissue plasminogen activator in menstruating patients) does not seem to be associated with increased bleeding, unless the patients are already suffering from menorrhagia[13,14].

Systemic diseases are more uncommon reasons for excessive menstrual bleeding. Women with hypothyroidism may develop menorrhagia that usually resolves with treatment of the thyroid disorder[15].

While 'unexplained' menorrhagia is a very appropriate term for the condition in the absence of any pathology it is commonly referred to less clearly as 'dysfunctional uterine bleeding', which implies endocrine abnormalities and anovulatory cycles. However, it must be emphasized that most cases of menorrhagia are associated with regular ovulatory cycles and anovulatory cycles tend to occur mainly soon after menarche or close to menopause.

In ovulatory cycles excessive menstrual bleeding has been ascribed to abnormal uterine levels of prostaglandins. A discrepancy between the vasoconstricting and aggregating actions of prostaglandin $F_{2\alpha}$ ($PGF_{2\alpha}$) and thromboxane A_2 and the vasodilating actions of prostaglandin E_2 (PGE_2) and prostacyclin (PGI_2) on the myometrial and endometrial vasculature is believed to cause a vascular imbalance predisposing to heavy menstrual bleeding[16]. In menorrhagic women the release of PGE_2, $PGF_{2\alpha}$ and PGI_2 is elevated in the endometrium and myometrium and higher levels of those cytokines are detected in menstrual fluid of those women when compared with women who have normal menses[17]. In addition, increased concentrations of PGE_2 and PGI_2 receptors are found in the myometrium from women with excessive menstrual bleeding predisposing to vasodilation[18].

The increase of vasodilatatory factors and their receptors may further enhance menstrual bleeding and vascular dysfunction by upregulating the cyclo-oxygenase–prostaglandin biosynthetic pathway via a positive feedback loop, and promote an autocrine–paracrine regulation of growth factors specific for vascular function (e.g. VEGF)[19].

Nitric oxide (NO) is a another potent vasodilator and a strong candidate for the cause of excessive blood loss as menorrhagic endometrium was recently found to overexpress the enzyme endothelial nitric oxide synthase (eNOS) and to contain significantly higher amounts of NO than normal endometrium[20].

Furthermore, a significantly elevated fibrinolytic activity in the endometrium, which is believed to be caused by a premenstrual rise in tissue plasminogen activator antigen production with delayed increase in plasminogen inhibitor type 1, is thought to be another underlying mechanism for menorrhagia[21].

There are now also increasing data to suggest that an imbalance between matrix metalloproteinases (MMPs), a family of matrix-degrading proteinases, and their physiological inhibitors (tissue inhibitors of metalloproteinases, TIMPs) might have an important role in abnormal menstrual bleeding[22,23].

Recent molecular research has focused on the identification of new local modulators involved in pathological menstrual bleeding. LEFTY-A, a novel member of the transforming growth factor-β family identified originally as an endometrial bleeding-associated factor (EBAF), was identified as a candidate for this local control. New data indicate that LEFTY-A may provide a crucial signal for endometrial breakdown and bleeding by triggering expression of several MMPs[24]. Further gene expression studies are certainly going to give more detailed insights into the molecular determinants of excessive menstrual bleeding.

INVESTIGATION

The evaluation of menorrhagia should focus on the:

- Morbidity of excessive blood loss
- Assessment of uterine pathology
- Exclusion of systemic disease

Symptoms related by the patient with menorrhagia can often be more revealing than laboratory tests or imaging. Considering the lengthy list of possible etiologies that contribute to menorrhagia, taking a detailed history is imperative. It should focus on length and subjective assessment of blood flow, intermenstrual interval, and changes from previous bleeding patterns. Women with ovulatory bleeding are likely to have heavy regular menstruation over several consecutive cycles without any intermenstrual bleeding. Presumptive evidence of ovulation can be gained from a history of premenopausal symptoms. Anovulatory bleeding is frequently not associated with any of these symptoms and occurs unpredictably.

The quantity of bleeding itself is a very subjective issue when considering vaginal bleeding. It has been estimated in clinical practice that only 40% of women complaining of menorrhagia have measured losses greater than 80 ml[25]. Furthermore, in many cases a discordance between patients' menstrual symptoms and the diagnosis of menorrhagia exists as many general practitioners are significantly biased and use the term menorrhagia as a blanket category[2]. In addition, the number of tampons or pads used or the duration of bleeding are unreliable indicators of blood loss[26].

Although not available routinely, objective measurement of menstrual blood loss is a valuable investigation in the assessment of excessive menstrual periods. The 'alkaline hematin method', where sanitary devices are soaked in 5% sodium hydroxide to convert the blood to alkaline hematin which is then quantified by photometry is a specialized, time-consuming technique and generally considered to be a research tool[27]. Better suited for the clinical practice are pictoral blood loss assessment charts. In this semiquantitive evaluation the patient scores the daily number

of lightly, moderately, or heavily soiled tampons or sanitary towels. However, the validity of this has been questioned[28]. Furthermore, recent technological changes in the manufacture of sanitary towels means that these pictorial methods need to be revalidated. The measurement of total menstrual fluid by means of a weighing technique was recently described as sufficiently accurate for clinical purposes[29]. However, this method is not yet widely used and requires further evaluation.

An abdominal, bimanual and speculum pelvic examination is mandatory in all women with menorrhagia. Papanicolaou (Pap) smear results of cervical cytology should be up to date in accordance with the local screening programs.

A full blood count is needed to determine the presence or absence of anemia. However, not all women with objective menorrhagia are anemic. Iron studies are not recommended in this setting. Testing for bleeding disorders should be undertaken if clinically indicated, e.g. menorrhagia since menarche or a history of bleeding after dental extractions and childbirth. Thyroid function tests should only be undertaken if clinically indicated. No other endocrine investigations are warranted[3,30].

Imaging

Transvaginal sonography (TVS) is usually the first-step investigation in patients with menorrhagia. It is a non-invasive, non-painful method which examines not only the endometrium, but also the myometrium and ovaries. TVS measures endometrial thickness and diagnoses polyps and myomata with a sensitivity of 80% and specificity of 69%[31]. However, unlike many other imaging techniques, TVS assessment is a dynamic procedure, and therefore its accuracy largely depends on the skill and experience of the sonographer.

It is now well established that endometrial thickness measured by TVS is indicative of pathology in postmenopausal women. The exact cut-off values for endometrial thickness measurement in premenopausal women to predict endometrial hyperplasia or cancer are a subject of continuing debate. While a thin endometrium probably predicts the absence of endometrial pathology, the physiologic changes of endometrial thickness during the menstrual cycle reduces the specificity of TVS. Therefore TVS should be performed after menstruation in the follicular phase of the menstrual cycle. The British 'Royal College of Gynaecologists' (RCOG) Guideline Development Group' analyzed a number of studies involving premenopausal women and concluded that 10–12 mm was a reasonable cut-off when using TVS as a method prior to more invasive procedures of endometrial assessment[32].

The limitations of simple TVS can sometimes be overcome with sonohysterography. By instillation of saline into the uterine cavity the interface between the fluid and endometrial masses can be visualized, which is very helpful in determining the presence or absence of polyps or intracavitary leiomyomas[33]. TVS in combination with color flow Doppler may assist in the detection of endometrial hyperplasia and cancer, as blood flow is known to be altered in malignancies[34]. Increased blood flow, however, has also been reported for benign pathologies and it is controversial whether Doppler sonography improves diagnosis of premalignant and malignant endometrial lesions[34].

Although TVS is very useful for visualizing uterine pathology in women with menorrhagia, in most cases it is insufficient on its own to establish a diagnosis. This warrants endometrial sampling.

Endometrial sampling

The purpose of performing endometrial sampling in women with menorrhagia is to exclude or diagnose endometrial cancer or hyperplasia. It is recommended in women with menorrhagia aged more than 40 years and in women with increased risk of endometrial malignancy. Significant risk factors for development of an endometrial carcinoma are obesity, diabetes mellitus, hypertension, chronic anovulation, nulliparity with a history of infertility, a family history of endometrial and/or colonic cancer and tamoxifen therapy[32]. In younger women endometrial sampling can also be indicated if abnormal bleeding does not resolve with medical treatment. In polycystic ovary syndrome in which endometrial hyperplasia is a common finding, endometrial assessment may be necessary if abnormal bleeding is a presenting symptom, or if suspicious sonographic endometrial features are observed[32].

The most common methods of endometrial sampling are:

- Endometrial biopsy
- Dilatation and curettage (D&C)
- Hysteroscopy

Endometrial biopsy can be performed in an outpatient setting. A variety of instruments for office endometrial biopsy have been developed. The two most commonly used are the Pipelle® (Unimar, USA) and the Vabra® aspiration biopsy device (Berkeley Medevices, USA). The Pipelle sampler is a flexible polypropylene suction catheter that uses an integral plastic piston to generate negative pressure to aspirate tissue. The Vabra curette is a stainless-steel cannula with a plastic chamber which is connected to a vacuum pump to obtain an endometrial sample by suction. In a meta-analysis by Dijkhuizen and colleagues, the Pipelle endometrial biopsy device, with detection rates of 91% for endometrial cancer and atypical endometrial hyperplasia in premenopausal women, was reported to be superior to D&C and hysteroscopy[35]. The 'RCOG Guideline Development Group' analyzed studies comparing the Pipelle sampler, D&C and other endometrial sampling devices, including the Vabra aspirator, and concluded that the Pipelle sampler was the preferable device in terms of diagnostic ability, patient acceptability and costs[32].

However, while a positive biopsy can save patients the inconvenience of more invasive procedures, a negative finding with continuing menorrhagia should be interpreted with caution as false-negative results of 10% and higher have been reported for patients with endometrial malignancies[36]. A repeated TVS and/or endometrial sampling is therefore recommended in these patients. In addition, while endometrial biopsy represents the method of choice for diagnosis or exclusion of endometrial hyperplasia or cancer, it is also well known that this blind procedure is unsuitable for diagnosing polyps or fibroids.

Dilatation and curettage has long been regarded as the gold standard for assessment of abnormal uterine bleeding. Despite this assertion, D&C is a blind procedure which does not sample the whole uterine cavity and it has

been estimated that it does not uncover endometrial pathology in more than 50% of cases[37]. Furthermore, D&C has erroneously been regarded to be a diagnostic as well as a therapeutic procedure. Objective menstrual blood loss assessment, however, has shown that while the first menstrual period after a D&C is lighter, following ones are unchanged to those before the procedure[25].

Increasing evidence suggests that traditional D&C no longer has a place either in diagnosis or in the treatment of excessive menstrual bleeding. D&C should be limited to the few cases in which an office endometrial biopsy is not appropriate.

Hysteroscopy enables direct visualization of the endometrial cavity and it is the principal technique of investigating the uterine cavity to detect polyps and fibroids. Hysteroscopy can be performed either as an out-patient procedure with or without local anesthesia or as an in-patient procedure with local or general anesthesia. The procedure may be carried out either with rigid or fiberoptic instruments. The uterine cavity is distended either with carbon dioxide or sterile isotonic fluids, with a satisfactory view of the cavity being obtained in more than 90% of cases. As the hysteroscope is inserted under vision, major complications are extremely rare and minor complications occur in fewer than 2% of patients[38]. Hysteroscopy in an out-patient setting is safe and successful in the diagnosis of uterine pathology. There appears to be no loss in diagnostic sensitivity for endometrial lesions when compared to inpatient examination or any reduction in the percentage of endometrial biopsies suitable for histological analysis[39]. The main limiting factor to a large-scale use of office hysteroscopy is the level of pain or discomfort a patient feels during or soon after the procedure, which is often caused by the insertion of the hysteroscope. The development of small-diameter hysteroscopes enabling a so called 'mini-hysteroscopy' have led to remarkable progress and higher acceptance of office hysteroscopy.

Hysteroscopy has been advocated by many to be the standard for the diagnosis of abnormal uterine bleeding. Results of various groups, however, have shown that hysteroscopy alone without biopsy carries low sensitivity and positive predictive value in the diagnosis of endometrial carcinoma and hyperplasia. An endometrial biopsy or D&C should therefore be performed during hysteroscopy for accurate diagnosis of endometrial histopathology[40]. Furthermore, caution is advised in the uncritical use of hysteroscopy in patients suspected of having an endometrial malignancy. It has been shown that hysteroscopy can cause dissemination of viable malignant cells from carcinomatous uteri into the abdominal cavity[41].

MEDICAL MANAGEMENT

Background and treatment options

A wide variety of drugs for the treatment of menorrhagia have been developed over the last decade. Medical treatment avoids morbidity and mortality of major surgery, but may have side-effects and has to be taken long term. It is important to evaluate drug therapies in terms of reduction of measured menstrual blood loss, because, as mentioned earlier, there is poor correlation between objective and subjective assessment. Well-designed randomized controlled trials with objective measurement of menstrual blood loss, although rarely performed, provide the best evidence of the efficacy of any intervention.

Menorrhagia is the commonest cause of iron-deficiency anemia in Western women. In many cases, the principal symptom experienced by women with menorrhagia is fatigue. This may be successfully treated with iron and a daily dose of 60–180 mg elemental iron might be the only necessary treatment. It could be argued that menstrual blood loss should be reduced within the normal range (i.e. < 80 ml per period). Women who want to avoid surgery, however, may accept a higher loss if they can cope with the flow and the anemia is controlled with iron.

The aims of medical therapy are to reduce blood loss and the risk of anemia and improve quality of life. Medical treatment of menorrhagia can be divided into non-hormonal and hormonal therapy (Table 2). The choice of therapy has also to be considered in relation to the following factors: (a) Does the woman suffer from dysfunctional bleeding or is a uterine pathology the reason for menorrhagia? (b) Does the woman wish to retain her fertility? (c) Does the woman require contraception? (d) Does the woman have an irregular cycle? (e) Is dysmenorrhea a significant symptom? (f) Are there any contraindications to treatment? and (g) What are the patients preferences? It is important to properly inform patients about the different treatment options to enable them to make informed choices. It has been shown that the provision of information to patients can alter their choices about treatment and may improve outcomes of care[42].

Table 2 Medical treatment options for menorrhagia

Non-hormonal treatment options for menorrhagia
Non-steroidal anti-inflammatory drugs
    mefenamic acid
    meclofenamic acid
    naproxen
    ibuprofen
    flurbiprofen
    diclofenac
Antifibrinolytics
    tranexamic acid
Reducers of capillary fragility
    etamsylate
Stimulators of endogenous hemostasis
    desmopressin (DDAVP)

Hormonal treatment options for menorrhagia
Oral progestogens
    norethisterone
    medroxyprogesterone acetate
    dydrogestrone
Intrauterine progestogens:
    levonorgestrel-releasing intrauterine device (Mirena®)
    progesterone-releasing intrauterine device
      (Progestasert®)
Combined estrogen/progestogens
    oral contraceptives
Other
    danazol
    gestrinone
    gonadotropin releasing hormone analogs

Non-hormonal treatments of menorrhagia

Non-steroidal anti-inflammatory drugs

The cyclo-oxygenase (COX) pathway with its two enzymes COX-1 and COX-2 represents one of the major routes for oxidative metabolism of arachidonic acid to prostaglandins. The demonstrated involvement of prostaglandins in the genesis of menorrhagia pointed to COX inhibitors as a potentially effective treatment. COX inhibitors, commonly referred to as non-steroidal anti-inflammatory drugs (NSAIDs), can be chemically classified into two main groups – COX-1 inhibitors: salicytes (aspirin), indolacetic acid analogs (indometacin), aryl proprionic acid derivates (naproxen, ibuprofen), fenamates (mefenamic acid, flufenamic acid, meclofenamic acid), and COX-2 inhibitors: coxibs (celecoxib).

Various NSAIDs have been evaluated in a number of randomized trials, which to date, in regards to their efficacy in treating menorrhagia, have been limited to COX-1 inhibitors. In a Cochrane review, five of seven randomized trials showed that mean menstrual blood loss was less with NSAIDs than with placebo, and two showed no difference. Furthermore, there was no evidence that one NSAID (naproxen or mefenamic acid) was superior to the other[43]. The fenamates (e.g. mefenamic acid) are the most extensively studied NSAIDs. They have the unique property to inhibit prostaglandin synthesis as well as to bind to prostaglandin receptors, which, as previously mentioned, are significantly increased in the uteri from women with menorrhagia[18]. Reduction in menstrual blood flow ranges from 22–46% with this therapy. With regards to long-term therapy, a follow-up of 12–15 months after commencing treatment showed continuing efficacy of the NSAID mefenamic acid[44]. Reduction of menstrual blood loss has also been evaluated for other NSAIDs such as naproxen, ibuprofen, sodium diclofenac and flurbiprofen. The percentage of blood loss reduction varied from 25 to 47% depending on the agent and dosage used[43].

Optimal doses and schedules are difficult to define. Most studies, however, analyzed regimens that started with the first day of menses and continued for 5 days or until cessation of menstruation. Naproxen and mefanemic acid are typically prescribed in a dosage of 250–500 mg two to four times per day; ibuprofen has been studied in doses ranging from 600–1200 mg per day[43].

Common side-effects of NSAIDs are gastrointestinal complications and inhibition of platelet aggregation. NSAIDs are therefore contraindicated in women with peptic ulceration and bleeding diathesis or in those who want to undergo a surgical procedure. Apart from that, NSAIDs have a low profile of adverse effects in otherwise healthy women.

Specific inhibitors of COX-2 might also be effective in the treatment of menorrhagia, but their role has not yet been evaluated.

Randomized studies comparing NSAIDs with other agents for menorrhagia suggest that both tranexamic acid and danazol are more effective with regards to decreasing blood loss. However, tranexamic acid and danazol cause more side-effects when compared with NSAIDs. In a limited number of small studies there was no statistically significant difference between NSAIDs and other treatments (oral progestogen, etamsylate, progesterone-releasing intrauterine system (IUS), oral contraceptive pill). However, most of these studies were underpowered.

In summary, NSAIDs should be considered as a first-line therapy in essential menorrhagia. The degree of reduction of menstrual blood loss is modest, but NSAIDs are well tolerated and suitable for long-term treatment. Furthermore, they are also effective in women with a copper or non-hormonal intrauterine contraceptive device. An additional beneficial effect is that these drugs will also alleviate symptoms from dysmenorrhea.

Antifibrinolytics

As mentioned before, significantly elevated fibrinolytic activity in the endometrium caused by a premenstrual rise in tissue plasminogen activators is believed to be an underlying mechanism for menorrhagia[21]. Plasminogen activator inhibitors (antifibrinolytic agents) have therefore been promoted as a treatment for menorrhagia.

Tranexamic acid is a synthetic lysine derivate that exerts its antifibrinolytic effect by reversibly blocking lysine binding sites on plasminogen and thus preventing fibrin degradation[45]. In a number of small clinical studies in women with dysfunctional bleeding, tranexamic acid 2–4.5 g/day for 4–7 days reduced menstrual blood flow by 34–59% over two to three cycles. The effect was shown to be superior to placebo, mefenamic acid, flurbiprofen, etamsylate and oral luteal phase norethisterone at clinically relevant dosages[46].

Tranexamic acid is usually well tolerated. Reported side-effects have been limited to mild gastrointestinal complaints, including nausea, vomiting or diarrhea. However, there was no significant increase in reported events with antifibrinolytic therapy in comparison to placebo or other treatments in a Cochrane analysis[46]. Earlier theoretical concerns about thromboembolism caused by antifibrinolytic action of tranexamic acid have been refuted by long-term studies. The incidence of thrombosis in women treated with tranexamic acid was shown to be comparable to the spontaneous frequency of the condition in the general population.

In conclusion, antifibrinolytic agents are an effective treatment of menorrhagia and should be considered as a first-line therapy for dysfunctional bleeding. Antifibrinolytics are also effective in women with copper or non-hormonal intrauterine devices[45,46].

Reducers of capillary fragility

Etamsylate (epsilono-caproic acid) is believed to act by reducing capillary fragility, but the precise mechanism is unknown. Although results are conflicting, studies with an objective menstrual blood loss measurement using the recommended doses showed that etamsylate is inferior to other medications like NSAIDs or antifibrinolytics and might not reduce menstrual blood loss at all. Its use is not recommended in the UK[2].

Stimulators of endogenous hemostasis

Desmopressin (DDAVP) is a synthetic analog of the natural hormone vasopressin. It has an established role in the management of patients with bleeding disorders such as vWD and hemophilia A, because of its ability to induce an increase in plasma concentration of von Willebrand factor (vWF) and factor VIII (FVIII). In cases of severe menorrhagia in women with vWD, DDAVP is given intravenously in a dosage of $0.3\,\mu g/kg$ body weight, which will rapidly increase the recipients FVIII and vWF levels by three- to five-fold. For home use, a highly concentrated intranasal spray formulation ($150–300\,\mu g$ per intranasal spray) can be used. It is usually taken at the onset of menstrual bleeding, with a second dose being taken the following day. Nevertheless, despite convincing results based on women's subjective assessment, no data from properly powered randomized studies, objectively evaluating the effect of nasal DDAVP, have been published yet[47].

DDAVP is also known to increase tissue plasminogen activator expression and platelet adhesiveness as well as vasoconstriction. These properties might explain the results of a recent study showing an improvement of IUD-related menorrhagia in women treated with DDAVP tablets[48]. However, larger randomized studies are required to confirm the results.

Hormonal treatments of menorrhagia

Progestogens

Progestogens are the commonest prescription for women with unexplained menorrhagia. The use of progestogens is based on the erroneous concept that women with menorrhagia principally have anovulatory cycles and that progestogens co-ordinate regular shedding when given as late luteal phase supplements on days 15–26 of the cycle. However, many studies have shown that most women with regular excessive menstrual bleeding have normal ovulatory cycles[25]. Therefore, the role and efficacy of progestogens in treating all cases of unexplained menorrhagia remains controversial and there is little objective evidence to support the use of this therapy.

A variety of routes of administration and dosage schedules exist. These range from intermittent luteal phase oral administration, through intramuscular injection, to continuous local administration by an intrauterine device, each of which has different efficacy in distinct clinical situations.

Systemic administration The value of systemic progestogen administration for the treatment of menorrhagia is difficult to determine, as there have been no randomized trials comparing these agents with placebo. However, numerous trials have compared progestogens with other medical therapies.

Women with regular excessive menstrual loss do not benefit from cyclical oral progestogens for short duration (5–10 days). This treatment was even reported to increase menstrual bleeding[49]. A Cochrane meta-analysis on cyclic progestogen therapy concluded that luteal phase progestogens were less effective at reducing menstrual blood loss when compared with tranexamic acid, danazol and the progesterone-releasing IUD[50]. Longer regimens (5 mg norethisterone three times/day on days 5–26 of the menstrual cycle) have been reported to produce a significant reduction in menstrual blood loss (by 87%) when compared with pretreatment levels. However, the rate of satisfaction of women under this regimen is poor, with only 22% willing to continue with the treatment after three cycles[51]. High-dose progestogens such as 30 mg daily can be administered to control excessive bleeding. This is usually effective within 24–48 h. After this, the dose of the progestogen can be reduced and finally stopped after a few days when another bleeding, usually lighter, will occur. Side-effects of oral progestogens vary according to the type, dose and duration of administration. They include weight gain, headache, depression and a premenstrual-like syndrome (bloating, fluid retention, breast tenderness). Patients treated with oral progestogen therapy must be informed that this is not a form of contraception.

Intrauterine administration Intrauterine coil devices were originally developed for contraception. While menstrual loss is usually increased after insertion of inert or copper-containing intrauterine contraceptive devices, it is largely reduced when they are impregnated with progestogens. There are currently two progestogen–impregnated intrauterine systems (IUS) on the market: the Mirena® IUS (Schering, Germany) that delivers 20 μg of levonorgestrel (LNG) over 24 h for about 5 years, and the Progestasert® IUS (Alza Pharmaceuticals, USA) that releases approximately 65 μg of progesterone over 24 h for about 16 months. Other newer so-called 'frameless' IUDs are currently being evaluated in clinical trials.

The Mirena IUS (LNG-IUS) reduces menstrual blood loss by up to 96% and 20% of women using the LNG-IUS are reported to be amenorrheic after 1 year[52]. Over a 3-year period 65% of women with a LNG-IUS continue to report improved menstrual bleeding. Apart from lowering menstrual blood loss, LNG-IUSs may alleviate symptoms of dysmenorrhea and reduce the incidence of pelvic inflammatory disease. Furthermore, LNG-IUS provides very effective contraception and appears to have the greatest impact on bleeding volume of all medical therapies. There have also been comparisons with surgical therapies. Endometrial resection, along with balloon ablation, proved to be about 10% more effective than the LNG-IUS in controlling bleeding at 1 year in a randomized controlled study[53]. To assess if the LNG-IUS could provide a conservative alternative to hysterectomy in the treatment of excessive uterine bleeding, a Finnish trial randomized a cohort of women with ovulatory dysfunctional bleeding scheduled for hysterectomy, for continuation of their medical treatment or a LNG-IUS. Although there was a significant bias in the study, the primary outcome was the women's decision to undergo surgery. In the IUS group 64% decided to cancel surgery versus 14% in the medical treatment group[54].

The main adverse effects associated with LNG-IUS are frequently occurring variable bleeding and spotting, particularly within the first few months of use. It is very important to counsel women before the IUS is fitted about the changes in bleeding pattern that will occur. This also includes, the possibility of amenorrhea which, may be undesirable or even unacceptable for others on cultural, moral or religious grounds. LNG-IUS are also sometimes associated with the development of ovarian cysts, but these are usually symptomless and show a high rate of spontaneous resolution.

When compared with other medications the LNG-IUS is much cheaper per menstrual cycle unless it is removed before 5 years. Therefore long-term acceptability is crucial. Cost-effectiveness in comparison with hysterectomy has also been evaluated. The LNG-IUS showed similar efficacy and patient satisfaction at much lower costs ($1530 for IUS vs. $4222 for hysterectomy)[55].

In conclusion, LNG-IUS can now be considered to be a serious alternative to conventional medical and surgical treatment of dysfunctional uterine bleeding. It has less morbidity and is more cost-effective than surgery and preserves fertility while providing contraception. Furthermore, the LNG-IUS may be discontinued when the patient becomes menopausal, or its use may be continued for hormone replacement therapy.

The Progestasert, which was the first hormonally impregnated device on the market, has been reported to produce reductions in menstrual blood loss and decrease length of bleeding time in various small case studies[56]. However, due to the lack of prospective randomized studies no objective conclusions can be drawn. The main disadvantage of this device is its association with an increased risk of ectopic pregnancy. Furthermore, Progestasert requires re-insertion every 18 months.

Estrogen/progestogen combinations

Estrogen/progestogen combinations in the form of oral contraceptive pills (COCs) are widely used in the management of irregular or excessive menstrual bleeding. While sequential hormone replacement therapy is used clinically there are no published clinical trials to date for the treatment of menorrhagia[32]. When taken in a cyclical fashion, COCs induce regular shedding of a thinner endometrium and inhibit ovulation. The exact endometrial mode of contraceptive pills is unknown, and probably involves induction of endometrial atrophy.

From clinical experience COCs are generally considered to be effective in the management of dysfunctional menstrual bleeding. However, there are few available data to support this observation as randomized-controlled trials with adequate patient number, duration of at least three to six cycles and adequate follow-up have not been conducted[57]. Consequently, due to the paucity of data, a Cochrane analysis was unable to analyze if COCs are an effective medical therapy to reduce menorrhagia[57].

Although there is some indication that the frequency of menstrual disturbances, such as spotting and breakthrough bleeding, is reduced when the COCs contains a relatively high dose of progestogen, no evidence exists suggesting that changing the progestogen component influences menstrual blood loss. Similarly, it is unclear whether low-dose ethinylestradiol preparations are as effective in reducing menstrual blood loss as higher doses. Many of the studies used a higher dose than the 30–35 µg ethinylestradiol of preparations currently in use.

To take the COCs for longer time spans with shorter periods might be beneficial in improving excessive menstrual bleeding. An extended–cycle levonorgestrel–/ethinylestradiol-containing oral contraceptive (Seasonale®, Duramed Pharmaceuticals, USA) has been developed recently that produces a menstrual period every 3 months only[58]. Its use in menorrhagia, however, remains to be evaluated.

Androgens

Danazol Danazol is an isoxazol deivative of 17α-ethinyl-testosterone which acts on the hypothalamic pituitary axis as well as on the endometrium to produce atrophy. Danazol was shown to reduce menstrual blood loss by up to 80% from baseline. Higher doses of Danazol (≥ 200 mg/day) seem to be more successful than low-dosage therapy, most likely because of an inhibitory effect on ovulation[32]. Danazol appears to be a more effective treatment for excessive menstrual bleeding than other medical treatments like NSAIDs, oral progestogens or OCPs. There have been no randomized trials comparing danazol with tranexamic acid or the LNG-IUD[59].

Although danazol is effective in the treatment of menorrhea its clinical use is limited by androgenic side-effects, e.g. acne, oily skin, weight gain and deepening of the voice that are experienced by up to three-quarters of the patients. It may also increase the risk for unhealthy cholesterol levels. No studies to date show the effects of long-term use of danazol.

Furthermore, women must be advised to use barrier methods for contraception because of the potential virilization of the fetus if pregnancy occurs while on danazol treatment. Due to these side-effects, danazol is best restricted to women awaiting surgery or as a short-term endometrial thinning agent prior to endometrial destruction.

Gestrinone Gestrinone is a 19-testosterone derivative which has antiprogestogenic, anti-estrogenic and androgenic activity. Gestrinone was shown in a placebo-controlled study to successfully reduce menstrual blood loss in 79% patients suffering from excessive menstrual bleeding[60]. However, most women treated with gestrinone experience side-effects such as hirsutism, weight gain and acne which precludes long-term therapy[32].

Gonadotropin releasing hormone agonists

Gonadotropin releasing hormone (GnRH) agonists, administered continuously or in depot form, down-regulate expression of GnRH receptors, which blocks gonadotropin secretion from the anterior pituitary. This leads to subsequent suppression of ovarian function and causes a hypoestrogenic state. GnRH agonists can be used in various ways for the therapy of excessive menstrual bleeding but have been reported mainly for their effectiveness in treating bleeding associated with fibroids. GnRH analogs frequently induce amenorrhea in association with reduction of uterine volume by 40–60%[32,61].

However, there are significant side-effects from the hypoestrogenic state during GnRH analog therapy. These include menopausal symptoms such as hot flushes, night sweat, vaginal dryness, weight change and depression.

The most important concern is possible osteoporosis from estrogen withdrawal. The duration of treatment with GnRH analogs is therefore limited to 6 months. Most studies have shown that after GnRH agonist treatment is discontinued there is regrowth both of uteri and fibroids to nearly pretreatment size and recurrence of bleeding problems in most patients. Furthermore, GnRH agonist treatment does not necessarily prevent a pregnancy. As there is some risk for malformations after GnRH treatment in pregnancy, women should use non-hormonal birth control during therapy.

Concerns about bone loss and poor tolerability of GnRH agonists have led to the development of several approaches to preserve enough estrogen to minimize side-effects. In the add-back therapy estrogen/progestogen hormone replacement is used in conjunction with GnRH agonists. Hormone levels are usually high enough to protect from menopausal symptoms and osteoporosis but too low to offset the beneficial effects of the GnRH agonist[61]. Adding bisphosphonates as bone-protective agents to the GnRH agonist treatment is another strategy. Other agents which have been tested in combination with GnRH agonists to preserve bone density are parathyroid hormone and the selective estrogen-receptor modulator (SERM) tibolone.

The side-effects of GnRH agonists usually preclude their long-term use. However, they are highly effective in short-term therapies, e.g. preoperative endometrial thinning before endometrial destruction or fibroid/uterine shrinkage before myomectomy/hysterectomy. Similarly, GnRH agonist treatment for 2–3 months before surgery for uterine leiomyomas is known to limit side-effects and costs, and in certain cases avoids hysterectomy.

Antiprogestational agents

Mifepristone (RU–486) is a synthetic 19-norsteroid with antiprogestogen activity that is known to inhibit ovulation and to disrupt endometrial integrity. A recent trial has shown that mifepristone acts as a contraceptive agent and that it induces amenorrhea at a dosage of 5 mg per day in most women[62]. Mifepristone has also been used to a limited extent in the medical treatment of uterine fibroids[63].

As the endometrial effect of mifepristone is achieved without estrogen deprivation it might be a promising novel long-term approach to the treatment of excessive menstrual bleeding. However, clinical studies are required before its use in menorrhagia can be recommended.

PRACTICE POINTS

- Menorrhagia is a very common problem
- Most women with a complaint of heavy periods have no pathology
- Most women with menorrhagia have ovulatory cycles
- Investigations include transvaginal ultrasound, endometrial biopsy and hysteroscopy
- Effective treatments, e.g. mefenamic acid and tranexamic acid, can be taken only during the period and will not affect fertility
- The levonorgestrel IUCD is an effective treatment which can avoid women having a hysterectomy
- Treatment is long term and will have to be continued until the menopause

REFERENCES

1. Rees MC. Role of menstrual blood loss measurements in management of complaints of excessive menstrual bleeding. Br J Obstet Gynaecol 1991; 98: 327–8

2. Warner P, Critchley HO, Lumsden MA, et al. Referral for menstrual problems: cross sectional survey of symptoms, reasons for referral, and management. BMJ 2001; 323: 24–8

3. Royal College of Obstetricians and Gynaecologists. The Initial Management of Menorrhagia. Evidence-Based Clinical Guidelines, 1. London: RCOG Press, 1998

4. Hallberg L, Hogdahl AM, Nilsson L, Rybo G. Menstrual blood loss – a population study. Variation at different ages and attempts to define normality. Acta Obstet Gynecol Scand 1966; 45: 320–51

5. Clarke A, Black N, Rowe P, et al. Indications for and outcome of total abdominal hysterectomy for benign disease: a prospective cohort study. Br J Obstet Gynaecol 1995; 102: 611–20

6. Flake GP, Andersen J, Dixon D. Etiology and pathogenesis of uterine leiomyomas: a review. Environ Health Perspect 2003; 111: 1037–54

7. Hague S, Zhang L, Oehler MK, et al. Expression of the hypoxically regulated angiogenic factor adrenomedullin correlates with uterine leiomyoma vascular density. Clin Cancer Res 2000; 6: 2808–14

8. Jha RC, Takahama J, Imaoka I, et al. Adenomyosis: MRI of the uterus treated with uterine artery embolization. AJR Am J Roentgenol 2003; 181: 851–6

9. Kadir RA, Economides DL, Sabin CA, et al. Frequency of inherited bleeding disorders in women with menorrhagia. Lancet 1998; 351: 485–9

10. Dilley A, Drews C, Miller C, et al. von Willebrand disease and other inherited bleeding disorders in women with diagnosed menorrhagia. Obstet Gynecol 2001; 97: 630–6

11. Kouides PA. Menorrhagia from a haematologist's point of view. Part I: initial evaluation. Haemophilia 2002; 8: 330–8

12. van Eijkeren MA, Christiaens GC, Haspels AA, Sixma JJ. Measured menstrual blood loss in women with a bleeding disorder or using oral anticoagulant therapy. Am J Obstet Gynecol 1990; 162: 1261–3

13. Wein TH, Hickenbottom SL, Morgenstern LB, et al. Safety of tissue plasminogen activator for acute stroke in menstruating women. Stroke 2002; 33: 2506–8

14. Koch AZ, Abubaker J, Barnett VT, Chan LN. Use of thrombolytic therapy to treat heparin-refractory pulmonary embolism in a menstruating patient. Pharmacotherapy 2002; 22: 118–22

15. Krassas GE, Pontikides N, Kaltsas T, et al. Disturbances of menstruation in hypothyroidism. Clin Endocrinol (Oxf) 1999; 50: 655–9

16. Makarainen L, Ylikorkala O. Primary and myoma-associated menorrhagia: role of prostaglandins and effects of ibuprofen. Br J Obstet Gynaecol 1986; 93: 974–8

17. Rees MC, Anderson AB, Demers LM, Turnbull AC. Prostaglandins in menstrual fluid in menorrhagia and dysmenorrhoea. Br J Obstet Gynaecol 1984; 91: 673–80

18. Adelantado JM, Rees MC, Lopez Bernal A, Turnbull AC. Increased uterine prostaglandin E receptors in menorrhagic women. Br J Obstet Gynaecol 1988; 95: 162–5

19. Sales KJ, Jabbour HN. Cyclooxygenase enzymes and prostaglandins in pathology of the

endometrium. Reproduction 2003; 126: 559–67

20. Zervou S, Klentzeris LD, Old RW. Nitric oxide synthase expression and steroid regulation in the uterus of women with menorrhagia. Mol Hum Reprod 1999; 5: 1048–54

21. Gleeson NC. Cyclic changes in endometrial tissue plasminogen activator and plasminogen activator inhibitor type 1 in women with normal menstruation and essential menorrhagia. Am J Obstet Gynecol 1994; 171: 178–83

22. Vincent AJ, Zhang J, Ostor A, et al. Decreased tissue inhibitor of metalloproteinase in the endometrium of women using depot medroxyprogesterone acetate: a role for altered endometrial matrix metalloproteinase/tissue inhibitor of metalloproteinase balance in the pathogenesis of abnormal uterine bleeding? Hum Reprod 2002; 17: 1189–98

23. Curry TE Jr, Osteen KG. The matrix metalloproteinase system: changes, regulation, and impact throughout the ovarian and uterine reproductive cycle. Endocr Rev 2003; 24: 428–65

24. Cornet PB, Picquet C, Lemoine P, et al. Regulation and function of LEFTY-A/EBAF in the human endometrium. mRNA expression during the menstrual cycle, control by progesterone, and effect on matrix metallo-proteinases. J Biol Chem 2002; 277: 42496–504

25. Haynes PJ, Hodgson H, Anderson AB, Turnbull AC. Measurement of menstrual blood loss in patients complaining of menorrhagia. Br J Obstet Gynaecol 1977; 84: 763–8

26. Chimbira TH, Anderson AB, Turnbull A. Relation between measured menstrual blood loss and patient's subjective assessment of loss, duration of bleeding, number of sanitary towels used, uterine weight and endometrial surface area. Br J Obstet Gynaecol 1980; 87: 603–9

27. Hallberg L, Nilsson L. Determination of menstrual blood loss. Scand J Clin Lab Invest 1964; 16: 244–8

28. Reid PC, Coker A, Coltart R. Assessment of menstrual blood loss using a pictorial chart: a validation study. BJOG 2000; 107: 320–2

29. Fraser IS, Warner P, Marantos PA. Estimating menstrual blood loss in women with normal and excessive menstrual fluid volume. Obstet Gynecol 2001; 98: 806–14

30. Hope S. 10 minute consultation: menorrhagia. BMJ 2000; 321: 935

31. Vercellini P, Cortesi I, Oldani S, et al. The role of transvaginal ultrasonography and outpatient diagnostic hysteroscopy in the evaluation of patients with menorrhagia. Hum Reprod 1997; 12: 1768–71

32. Royal College of Obstetricians and Gynaecologists. The Management of Menorrhagia in Secondary Care. Evidence-Based Clinical Guidelines, 5. London: RCOG Press, 1999

33. Dijkhuizen FP, De Vries LD, Mol BW, et al. Comparison of transvaginal ultrasonography and saline infusion sonography for the detection of intracavitary abnormalities in premenopausal women. Ultrasound Obstet Gynecol 2000; 15: 372–6

34. Levine D. Pelvic Doppler. Semin Ultrasound CT MR 1999; 20: 239–49

35. Dijkhuizen FP, Mol BW, Brolmann HA, Heintz AP. The accuracy of endometrial sampling in the diagnosis of patients with endometrial carcinoma and hyperplasia: a meta-analysis. Cancer 2000; 89: 1765–72

36. Feldman S, Shapter A, Welch WR, Berkowith RS. Two-year follow-up of 263 patients with post/perimenopausal vaginal bleeding and negative initial biopsy. Gynecol Oncol 1994; 55: 56–9

37. Bettochi S, Ceci O, Vicino M, et al. Diagnostic approach of dilatation and curettage. Fertil Steril 2001; 75: 803–5

38. Symonds I. Ultrasound, hysteroscopy and endometrial biopsy in the investigation of endometrial cancer. Best Pract Res Clin Obstet Gynaecol 2001; 15: 381–91

39. Cicinelli E, Parisi C, Galantino P, et al. Reliability, feasibility, and safety of mini-hysteroscopy with a vaginoscopic approach: experience with 6,000 cases. Fertil Steril 2003; 80: 199–202

40. Ben-Yehuda OM, Kim YB, Leuchter RS. Does hysteroscopy improve upon the sensitivity of dilatation and curettage in the diagnosis of endometrial hyperplasia or carcinoma? Gynecol Oncol 1998; 68: 4–7

41. Lo KW, Cheung TH, Yim SF, Chung TK. Hysteroscopic dissemination of endometrial carcinoma using carbon dioxide and normal saline: a retrospective study. Gynecol Oncol 2002; 84: 394–8

42. Kennedy AD, Sculpher MJ, Coulter A, et al. Effects of decision aids for menorrhagia on treatment choices, health outcomes, and costs: a randomized controlled trial. JAMA 2002; 288: 2701–8

43. Lethaby A, Augood C, Duckitt K. Nonsteroidal anti-inflammatory drugs for heavy menstrual bleeding. Cochrane Database Syst Rev 2002; 2: CD000400

44. Fraser IS, McCarron G, Markham R, et al. Long-term treatment of menorrhagia with mefenamic acid. Obstet Gynecol 1983; 61: 109–12

45. Wellington K, Wagstaff AJ. Tranexamic acid: a review of its use in the management of menorrhagia. Drugs 2003; 63: 1417–33

46. Lethaby A, Farquhar C, Cooke I. Antifibrinolytics for heavy menstrual bleeding. Cochrane Database Syst Rev 2000; 2: CD000249

47. Kadir RA, Lee CA, Sabin CA, et al. DDAVP nasal spray for treatment of menorrhagia in women with inherited bleeding disorders: a randomized placebo-controlled crossover study. Haemophilia 2002; 8: 787–93

48. Mercorio F, Simone RD, Carlo CD, et al. Effectiveness and mechanism of action of desmopressin in the treatment of copper intrauterine device-related menorrhagia: a pilot study. Hum Reprod 2003; 18: 2319–22

49. Preston JT, Cameron IT, Adams EJ, Smith SK. Comparative study of tranexamic acid and norethisterone in the treatment of ovulatory menorrhagia. Br J Obstet Gynaecol 1995; 102: 401–6

50. Lethaby A, Irvine G, Cameron I. Cyclical progestogens for heavy menstrual bleeding. Cochrane Database Syst Rev 2000; 2: CD001016

51. Irvine GA, Campbell-Brown MB, Lumsden MA, et al. Randomised comparative trial of the levonorgestrel intrauterine system and norethisterone for treatment of idiopathic menorrhagia. Br J Obstet Gynaecol 1998; 105: 592–8

52. Lethaby AE, Cooke I, Rees M. Progesterone/progestogen releasing intrauterine systems versus either placebo or any other medication for heavy menstrual bleeding. Cochrane Database Syst Rev 2000; 2: CD002126

53. Crosignani PG, Vercellini P, Mosconi P, et al. Levonorgestrel-releasing intrauterine device versus hysteroscopic endometrial resection in the treatment of dysfunctional uterine bleeding. Obstet Gynecol 1997; 90: 257–63

54. Lahteenmaki P, Haukkamaa M, Puolakka J, et al. Open randomised study of use of levonorgestrel releasing intrauterine system as alternative to hysterectomy. BMJ 1998; 316: 1122–6

55. Hurskainen R, Teperi J, Rissanen P, et al. Quality of life and cost-effectiveness of levonorgestrel-releasing intrauterine system

versus hysterectomy for treatment of menorrhagia: a randomised trial. Lancet 2001; 357: 273–7

56. Bergqvist A, Rybo G. Treatment of menorrhagia with intrauterine release of progesterone. Br J Obstet Gynaecol 1983; 90: 255–8

57. Iyer V, Farquhar C, Jepson R. Oral contraceptive pills for heavy menstrual bleeding. The Cochrane Database Syst Rev 2000; 2: CD000154

58. Anderson FD, Hait H. A multicenter, randomized study of an extended cycle oral contraceptive. Contraception 2003; 68: 89–96

59. Beaumont H, Augood C, Duckitt K, Lethaby A. Danazol for heavy menstrual bleeding. Cochrane Database Syst Rev 2002; 2: CD001017

60. Turnbull AC, Rees MC. Gestrinone in the treatment of menorrhagia. Br J Obstet Gynaecol 1990; 97: 713–15

61. Moghissi KS. A clinician's guide to the use of gonadotropin-releasing hormone analogues in women. Medscape Womens Health 2000; 5: 5

62. Brown A, Cheng L, Lin S, Baird DT. Daily low-dose mifepristone has contraceptive potential by suppressing ovulation and menstruation: a double-blind randomized control trial of 2 and 5 mg per day for 120 days. J Clin Endocrinol Metab 2002; 87: 63–70

63. Kettel LM, Murphy AA, Morales AJ, Yen SS. Clinical efficacy of the antiprogesterone RU486 in the treatment of endometriosis and uterine fibroids. Hum Reprod 1994; 9: 116–20

Uterine fibroids

6

J. Morrison and I.Z. MacKenzie

INTRODUCTION

Uterine leiomyomas, or fibroids, are benign smooth muscle tumors and are the commonest pelvic tumor in women; it has been estimated that by the age of 40 approximately a third of women have at least one fibroid. Pathological studies show that they are present in 50–70% of hysterectomy specimens but around only 10% of hysterectomies are performed specifically because of fibroids[1,2]. This indicates that most women with fibroids are asymptomatic.

ETIOLOGY

Genetic factors

Despite their high prevalence, relatively little is known about the etiology of fibroids. From epidemiological data there is evidence for a genetic component. The incidence in women of African origin is three to nine times higher than for other ethnic groups[3,4] and twin studies of hysterectomy rates have demonstrated that monozygotic twins have twice the twin pair correlation of dizygotic twins[5]. As fibroids are one of the more common reasons for hysterectomy[2,6] this would suggest there is also a genetic component to the incidence of fibroids. Familial studies also indicate a genetic compo-

nent to the development of fibroids. Women with a first-degree relative with fibroids were more than twice as likely to have fibroids compared with women without this family history[7].

Studies looking at the cytogenetics of fibroids have demonstrated a pattern of chromosomal abnormality in 40% of fibroids[8] with mutations occurring commonly at six chromosomal sites. However, 60% of fibroids are chromosomally normal and X-chromosome inactivation studies show that these tumors also arise from a single cell[9]. Interestingly, different fibroids in the same uterus can have different chromosomal changes, suggesting that each fibroid arises separately, albeit on a background of increased genetic susceptibility in that individual[10].

Hormonal influences

Identification of hormonal risk factors that cause fibroids to develop in a genetically predisposed woman is hampered because many fibroids are asymptomatic. Studies are therefore skewed, as they tend to focus on women who are treated by hysterectomy. Age of menarche is significantly associated with development of fibroids, with an approximate two-fold increase with an early as opposed to late menarche[11]. Pathological studies have demonstrated a reduction in size and number of fibroids in postmenopausal compared to premenopausal women[1]. Number of live births is inversely related to the risk of developing fibroids and grand multiparae have a 70–80% reduced risk compared with nulliparae[12,13]. Indeed, there is evidence from animal models for a protective effect of pregnancy. Eker rats are predisposed to develop fibroids secondary to a mutation in the tuberous sclerosis 2 tumor suppressor gene. In female rats with a single litter 71% have fibroids compared with 10% of females with multiple pregnancies[14]. Even a pseudo-pregnancy has been shown to be partially protective, supporting the role of hormonal changes.

All of these risk groups suggest an association with ovarian steroids. Gonadotropin releasing hormone (GnRH) agonists cause fibroid regression[15] by suppression of ovarian hormone production. The role of the combined oral contraceptive pill is unclear with various studies demonstrating either increased, reduced or no risk for developing fibroids. However, as combined oral contraceptives are often used to treat menorrhagia, it is difficult to determine whether these are having an effect on menstrual loss, rather than fibroid development or regression, and a randomized controlled trial would be needed to exclude these confounding effects. Studies of long-term depot medroxy-progesterone acetate (DepoProvera®) do indicate a significant reduction in development of fibroids (relative risk (RR) 0.4)[16]. However, the antiprogesterone, mifepristone, has also been shown to cause fibroid regression[17]. Thus it is unclear exactly how estrogen and progesterone affect fibroid growth, but it appears that cycling levels sufficient to stimulate and modify endometrial morphology are necessary for their development.

PRESENTATION

Fibroids are very prevalent in the population and many women are asymptomatic. They are often found incidentally during clinical or ultrasonic pelvic examination. Table 1 illustrates the frequency with which fibroids were reported following hysterectomy, performed for a variety of preoperative indications, over a 3-year period in Oxford[2]. It is therefore important to explain to women the nature and usual natural history of fibroids and to reassure them that no action is necessary unless symptoms develop.

The symptoms produced by fibroids often depend on their size and position. Fibroids may be categorized into three groups: intramural, submucosal, and subserosal (Figure 1). Intramural fibroids lie within the uterine wall and do not encroach upon the endometrial cavity, although they can cause some distortion leading to an increased endometrial surface area from which menstruation will occur. Sub-mucosal fibroids protrude into the endometrial cavity and are covered with endometrium on their intracavity surface, increasing endometrial surface area and distorting the endometrial cavity. They can fill the endometrial cavity and are attached to the underlying myometrium by a broad sessile stalk or by a narrow pedicle. Subserosal fibroids are situated immediately beneath the visceral peritoneum and either lead to an irregular uterine outline or form large tumors protruding from the surface in a sessile form or attached by a thin, pedunculated stalk. Fibroids may develop within one or other broad ligament and others can develop within the uterine cervix or have an attachment to the cervix. Occasionally they can derive a second blood supply from distant sites. If they then become separated from the body of the uterus they are called 'parasitic fibroids'.

Table 1 Frequency with which fibroids were found at histological section of 1170 uteri removed for different preoperative reasons. From reference 2

Preoperative reason for hysterectomy	Fibroids not present	Fibroids present	Total cases
Endometriosis	18	10	28
Fibroids	3	115	118
Suspected or proven malignancy	87	57	144
Menstrual symptoms	194	251	445
Pelvic or menstrual pain	40	27	67
Obstetric delivery complication	6	0	6
Pre-malignant condition e.g. atypical hyperplasia	19	14	33
Uterovaginal prolapse	115	85	200
Pelvic tumor of uncertain origin	55	74	129
Total	537	633	1170

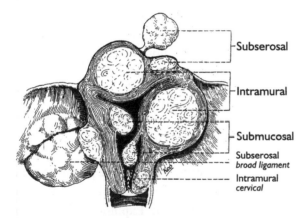

Figure 1 Diagrammatic representation of anatomical positions of fibroids

Menstrual symptoms

Menstrual blood loss can be abnormal because it is either excessively heavy or prolonged. Fibroids can cause either heavy or prolonged menstruation (Figure 2). They do not cause irregular menstrual, intermenstrual or post-menopausal bleeding unless they are the seat of malignant change or are placed intraluminally and become traumatized or thrombosed by prolapsing through the cervix. One ultrasound study found that submucosal and intramural fibroids were more common in women with abnormal menstruation than in asymptomatic women[18]; 58% of the women with abnormal bleeding had an intramural fibroid and 21% had a submucosal fibroid. These results reinforce the view that fibroids that distort the endometrial cavity can be asymptomatic since 13% of the asymptomatic women had an intramural fibroid and 1% had a submucosal fibroid. These data suggest that although submucosal fibroids are relatively uncommon compared with other types of fibroids, when present they usually cause symptoms. The mechanism for causing abnormal menstrual bleeding is not understood, but theories include: increasing the endometrial surface area, interfering with uterine blood supply, interfering with uterine contractility, ulceration of the endometrium overlying the fibroid, and causing venous stasis by a direct pressure effect. Submucosal fibroids that prolapse through the cervix (Figure 3) and become infarcted, not only cause heavy

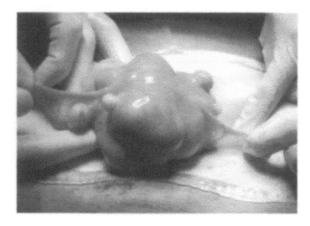

Figure 2 A uterus distorted with subserosal, pedunculated, and intramural fibroids leading to pressure and menstrual symptoms

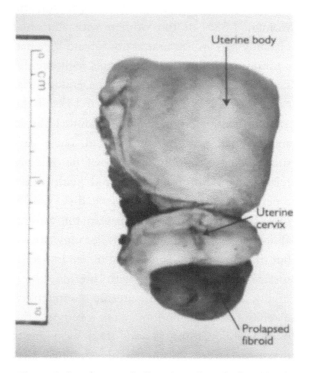

Figure 3 A submucosal fibroid prolapsed through the cervix in a hysterectomy specimen

bleeding, but also commonly lead to a marked discharge and severe cramping pains mimicking spontaneous miscarriage, especially if the fibroid is passed.

Pressure symptoms

A large fibroid uterus can fill the pelvis and cause compression of surrounding structures, commonly presenting as urinary frequency, by mechanically reducing bladder capacity, and occasionally as urinary urgency, urge and stress incontinence. Urinary retention may occur, but this is rare and usually associated with a cervical or low anterior fibroid. The ureters can be compressed or obstructed, resulting in a hydroureter or even hydronephrosis and renal compromise. Rarely, fibroids can cause problems with defecation or pressure on pelvic nerves, leading to pain.

Pain

Fibroids rarely cause pain outside pregnancy and other causes for the pain should be considered if fibroids are also present. Expulsion of a cervical fibroid can cause cramping pain and bleeding, as noted above. Pedunculated fibroids may also undergo torsion or degeneration and present with an acute abdomen, which can be confused clinically with an ovarian cyst accident, although the two can be differentiated by ultrasound appearance. Hyaline degeneration of a fibroid very occasionally occurs and can lead to a difficult diagnostic problem. Red degeneration occurs in pregnancy when there is hemorrhage within the fibroid. This causes an acute onset of pain, which may be misinterpreted as a concealed abruption. However, the fetus is not normally compromised and the pain usually settles with conservative management.

Fertility

Fibroids are more common in nulliparae, suggesting that pregnancy may have a protective effect. The relationship between fibroids and infertility is therefore complex and opinions differ. A systematic review of the evidence found that women with submucous fibroids had lower pregnancy rates compared with infertile controls (RR 0.32; 95% confidence interval (CI) 0.13–0.70) following *in vitro* fertilization (IVF) or spontaneous conception[19]. Non-cavity distorting fibroids had no effect on pregnancy rates following IVF (RR 0.96; 95% CI 0.96). There are no randomized trials comparing fertility rates of women who have had submucosal fibroids resected versus those without intervention. However, in one study resection of submucous fibroids increased the pregnancy rate compared with the non-fibroid infertile controls (RR 1.72; 95% CI 2.58) although the delivery rates were similar (RR 0.98; 95% CI 0.45–2.41). This would suggest that resecting submucosal fibroids may be beneficial, but as there is little to support an adverse effect of non-cavity distorting fibroids on fertility then, equally, there would be little to recommend their removal, and the potential for much harm. However, a subsequent prospective study examined 112 women with intramural fibroids and compared them with 322 women without intramural fibroids, all of whom underwent IVF or intracytoplasmic sperm injection[20]. Pregnancy rates were reduced in women with intramural fibroids compared to non-fibroid controls (23.3% vs. 34.1%; $p = 0.016$). However, the fibroid group were on average 2 years older than the non-fibroid group and a randomized controlled trial has been recommended to assess accurately the benefit of myomectomy on these patients.

Pregnancy

During pregnancy there is a rise in estrogens and progestogens produced primarily by the placenta, which may have a protective effect on the development of new fibroids. Existing fibroids can grow during pregnancy, although studies have found this to be the case in only 20–30% of fibroids, with only a 25% or less increase in volume of individual fibroids[21,22]. Nevertheless, this can result in a significant enlargement of the uterus for some women, and can lead to extreme discomfort due to the combined pressure effects of fibroids and a pregnancy (Figure 4).

A population-based study in the USA found that women with fibroids were more at risk of first-trimester bleeding, premature rupture of membranes, abruption, malpresentation, cesarean section, prolonged labor, low Apgar scores and low birth weight compared with controls matched for age, race, weight, etc.[23] Part of the increase in cesarean section rate for women with fibroids is due to complications with fetal lie/presentation. A low uterine or cervical fibroid blocking the presenting part from entering the pelvis makes breech or compound presentations more likely. A fibroid in this position has also been associated with incarceration of the retroverted gravid uterus, with potentially serious consequences An example of such a case is illustrated in Figure 4[24]. In addition, just as a cornual placental site can lead to a breech presentation, so a fibroid lying higher in the uterus may obstruct fetal

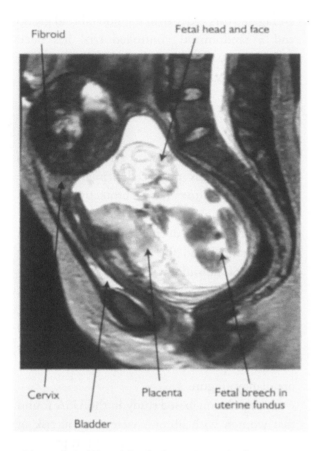

Fibroid

Fetal head and face

Cervix

Placenta

Fetal breech in uterine fundus

Bladder

Figure 4 A T2-weighted fast spin sagittal magnetic resonance image at 20 weeks' gestation showing an incarcerated retroverted uterus with a large fibroid superiorly on the lower portion of the anterior wall of the uterus with the cervix just below, above the level of the symphysis pubis. The uterine fundus containing the fetal breech is in the pouch of Douglas and the placenta is attached to the posterior uterine wall. Reproduced from reference 24 with permission

rotation to a cephalic position. The cesarean section may be complicated by fibroids, especially if they lie in the region of the anterior lower segment. The alternative upper segment 'classical' uterine incision may be required to avoid the fibroid.

Red degeneration of a fibroid, as described above, can occur during pregnancy and usually presents with pain and may mimic placental abruption or preterm labor. Once other pathologies have been excluded, conservative management is usually adequate, including analgesics, anti-emetics, and antipyretics.

Atonic post-partum hemorrhage is associated with fibroids. The mechanism for this is probably multifactorial and includes a disturbance to the vascular pattern within the myometrium, compromised placentation, with an increased risk of retained placenta following delivery and possibly altered uterine polarity, compromising physiological contractions and retraction following delivery. It is important to remember that most women with fibroids will have pregnancies uncomplicated by their fibroids.

Malignant change

Uterine sarcomas represent less than 1% of gynecological malignancies with an incidence of 1–2 per 100 000 women[25]. Since around 40% of these sarcomas are leiomyosarcomas[26], the incidence falls to 4–8 per million women. The risk of sarcomatous transformation is therefore exceedingly rare. An estimate of 0.1% lifetime risk per fibroid was based on the recorded incidence of fibroids in a study population[27], a rate that is almost certainly exaggerated since the true incidence of fibroids is likely to have been significantly higher. In addition, it is unclear what proportion of uterine leiomyosarcomas arise *de novo*, rather than from existing benign fibroids. Nevertheless, unexpected malignant tumors might be treated medically[27] in the first instance, and unexpected growth should alert the clinician to this possibility.

Intravenous or intravascular leiomyomatosis is a rare benign myomatous tumor present in the pelvic veins; even more rare, such tumors can grow within the venous tree and reach the right atrium causing cardiorespiratory symptoms (Figure 5). The lesion presents a typical gross appearance with cords of tumor extending through the myometrium and into the broad ligaments. From personal experience the diagnosis may only be made some years after a hysterectomy has removed the fibroid uterus. There can be difficulty distinguishing the condition from certain malignant processes such as endometrial sarcoma or stromatosis[28].

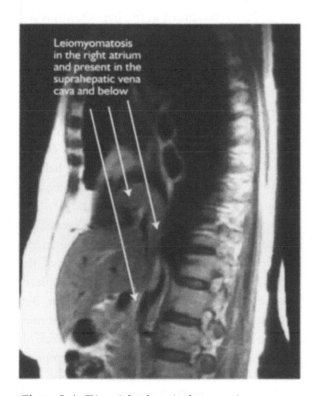

Figure 5 A T1-weighted sagittal magnetic resonance image of intravascular leiomyomatosis showing a tumor that arose within the pelvis and extending into the inferior vena reaching the right atrium in a woman presenting with a pelvic tumor and respiratory symptoms. By kind permission of Dr Zoë Traille

INVESTIGATION

Most women with fibroids will be asymptomatic and require no further investigation or treatment. However, if a woman presents with either menstrual or pressure symptoms or an awareness of a pelvic mass then further investigation is justified.

A full blood count is required to exclude anemia secondary to menorrhagia. Occasionally fibroids cause polycythemia thought to be due to fibroid production of erythropoietin[29,30]; rarely, preoperative venesection is required if the red cell count is very elevated. In cases presenting with a pelvic mass, apart from considering an unrecognized pregnancy, ovarian tumor markers and pelvic imaging may be useful to aid diagnosis.

Ultrasound examination is used to confirm a clinical diagnosis of a cystic or solid tumor, although on rare occasions differentiation between a fibroid uterus and solid ovarian tumor may prove difficult. Clinical examination should allow differentiation by eliciting the greater mobility of the ovarian tumor compared with that usually found within the fibroid uterus. Transvaginal ultrasound may be able to measure the endometrial thickness, but this is often technically difficult with fibroids. Magnetic resonance imaging (MRI) is useful for investigating pelvic masses, particularly where there is a diagnostic dilemma.

In women over 40 years with menorrhagia, investigation of the endometrium is indicated to exclude other endometrial causes of excessive blood loss, especially if there is any irregular bleeding. Outpatient endometrial curettage can be used, providing that the endometrial cavity is sounded first to ensure that the cavity has been adequately investigated. This approach will not usually identify submucosal fibroids or endometrial polyps. If either of these pathologies are suspected, outpatient or inpatient hysteroscopy should be considered.

In women in whom a rapidly developing pelvic mass is identified that is clinically consistent with a fibroid uterus, the possibility of malignant change should be considered. While imaging with MRI may be helpful, the diagnosis can only be confirmed by histological examination.

MEDICAL MANAGEMENT

For women troubled by menstrual symptoms and who have a fibroid uterus, medical treatment is worth using initially to try to relieve the symptoms. Mefenamic acid and tranexamic acid are recommended for treatment of dysfunctional uterine bleeding. It would not be unreasonable to try either of these in the presence of fibroids, as side-effects are minimal, but there is little evidence for their efficacy. In a small longitudinal prospective study of tranexamic acid and menorrhagia there was a significant reduction in blood loss in women without fibroids. This was accompanied by a reduction in uterine blood flow on Doppler ultrasound[31]. However, there was neither a significant reduction in blood loss nor uterine blood flow in women with fibroids (see Chapter 5).

Depot medroxyprogesterone acetate in case–control studies is associated with a protective effect on development of fibroids[16]. However, there are no randomized controlled trials to support its use in the treatment of menorrhagia secondary to fibroids, although it is effective for dysfunctional uterine bleeding. Increasingly the intrauterine levonorgestrel drug delivery system has been used for treatment of menorrhagia. Although there are no large randomized controlled trials, small clinical trials show an improvement in the reported menstrual blood loss as well as improvement in hemoglobin levels in women with menorrhagia secondary to fibroids[32]. Expulsion rate of the coil may be higher in women with an endometrial cavity distorted by fibroids, but a large cavity should not in itself be a contraindication to an intrauterine levonorgestrel-releasing drug delivery system. More recently a 'frameless' intrauterine levonorgestrel-releasing drug delivery system has been developed and initial pilot studies suggest that it is effective at treating fibroid-induced menorrhagia, despite having no effect on the overall size of the fibroids[33].

GnRH is produced in the hypothalamus and released in short pulses to stimulate follicle stimulating hormone (FSH) and luteinizing hormone (LH) release. If GnRH is given continuously the receptors are internalized and down-regulated, resulting in a block of FSH and LH release. This follows an initial increase in levels and leads to reversible ovarian failure. GnRH analogs have a much longer half-life than endogenous GnRH and shrink fibroids by stopping ovarian steroid production[15]. The reduction in size varies between women and between fibroids, but is reported to be in the region of 35–61% on average[34]. Most of the reduction in size is seen in the first couple of months, with little extra reduction after 3–6 months. However, following treatment, fibroids will re-grow rapidly to their original size[35]. If given prior to surgery GnRH analogs improve hemoglobin, reduce intraoperative blood loss and enable either Pfannenstiel's incision to be used or a vaginal hysterectomy to be performed[36].

GnRH agonists, such as goserelin 3.6 g by subcutaneous depot injection or buserelin

900–1200 µg by daily intranasal spray, work by inducing a hypogonadal state. Side-effects of treatment therefore include menopausal symptoms, such as hot flushes and vaginal dryness, in addition to the more serious reduction in bone density. The concept of 'add-back' therapy, adding low-dose estrogen/progestogen therapy to the GnRH treatment has been introduced to counteract these disadvantages. A randomized controlled trial of tibolone plus a GnRH agonist compared to GnRH agonist plus placebo showed no adverse effect on fibroid shrinkage, with maintenance of bone density and improvement in symptoms[37]. However, GnRH analogs are not yet licensed for long-term use.

Newer medical alternatives for treating fibroids have been explored. GnRH antagonists, cetrorelix and ganirelix are becoming commercially available and produce rapid gonadal suppression. Kettel et al.[34] demonstrated that daily subcutaneous injections provoked a rapid decrease in uterine size with instantaneous onset of amenorrhea. This approach has not received further investigation. Mifepristone, the progesterone receptor blocker, is a partial agonist and in the absence of progesterone has a progestogenic and anti-estrogenic effect. In two small pilot studies using mifepristone continuously at a dose of 25–50 mg daily fibroids shrank by almost 50% with improvement in menstrual loss and hemoglobin concentrations[17,38]. Estrogen levels were adequate to maintain bone density, but not to prevent hot flushes. However, there was simple endometrial hyperplasia in 28% of subjects treated with 5 mg or 10 mg per day for 6 months. While premalignant atypical hyperplasia was not observed in any of the study subjects, this finding does suggest that long-term mifepristone might provoke an 'unopposed estrogen' effect and therefore increase the risk of endometrial carcinoma. Further long-term studies are required before this approach to management can be recommended.

SURGICAL MANAGEMENT

As fibroids are often asymptomatic no further management may be required once other significant pathology has been excluded. Even large fibroids are likely to regress following the menopause although they are unlikely to disappear and the routine removal of large asymptomatic fibroids cannot be justified if the diagnosis is secure[39]. In the presence of symptoms of abnormal bleeding hysterectomy compares favorably with conservative approaches. In a prospective study of patients with fibroids undergoing surgical and medical treatment, hysterectomy was most likely to be associated with improvement in symptoms and quality of life. There was no change in the medically managed group[40]. Hysterectomy is therefore the definitive treatment for fibroids, but can only be considered in those who do not wish to preserve their fertility. The route of hysterectomy will depend on the size and site of the fibroids as well as the surgeon. GnRH agonists prescribed for 3 months preoperatively may shrink fibroids sufficiently to reduce the size of the uterus and permit hysterectomy by the vaginal route or reduce the length of abdominal incision required for the surgery. This approach has been recommended prior to performing a myomectomy (removing fibroids and conserving the uterus). Experience to date remains relatively limited, but the procedure of enucleation of the fibroids does not appear to be enhanced and blood loss is not reduced even though a reduction in size of the fibroid has been produced. More recently laparoscopic techniques have been employed. A small randomized controlled trial suggests that short-term recovery and immediate postoperative pain are improved with laparoscopically assisted vaginal hysterectomy, compared with abdominal hysterectomy[41]. However, there are no longer-term trials comparing laparoscopic and conventional routes for fibroid hysterectomy.

Myomectomy is a fertility-sparing procedure but there is the potential for significant hemorrhage that may require a hysterectomy as a life-saving procedure. Also, there can be significant adhesion formation following myomectomy, which may have an adverse impact on fertility. Myomectomies can be performed by laparotomy, laparoscopically or hysteroscopically. Two small randomized controlled trials suggested that laparoscopic surgery is associated with a shorter recovery period and less postoperative pain and fever[42,43]. In cases where a second-look laparoscopy has been performed adhesion rates were around 50% following laparoscopic resection[44]; whether this is significantly different to open myomectomy for similar patients is still to be determined.

As operative times are much longer with laparoscopic myomectomy there is increased potential for nerve damage and venous thrombosis to develop during surgery. In addition, there is some evidence to suggest that uterine scar rupture is a risk in a future labor, which would appear to be less frequent following myomectomy performed by laparotomy[45–47]. It is unclear whether this apparent difference relates to the technique usually adopted for repairing the defect in the myometrium following myomectomy or to some other unrecognized factor.

Menstrual symptoms due to fibroids are associated with those situated in submucosal or intraluminal positions. Hysteroscopic removal may improve menstrual loss, as well as fertility. If fertility is not an issue, ablation of the remaining endometrial surface could be performed at the same time. The chance of successful symptomatic improvement with endometrial ablation for women with fibroids is unfortunately lower than for women with an otherwise normal uterus, probably because the endometrial cavity is enlarged.

UTERINE ARTERY EMBOLIZATION

Uterine artery embolization (UAE) was first developed as a treatment for massive obstetric hemorrhage[48]. It was then used for a variety of similar emergencies. It was noted that, following the procedure women's fibroids reduced in size and the symptoms previously caused by their fibroids improved[49]. From the mid-1990s, the technique has been used as treatment for fibroids and a number of case series have been published[50,51].

UAE involves catheterization of the femoral artery. Using angiography to direct a guide-wire, a catheter is then passed into the uterine arteries and polyvinyl alcohol particles and small pieces of gelatin sponge are used to embolize and occlude the vessels.

The fibroids then undergo ischemic necrosis, which is accompanied by a variable amount of pain, often requiring opioid analgesia as an inpatient for 24–48 h. Around 15% of women will experience a post-embolization syndrome, secondary to tissue necrosis. Symptoms of fever, nausea and vomiting may mimic infection. These symptoms normally settle within a week. As with hysterectomy and myomectomy, there are infrequent risks of major complications, including sepsis, thromboembolism, disseminated intravascular coagulation and the need for urgent hysterectomy. In most cases there remains some uncertainty about the histological diagnosis at the time of treatment. Another short-term complication is hemorrhage around the arterial access sites, though this rarely results in serious vascular damage.

One medium-term complication is fibroid sloughing into the endometrial cavity, with passage through the cervix (5%)[52]. Surgery may be needed to remove it if the tissue becomes stuck in the uterine cavity. Another medium-term complication is ovarian failure secondary to embolization of collateral arteries that supply the ovary (5%). Patients hoping to retain their fertility should be warned about this complication. No studies have looked directly at fertility following UAE, although cases of pregnancy have been reported[53]. There is concern about the development of intrauterine fetal growth restriction in subsequent pregnancies and the incidence of uterine rupture in labor, and insufficient data exist to recommend this as a fertility-sparing procedure.

In some women a dramatic reduction in fibroid size is achieved, with apparent removal of the fibroid from the uterus as shown in Figure 6. What is unclear is the impact on future fibroid development after embolization. While hysterectomy has long-term benefits in this regard, myomectomy does not exclude the

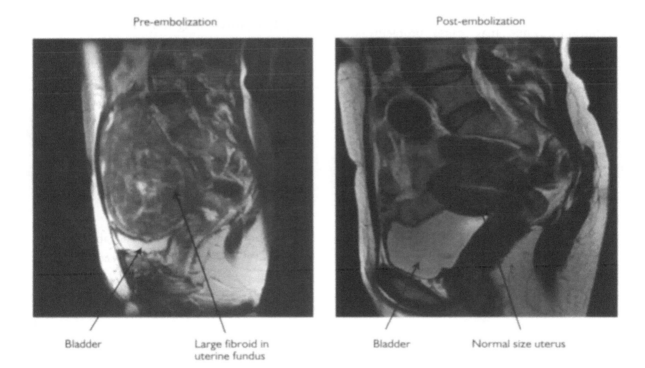

Pre-embolization

Post-embolization

Bladder   Large fibroid in uterine fundus

Bladder   Normal size uterus

Figure 6 Sagittal magnetic resonance images of a large uterine fibroid before and 3 months after successful embolization, showing a dramatic reduction in the size of the tumor. By kind permission of Dr Nigel Cowan

development and growth of further fibroids during a woman's remaining menstrual years. The National Institute for Clinical Excellence guidelines and those from the Royal College of Obstetricians and Gynaecologists (RCOG), state that the safety of UAE has not been proven and that all women should be appropriately counseled. Data from all cases should be sent to the British Society of Interventional Radiology register in addition to local audit. The RCOG guidelines also state that effects on pregnancy and subsequent offspring are unknown and that there may be long-term effects on children, and so advise that pregnancy should be avoided[54,55].

CONCLUSION

Fibroids are common benign tumors that can cause increased menstrual bleeding or pressure symptoms. They may cause problems with fertility, most probably if they are having an impact on the endometrial cavity and can affect pregnancy outcome. Long-term medical treatment is limited at present, although the levonorgestrel intrauterine drug delivery system looks promising. Hysterectomy is a major operation but has long-term benefits for quality of life and patient satisfaction, while myomectomy, often a more major surgical procedure than hysterectomy, provides the opportunity to preserve fertility. UAE is an alternative to major surgery, but long-term results are not yet available and it cannot presently be recom-

mended for women hoping to preserve their fertility. Sarcomatous change within an existing fibroid is extremely rare and, in the absence of symptoms and a rapidly growing tumor, intervention is not essential, with the expectation that fibroids usually regress following the menopause.

PRACTICE POINTS

- Fibroids are common and often asymptomatic
- Pregnancy, the oral contraceptive pill and Depo-Provera may be protective
- Fibroids usually regress after the menopause
- Submucous fibroids are associated with infertility
- No proven long-term medical treatment exists, but the levonorgestrel intrauterine drug delivery systems look promising
- GnRH agonists are useful in the short term prior to surgery
- Hysterectomy is currently the definitive treatment
- Myomectomy offers a potentially fertility-sparing alternative
- Uterine artery embolization needs further evaluation
- Transcervical endometrial ablative procedures may not be appropriate to relieve menstrual symptoms

REFERENCES

1. Cramer SF, Patel A. The frequency of uterine leiomyomas. Am J Clin Pathol 1990; 94: 435–8

2. MacKenzie IZ, Naish C, Rees M, Manek S. 1170 consecutive hysterectomies: indications and pathology. J Br Menopause Soc 2004; 10: 108–12

3. Vollenhoven BJ, Lawrence AS, Healy DL. Uterine fibroids: a clinical review. Br J Obstet Gynaecol 1990; 97: 285–98

4. Marshall LM, Spiegelman D, Barbieri RL, et al. Variation in the incidence of uterine leiomyoma among premenopausal women by age and race. Obstet Gynecol 1997; 90: 967–73

5. Treloar SA, Martin NG, Dennerstein L, et al. Pathways to hysterectomy: insights from longitudinal twin research. Am J Obstet Gynecol 1992; 167: 82–8

6. Lepine LA, Hillis SD, Marchbanks PA, et al. Hysterectomy surveillance – United States, 1980–1993. MMWR CDC Surveill Summ 1997; 46: 1–15

7. Vikhlyaeva EM, Khodzhaeva ZS, Fantschenko ND. Familial predisposition to uterine leiomyomas. Int J Gynaecol Obstet 1995; 51: 127–31

8. Rein MS, Friedman AJ, Barbieri RL, et al. Cytogenetic abnormalities in uterine leiomyomata. Obstet Gynecol 1991; 77: 923–6

9. Townsend DE, Sparkes RS, Baluda MC, McClelland G. Unicellular histogenesis of uterine leiomyomas as determined by electrophoresis by glucose-6-phosphate dehydrogenase. Am J Obstet Gynecol 1970; 107: 1168–73

10. Nilbert M, Heim S, Mandahl N, et al. Different karyotypic abnormalities, t(1;6) and del(7), in two uterine leiomyomas from the same patient. Cancer Genet Cytogenet 1989; 42: 51–3

11. Marshall LM, Spiegelman D, Goldman MB, et al. A prospective study of reproductive factors and oral contraceptive use in relation to the risk of uterine leiomyomata. Fertil Steril 1998; 70: 432–9

12. Parazzini F, Negri E, La Vecchia C, Chatenoud, et al. Reproductive factors and risk of uterine fibroids. Epidemiology 1996; 7: 440–2

13. Ross RK, Pike MC, Vessey MP, et al. Risk factors for uterine fibroids: reduced risk associated with oral contraceptives. Br Med J 1986; 293: 359–62

14. Walker CL, Cesen-Cummings K, Houle C, et al. Protective effect of pregnancy for development of uterine leiomyoma. Carcinogenesis 2001; 22: 2049–52

15. Filicori M, Hall DA, Loughlin JS, et al. A conservative approach to the management of uterine leiomyoma: pituitary desensitization by a luteinizing hormone-releasing hormone analogue. Am J Obstet Gynecol 1983; 147: 726–7

16. Lumbiganon P, Rugpao S, Phandhu-fung S, et al. Protective effect of depot-medroxyprogesterone acetate on surgically treated uterine leiomyomas: a multicentre case-control study. Br J Obstet Gynaecol 1996; 103: 909–14

17. Murphy AA, Kettel LM, Morales AJ, et al. Regression of uterine leiomyomata in response to the antiprogesterone RU 486. J Clin Endocrinol Metab 1993; 76: 513–17

18. Clevenger-Hoeft M, Syrop CH, Stovall DW, et al. Sonohysterography in premenopausal women with and without abnormal bleeding. Obstet Gynecol 1999; 94: 516–20

19. Pritts EA. Fibroids and infertility: a systematic review of the evidence. Obstet Gynecol Surv 2001; 56: 483–91

20. Hart R, Khalaf Y, Yeong CT, et al. A prospective controlled study of the effect of intramural

uterine fibroids on the outcome of assisted conception. Hum Reprod 2001; 16: 2411–17

21. Aharoni A, Reiter A, Golan D, et al. Patterns of growth of uterine leiomyomas during pregnancy. A prospective longitudinal study. Br J Obstet Gynaecol 1988; 95: 510–13

22. Rosati P, Exacoustos C, Mancuso S. Longitudinal evaluation of uterine myoma growth during pregnancy. A sonographic study. J Ultrasound Med 1992; 11: 511–15

23. Coronado GD, Marshall LM, Schwartz SM. Complications in pregnancy, labor, and delivery with uterine leiomyomas: a population-based study. Obstet Gynecol 2000; 95: 764–9

24. Hamoda H, Chamberlain PF, Moore NR, et al. Conservative treatment of an incarcerated gravid uterus. Br J Obstet Gynaecol 2002; 109: 1074–5

25. Arrastia CD, Fruchter RG, Clark M, et al. Uterine carcinosarcomas: incidence and trends in management and survival. Gynecol Oncol 1997; 65: 158–63

26. Riddle PJ, Echeta CB, Manek S, et al. Retrospective study of the management of uterine sarcomas at Oxford 1990–1998. Role of adjuvant treatment. Clin Oncol 2002; 14: 54–61

27. Murphy NJ, Wallace DL. Gonadotropin releasing hormone (GnRH) agonist therapy for reduction of leiomyoma volume. Gynecol Oncol 1993; 49: 266–7

28. Harper RS, Scully RE. Intravenous leiomyomatosis of the uterus. A report of four cases. Obstet Gynecol 1961; 18: 519–29

29. Kohama T, Shinohara K, Takahura M, et al. Large uterine myoma with erythropoietin messenger RNA and erythrocytosis. Obstet Gynecol 2000; 96: 826–8

30. Suzuki M, Takamizawa S, Nomaguchi K, et al. Erythropoietin synthesis by tumor tissues in a patient with uterine myoma and erythrocytosis. Br J Haematol 2001; 113: 49–51

31. Lakhani KP, Marsh MS, Purcell W, Hardiman P. Uterine artery blood flow parameters in women with dysfunctional uterine bleeding and uterine fibroids: the effects of tranexamic acid. Ultrasound Obstet Gynecol 1998; 11: 283–5

32. Starczewski A, Iwanicki M. Intrauterine therapy with levonorgestrel releasing IUD of women with hypermenorrhea secondary to uterine fibroids. Ginekol Pol 2000; 71: 1221–5

33. Wildemeersch D, Schacht E. The effect on menstrual blood loss in women with uterine fibroids of a novel 'frameless' intrauterine levonorgestrel-releasing drug delivery system: a pilot study. Eur J Obstet Gynecol Reprod Biol 2002; 102: 74–9

34. Kettel LM, Murphy AA, Morales AJ, et al. Rapid regression of uterine leiomyomas in response to daily administration of gonadotropin-releasing hormone antagonist. Fertil Steril 1993; 60: 642–6

35. Matta WH, Shaw RW, Nye M. Long-term follow-up of patients with uterine fibroids after treatment with the LHRH agonist buserelin. Br J Obstet Gynaecol 1989; 96: 200–6

36. Lethaby A, Vollenhoven B, Sowter M. Preoperative GnRH analogue therapy before hysterectomy or myomectomy for uterine fibroids (Cochrane Review). In The Cochrane Library, Issue 4. Oxford: Update Software, 2003

37. Hammar M, Christau S, Nathorst-Boos J, et al. A double-blind, randomised trial comparing the effects of tibolone and continuous combined hormone replacement therapy in postmenopausal women with menopausal symptoms. Br J Obstet Gynaecol 1998; 105: 904–11

38. Eisinger SH, Meldrum S, Fiscella K, et al. Low-dose mifepristone for uterine leiomyomata. Obstet Gynecol 2003; 101: 243–50

39. Reiter RC, Wagner PL, Gambone JC. Routine hysterectomy for large asymptomatic uterine

leiomyomata: a reappraisal. Obstet Gynecol 1992; 79: 481–4

40. Carlson KJ, Miller BA, Fowler FJ Jr. The Maine Women's Health Study: II. Outcomes of non-surgical management of leiomyomas, abnormal bleeding, and chronic pelvic pain. Obstet Gynecol 1994; 83: 566–72

41. Ferrari MM, Berlanda N, Mezzopane R, et al. Identifying the indications for laparoscopically assisted vaginal hysterectomy: a prospective, randomised comparison with abdominal hysterectomy in patients with symptomatic uterine fibroids. Br J Obstet Gynaecol 2000; 107: 620–5

42. Mais V, Ajossa S, Guerriero S, et al. Laparoscopic versus abdominal myomectomy: a prospective, randomized trial to evaluate benefits in early outcome. Am J Obstet Gynecol 1996; 174: 654–8

43. Seracchioli R, Rossi S, Govoni F, et al. Fertility and obstetric outcome after laparoscopic myomectomy of large myomata: a randomized comparison with abdominal myomectomy. Hum Reprod 2000; 15: 2663–8

44. Milad MP, Morrison K, Sokol A, et al. A comparison of laparoscopic supracervical hysterectomy vs. laparoscopically assisted vaginal hysterectomy. Surg Endosc 2001; 15: 286–8

45. Palerme GR, Friedman EA. Rupture of the gravid uterus in the third trimester. Am J Obstet Gynecol 1966; 94: 571–6

46. Nezhat CH, Nezhat F, Roemisch M, et al. Pregnancy following laparoscopic myom-ectomy: preliminary results. Hum Reprod 1999; 14: 1219–21

47. Dubuisson JB, Fauconnior A, Deffarges JV, et al. Pregnancy outcome and deliveries following laparoscopic myomectomy. Hum Reprod 2000; 15: 869–73

48. Heaston DK, Mineau DE, Brown BJ, Miller FJ Jr. Transcatheter arterial embolization for control of persistent massive puerperal hemorrhage after bilateral surgical hypogastric artery ligation. Am J Roentgenol 1979; 133: 152–4

49. Ravina JH, Merland JJ, Herbreteau D, et al. Preoperative embolization of uterine fibroma. Preliminary results (10 cases). Presse Med 1994; 23: 1540

50. Ravina JH, Herbreteau D, Ciraru-Vigneron N, et al. Arterial embolisation to treat uterine myomata. Lancet 1995; 346: 671–2

51. Reidy JF, Bradley EA. Uterine artery embolization for fibroid disease. Cardiovasc Intervent Radiol 1998; 21: 357–60

52. Bradley EA, Reidy JF, Forman RG, et al. Transcatheter uterine artery embolisation to treat large uterine fibroids. Br J Obstet Gynaecol 1998; 105: 235–40

53. Ravina JH, Vigneron NC, Aymard A, et al. Pregnancy after embolization of uterine myoma: report of 12 cases. Fertil Steril 2000; 73: 1241–3

54. National Institute for Clinical Excellence. Uterine Artery Embolisation for Fibroids. London: National Institute for Clinical Excellence, 2003

55. Royal College of Obstetricians and Gynaecologists and Royal College of Radiologists. Clinical Recommendations on the Use of Uterine Artery Embolisation in the Management of Fibroids. Report of a Joint Working Party of the RCOG and RCR. London: RCOG Press, 2001

The irregular cycle: polycystic ovary syndrome

7

A. Balen

INTRODUCTION

Many women are troubled by an erratic or unpredictable menstrual cycle. In the 'developed world' the commonest cause is polycystic ovary syndrome (PCOS). Overall, PCOS is also the commonest endocrine disturbance affecting women. The classical symptoms of 'Stein–Leventhal syndrome' as it was eponymously referred to for many years – namely menstrual disturbance (amenorrhea or oligomenorrhea, hyperandrogenism and obesity) – are now known to describe the extreme end of the spectrum of what we believe to be a very heterogeneous condition, whose pathophysiology appears to be multifactorial and polygenic. The definition of the syndrome has been much debated. Key features include menstrual cycle disturbance, hyperandrogenism and obesity. There are many extra-ovarian aspects to the pathophysiology of PCOS yet ovarian dysfunction is central. At a recent joint American Society of Reproductive Medicine/European Society of Human Reproduction and Embryology (ASRM/ESHRE) consensus meeting a refined definition of PCOS was agreed, namely the presence of two out of the following three criteria:

(1) Oligo- and/or anovulation;

(2) Hyperandrogenism (clinical and/or biochemical);

(3) Polycystic ovaries, with the exclusion of other etiologies[1].

The morphology of the polycystic ovary, which has been redefined as an ovary with 12 or more follicles measuring 2–9 mm in diameter and/or increased ovarian volume ($> 10 \, cm^3$)[2].

There is considerable heterogeneity of symptoms and signs amongst women with PCOS and for an individual these may change over time[3]. PCOS is familial and various aspects of the syndrome may be differentially inherited. Polycystic ovaries can exist without clinical signs of the syndrome, which may then become expressed over time. There are a number of interlinking factors that affect expression of PCOS. A gain in weight is associated with a worsening of symptoms whilst weight loss will ameliorate the endocrine and metabolic profile and symptomatology[4].

Elevated serum concentrations of insulin are more common both in lean and obese women with PCOS when compared with weight-matched controls. Indeed it is hyperinsulinemia that appears to be the key to the pathogenesis of the syndrome as insulin stimulates androgen secretion by the ovarian stroma and appears to affect the normal development of ovarian follicles, both by the adverse effects of androgens on follicular growth and possibly also by suppressing apoptosis and permitting the survival of follicles otherwise destined to disappear.

WHAT IS POLYCYSTIC OVARY SYNDROME?

Polycystic ovaries are commonly detected by ultrasound or other forms of pelvic imaging, with an estimated 20–33% prevalence in the general population[5,6]. However, not all women with polycystic ovaries demonstrate the clinical and biochemical features that define polycystic ovary syndrome. The biochemical disturbance includes elevated serum concentrations of luteinizing hormone (LH), testosterone, androstenedione, and insulin.

The polycystic ovary

Transabdominal and/or transvaginal ultrasound have become the most commonly used

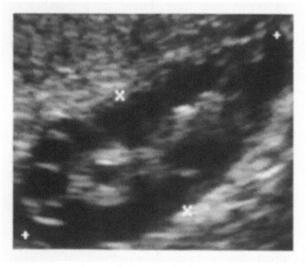

Figure 1 Transvaginal ultrasound of a polycystic ovary

diagnostic methods for the identification of polycystic ovaries (Figure 1). Although the ultrasound criteria for the diagnosis of polycystic ovaries have never been universally agreed, the characteristic features are accepted as being an increase in the number of follicles and the amount of stroma as compared with normal ovaries. The transabdominal ultrasound criteria of Adams and colleagues[7] defined a polycystic ovary as one which contains, in one plane, at least ten follicles (usually between 2 and 8 mm in diameter) arranged peripherally around a dense core of ovarian stroma. Such criteria have been used for many years but at a recent joint ASRM/ESHRE consensus meeting a refined definition of PCOS was agreed, encompassing a description of the morphology of the polycystic ovary. According to the available literature, the criteria fulfilling sufficient specificity and sensitivity to define the polycystic ovary are the presence of 12 or more follicles measuring 2–9 mm in diameter and/or increased ovarian volume ($> 10\,cm^3$)[2]. If there is a follicle greater than 10 mm in diameter, the scan should be repeated at a time of ovarian quiescence in order to calculate volume and area. The presence of a single polycystic ovary is sufficient to provide the diagnosis. The distribution of the follicles and the description of the stroma are not required in the diagnosis. Increased stromal echogenicity and/or stromal volume are specific to polycystic ovary, but it has been shown that the measurement of the ovarian volume (or area) is a good surrogate for the quantification of the stroma in clinical practice. A woman having polycystic ovary in the absence of an ovulation disorder or hyperandrogenism ('asymptomatic polycystic ovary') should not be considered as having PCOS, although she may develop symptoms over time, for example, if she gains weight.

The term 'polycystic ovary' in some respects adds to the confusion that surrounds its diagnosis. The 'cysts' are not cysts as they contain oocytes so, in reality the ovary should be termed polyfollicular, and thus reflect the finding that the 'cysts' are actually follicles whose development has been arrested. Indeed the prerequisite of a certain number of cysts may be of less relevance than the volume of ovarian stroma, which has been shown to closely correlate with serum testosterone concentrations[8].

Defining the 'syndrome'

While it is now clear that ultrasound provides an excellent technique for the detection of polycystic ovarian morphology, identification of polycystic ovaries by ultrasound does not automatically confer a diagnosis of PCOS. Controversy still exists over a precise definition of the 'syndrome' and whether or not the diagnosis requires confirmation of polycystic ovarian morphology. The generally accepted view in Europe is that a spectrum exists, ranging from women with polycystic ovarian morphology and no overt abnormality at one end, to those with polycystic ovaries associated with severe clinical and biochemical disorders at the other end. Using a combination of clinical, ultrasonographic, and biochemical criteria, the diagnosis of PCOS is usually reserved for those women who exhibit an ultrasound picture of polycystic ovaries, and who display one or more of the clinical symptoms (menstrual cycle disturbances, hirsutism, obesity, hyperandrogenism), and/or one or more of the recognized biochemical disturbances (elevated LH, testosterone, androstenedione, or insulin)[3]. A

joint ASRM/ESHRE consensus meeting on PCOS was held in Rotterdam, in May 2003. At this meeting a refined definition of PCOS was agreed[1], which, for the first time, includes a description of the morphology of the polycystic ovary. The new definition requires the presence of two out of the following three criteria:

(1)   Oligo- and/or anovulation;
(2)   Hyperandrogenism (clinical and/or biochemical);
(3)   Polycystic ovaries, with the exclusion of other etiologies[1].

National and racial differences in expression of polycystic ovary syndrome

The highest reported prevalence of polycystic ovary has been 52% amongst South Asian immigrants in Britain, of whom 49.1% had menstrual irregularity[9]. Rodin and co-workers[9] demonstrated that South Asian women with polycystic ovary had a comparable degree of insulin resistance to controls with established type 2 diabetes mellitus. Generally, there has been a paucity of data of the prevalence of PCOS among women of South Asian origin, both among migrant and native groups. Type 2 diabetes and insulin resistance have a high prevalence among indigenous populations in South Asia, with a rising prevalence among women. Insulin resistance and hyperinsulinemia are common antecedents of type 2 diabetes, with a high prevalence in South Asians. Type 2 diabetes also has a familial basis, inherited as a complex genetic trait that interacts with environmental factors, chiefly nutrition, commencing from fetal life. We have already found that South Asians with anovular PCOS have greater insulin resistance and more severe symptoms of the syndrome than Caucasians with anovular

PCOS[10]. Furthermore, it is known that women from South Asia, living in the UK appear to express symptoms at an earlier age than their Caucasian British counterparts.

Health consequences of polycystic ovary syndrome

Obesity and metabolic abnormalities are recognized risk factors for the development of ischemic heart disease (IHD) in the general population, and these are also recognized features of PCOS. The questions are whether women with PCOS are at an increased risk of IHD, and whether this will occur at an earlier age than women with normal ovaries? The basis for the idea that women with PCOS are at greater risk for cardiovascular disease is that these women are more insulin resistant than weight-matched controls, and metabolic disturbances associated with insulin resistance are known to increase cardiovascular risk in other populations.

Insulin resistance is defined as a diminution in the biological responses to a given level of insulin. In the presence of an adequate pancreatic reserve, normal circulating glucose levels are maintained at higher serum insulin concentrations. In the general population cardiovascular risk factors include insulin resistance, obesity, glucose intolerance, hypertension, and dyslipidemia.

Hyperinsulinemia has been demonstrated both in obese and non-obese women with PCOS, suggesting that a form of insulin resistance is specific to PCOS in addition to that caused by obesity. Obese women with PCOS have consistently been shown to be more insulin resistant than weight-matched controls. It appears that obesity and PCOS have an additive effect on the degree and severity of the

insulin resistance and subsequent hyper-insulinemia in this group of women.

Insulin sensitivity varies depending upon menstrual pattern. Women with PCOS who are oligomenorrheic are more likely to be insulin resistant than those with regular cycles – irrespective of their body mass index (BMI). Insulin resistance is restricted to the extra-splanchnic actions of insulin on glucose dispersal. The liver is not affected (hence the fall in sex hormone binding globulin (SHBG) and high-density lipoprotein (HDL)), neither is the ovary (hence the menstrual problems and hypersecretion of androgens), nor the skin (hence the development of acanthosis nigricans). The insulin resistance causes compensatory hypersecretion of insulin, particularly in response to glucose, so euglycemia is usually maintained at the expense of hyperinsulinemia.

Central obesity

Simple obesity is associated with greater deposition of gluteo femoral fat while central obesity involves greater truncal abdominal fat distribution. Obesity is observed in 35–60% of women with PCOS. Hyperandrogenism is associated with a preponderance of fat localized to truncal abdominal sites. Women with PCOS have a greater truncal abdominal fat distribution as demonstrated by a higher waist:hip ratio. The central distribution of fat is independent of BMI and associated with higher plasma insulin and triglyceride concentrations, and reduced HDL cholesterol concentrations.

Impaired glucose tolerance and diabetes

Known risk factors for cardiovascular disease are impaired glucose tolerance and diabetes. It is reported that 18–20% of obese women with PCOS demonstrate impaired glucose tolerance. Dahlgren and colleagues[11], noted the prevalence of type 2 diabetes was 15% in women with PCOS compared with 2% in the controls. Most women with type 2 diabetes under the age of 45 years have PCOS. Insulin resistance combined with abdominal obesity is thought to account for the higher prevalence of type 2 diabetes in PCOS. There is a concomitant increased risk of gestational diabetes.

Hypertension

The prevalence of treated hypertension is three times higher in women with PCOS between the ages of 40 and 59 years compared with controls[11]. In his series, Gjonnaess[12] reported the incidence of pre-eclampsia in obese women with PCOS conceiving after ovarian electro-cautery to be 12.9% compared with 3.8% in the general pregnant population.

Dyslipidemia

Women with PCOS have high concentrations of serum triglycerides and suppressed HDL levels, particularly a lower HDL_2 subfraction. HDLs play an important role in lipid metabolism and are the most important lipid parameter in predicting cardiovascular risk in women. Performing the task of 'reverse cholesterol transport', HDLs remove excess lipids from the circulation and tissues to transport them to the liver for excretion, or transfer them to other lipoprotein particles. Cholesterol is only one component of HDL, a particle with constantly changing composition forming HDL_3 then HDL_2, as unesterified cholesterol is taken from tissue, esterified and exchanged for triglyceride

with other lipoprotein species. Consequently, measurement of a single constituent in a particle involved in a dynamic process gives an incomplete picture[13].

Thus, in examining the surrogate risk factors for cardiovascular disease, there is evidence that insulin resistance, central obesity and hyper-androgenemia are features of PCOS and have an adverse effect on lipid metabolism. Women with PCOS have been shown to have dyslipidemia, with reduced HDL cholesterol and elevated serum triglycerides concentrations, along with elevated serum plasminogen activator inhibitor-I concentrations. The evidence is therefore mounting to suggest that women with PCOS may have an increased risk of developing cardiovascular disease and diabetes later in life, which has important implications regarding their management.

However, in another study Pierpoint and co-workers[14], reported the mortality rate in 1028 women diagnosed as having PCOS between 1930 and 1979. All the women were older than 45 years, and 770 women had been treated by wedge resection of the ovaries. In all, 786 women were traced; the mean age at diagnosis was 26.4 years and the average duration of follow-up was 30 years. There were 59 deaths, of which 15 were from circulatory disease (13 of these were from ischemic heart disease). There were six deaths from diabetes as an underlying or contributory cause compared with the expected 1.7 deaths. The standard mortality rate both overall and for cardiovascular disease was not higher in the women with PCOS compared with the national mortality rates in women, although the observed proportion of women with diabetes as a contributory or underlying factor leading to death was significantly higher than expected (odds ratio 3.6; 95% confidence interval (CI) 1.5–8.4). Thus, despite surrogate markers for cardiovascular disease, in this study, no increased rate of death from this disease could be demonstrated.

Polycystic ovary syndrome in younger women

At what stage do the risk factors for cardiovascular disease become apparent in women with PCOS? The majority of studies that have identified the risk factors of obesity and insulin resistance in women with PCOS have investigated adult populations, commonly including women who have presented to specialist endocrine or reproductive clinics. However, PCOS has been identified in much younger populations[6], in which women with increasing symptoms of PCOS, were found to be more insulin resistant. These data emphasize the need for long-term prospective studies of young women with PCOS in order to clarify the natural history, and to determine which women will be at risk of diabetes and cardiovascular disease later in life. A study of women with PCOS and a mean age of 39 years followed over a period of 6 years, found that 9% of those with normal glucose tolerance developed impaired glucose tolerance (IGT) and 8% developed non-insulin dependent diabetes (NIDDM)[15]. Fifty-four per cent of women with IGT at the start of the study had NIDDM at follow-up. Not surprisingly, the risks of disease progression were greatest in those who were overweight.

Endometrial cancer

Endometrial adenocarcinoma is the second most common female genital malignancy but only 4% of cases occur in women less than 40 years of age. The risk of developing endometrial cancer has been shown to be adversely influenced by a number of factors including obesity, long-term use of unopposed estrogens, nulliparity and infertility. Women with endometrial carcinoma have had fewer births compared with controls and it has also been demonstrated that infertility *per se* gives a relative risk of 2. Hypertension and type 2 diabetes mellitus have long been linked to endometrial cancer, with relative risks of 2.1 and 2.8, respectively[16] – conditions that are now known also to be associated with PCOS. The true risk of endometrial carcinoma in women with PCOS, however, is difficult to ascertain.

Endometrial hyperplasia may be a precursor to adenocarcinoma, with cystic glandular hyperplasia progressing in perhaps 0.4% of cases and adenomatous hyperplasia in up to 18% of cases over 2–10 years. Precise estimation of rate of progression is impossible to determine. Some authors have reported conservative management of endometrial adenocarcinoma in women with PCOS with a combination of curettage and high-dose progestogens. The rationale is that cancer of the endometrium often presents at an early stage, is well differentiated, with low risk of metastasis and, therefore, is not perceived as being life-threatening, whilst poorly differentiated adenocarcinoma in a young woman has a worse prognosis and warrants hysterectomy. In general, however, the literature on women with PCOS and endometrial hyperplasia or adenocarcinoma suggests that this group of patients has a poor prognosis for fertility. This may be because of the factors that predisposed to the endometrial pathology – chronic anovulation combined often with severe obesity – or secondary to the endometrial pathology disrupting potential embryonic implantation. Thus, a more traditional and radical surgical approach (i.e. hysterectomy) is suggested as the safest way to prevent progression of the cancer. Early-stage disease may permit ovarian conservation and the possibility of pregnancy by surrogacy.

Although the degree of risk has not been clearly defined, it is generally accepted that for women with PCOS who experience amenorrhea, or oligomenorrhea, the induction of artificial withdrawal bleeds to prevent endometrial hyperplasia is prudent manage-ment. There are no data on the frequency with which women with PCOS should shed their endometrium. It seems prudent to induce a withdrawal bleed either monthly or at least every 3 months, not only to prevent endometrial hyperplasia but also to enable the bleed to be acceptable when it occurs – as progressive endometrial development may lead to a prolonged and heavy bleed when it does occur. For those with oligo-/amenorrhea who do not wish to use cyclical hormone therapy we recommend an ultrasound scan to measure endometrial thickness and morphology every 6–12 months (depending upon menstrual history). An endometrial thickness greater than 10 mm in an amenorrheic woman warrants an artificially induced bleed, that should be followed by a repeat ultrasound scan and endometrial biopsy if the endometrium has not been shed. Another option is to consider a progestogen-releasing intrauterine system, such as the Mirena®.

Breast cancer

Obesity, hyperandrogenism, and infertility occur frequently in PCOS, and are features known to be associated with the development of breast cancer. However, studies examining the relationship between PCOS and breast carcinoma have not always identified a significantly increased risk. The study by Coulam and colleagues[17] calculated a relative risk of 1.5 (95% CI 0.75–2.55) for breast cancer in their group of women with chronic anovulation which was not statistically significant. After stratification by age, however, the relative risk was found to be 3.6 (95% CI 1.2–8.3) in the postmenopausal age group. More recently, Pierpoint and associates[14] reported a series of 786 women with PCOS in the UK who were traced from hospital records after histological diagnosis of polycystic ovaries between 1930 and 1979. Mortality was assessed from the national registry of deaths and standardized mortality rates (SMR) calculated for patients with PCOS compared with the normal population. The average follow-up period was 30 years. The SMR for all neoplasms was 0.91 (95% CI 0.60–1.32) and for breast cancer 1.48 (95% CI 0.79–2.54). In fact, breast cancer was the leading cause of death in this cohort.

Ovarian cancer

In recent years there has been much debate about the risk of ovarian cancer in women with infertility, particularly in relation to the use of drugs to induce superovulation for assisted conception procedures. Inherently, the risk of ovarian cancer appears to be increased in women who have multiple ovulations – that is those who are nulliparous (possibly because of infertility) with an early menarche and late menopause. Thus, it may be that inducing multiple ovulations in women with infertility will increase their risk – a notion that is by no means proven. Women with PCOS who are oligo-/anovulatory might therefore be expected to be at low risk of developing ovarian cancer if it is lifetime number of ovulations rather than pregnancies that is critical. Ovulation induction to correct anovulatory infertility aims to induce unifollicular ovulation and so, in theory, should raise the risk of a woman with PCOS to that of a normal ovulating woman. The polycystic ovary, however, is notoriously sensitive to stimulation and it is only in recent years, with the development of high-resolution transvaginal ultrasonography, that the rate of unifollicular ovulation has attained acceptable levels. The use of clomiphene citrate and gonadotropin therapy for ovulation induction in the 1960s–1980s resulted in many more multiple ovulations (and indeed multiple pregnancies) than in recent times and might therefore present with an increased rate of ovarian cancer when these women reach their sixties – the age of greatest incidence.

There are a few studies that have addressed the possibility of an association between polycystic ovaries and ovarian cancer. The results are conflicting, and generaliztion is limited due to problems with the study designs. In the large UK study of Pierpoint and colleagues[14] the SMR for ovarian cancer was 0.39 (95% CI 0.01–2.17).

MANAGEMENT OF THE POLYCYSTIC OVARY SYNDROME

The management of the PCOS is symptom orientated. Whilst obesity aggravates the symptoms, the metabolic scenario conspires against weight loss. Diet and exercise are key to symptom control. Initial reports of the use of insulin-sensitizing agents (e.g. metformin)[4,18] have been encouraging and suggest an improvement in biochemistry, symptoms and an increase in fertility. Ovulation induction has traditionally involved the use of clomiphene citrate and then gonadotropin therapy or laparoscopic ovarian surgery in those who are clomiphene resistant. Patients with PCOS are not estrogen deficient and those with amenorrhea are at risk not of osteoporosis but rather of endometrial hyperplasia or adenocarcinoma. Cycle control and regular withdrawal bleeding is achieved with the combined oral contraceptive pill, which has the additional beneficial effect of suppressing serum testosterone concentrations and hence improving hirsutism and acne. Dianette® and Yasmin®, containing the anti-androgens cyproterone acetate and drospirenone, respectively, are usually recommended.

Investigations utilized to determine polycystic ovary syndrome are outlined in Table 1.

Glucose tolerance

Women who are obese, and also many slim women with PCOS, will have insulin resistance and elevated serum concentrations of insulin (usually < 30 mU/l fasting). We suggest that a 75 g oral glucose tolerance test (GTT) be performed in women with PCOS and a BMI > 30 kg/m^2, with an assessment of the fasting and 2-h glucose concentration (Table 2). It has been suggested that South Asian women should have an assessment of glucose tolerance if their BMI is > 25 kg/m^2 because of the greater risk of insulin resistance at a lower BMI than seen in the Caucasian population.

Table 1 Investigations for polycystic ovary syndrome

Test	Normal range (may vary with individual assays)	Additional points
Pelvic ultrasound	to assess ovarian morphology and endometrial thickness	transabdominal scan satisfactory in women who are not sexually active
Testosterone (T)	0.5–3.5 nmol/l	
Sex hormone binding globulin (SHBG)	16–119 nmol/l	it is unnecessary to measure other androgens unless total testosterone is > 5 nmol/l, in which case referral is indicated
Free androgen index: T x 100/SHBG	< 5	insulin suppresses SHBG, resulting in a high free androgen index in the presence of a normal total T
Estradiol	measurement is unhelpful to diagnosis	estrogenization may be confirmed by endometrial assessment
Luteinizing hormone (LH)	2–10 IU/l	FSH and LH best measured during days 1–3 of a menstrual bleed. If oligo-/amenorrheic then random samples are taken
Follicle stimulating hormone (FSH)	2–8 IU/l	
Prolactin, thyroid function, thyroid stimulating hormone (TSH)	< 500 mU/l 0.5–5 IU/l	measure if oligo-/amenorrheic
Fasting insulin (not routinely measured; insulin resistance assessed by glucose tolerance test)	< 30 mU/l	

Table 2 Definitions of glucose tolerance after a 75 g glucose tolerance test (GTT)

	Diabetes mellitus	Impaired glucose tolerance	Impaired fasting glycemia
Fasting glucose (mmol/l)	≥ 7.0	< 7.0	≥ 6.1 and < 7.0
2-h glucose (mmol/l)	≥ 11.1	≥ 7.8	< 7.8
Action	refer to diabetic clinic	dietary advice; check fasting glucose annually	dietary advice; check fasting glucose annually

Obesity

The clinical management of a woman with PCOS should be focused on her individual problems. Obesity worsens both symptomatology and the endocrine profile and so obese women (BMI $> 30\,kg/m^2$) should therefore be encouraged to lose weight. Weight loss improves the endocrine profile, the likelihood of ovulation and a healthy pregnancy.

Much has been written about diet and PCOS. The right diet for an individual is one that is practical, sustainable and compatible with her lifestyle. It is sensible to keep carbohydrate content down and to avoid fatty foods. It is often helpful to refer to a dietician.

Anti-obesity drugs may help with weight loss. These can be prescribed by general practitioners and their use must be closely monitored. Metformin may improve with insulin resistance and may aid some women with weight loss, combined with a healthy diet and exercise program. Metformin therapy is discussed below.

Menstrual irregularity

The easiest way to control the menstrual cycle is the use of a low-dose combined oral contraceptive preparation. This will result in an artificial cycle and regular shedding of the endometrium. An alternative is a progestogen (such as medroxyprogesterone acetate (Provera®) or dydrogesterone (Duphaston®) for 12 days every 1–3 months to induce a withdrawal bleed. It is also important once again to encourage weight loss.

In women with anovulatory cycles the action of estradiol on the endometrium is unopposed because of the lack of cyclical progesterone secretion. This may result in episodes of irregular uterine bleeding, and in the long-term endometrial hyperplasia and even endometrial cancer (see above). An ultrasound assessment of endometrial thickness provides a bioassay for estradiol production by the ovaries and conversion of androgens in the peripheral fat. If the endometrium is thicker than 15 mm a withdrawal bleed should be induced and, if the endometrium fails to shed, then endometrial sampling is required to exclude endometrial hyperplasia or malignancy. The only young women to get endometrial carcinoma (< 35 years), which otherwise has a mean age of occurrence of 61 years in the UK, are those with anovulation secondary to PCOS or estrogen-secreting tumors.

Infertility

Ovulation can be induced with the anti-estrogens, clomiphene citrate (50–100 mg) or tamoxifen (20–40 mg), days 2–6 of a natural or artificially induced bleed. Whilst clomiphene is successful in inducing ovulation in over 80% of women, pregnancy only occurs in about 40%. Clomiphene citrate should only be prescribed in a setting where ultrasound monitoring is available (and performed) in order to minimize the 10% risk of multiple pregnancy and to ensure that ovulation is taking place[19]. A daily dose of more than 100 mg rarely confers any benefit and can cause thickening of the cervical mucus, which can impede passage of sperm through the cervix. Once an ovulatory dose has been reached, the cumulative conception rate continues to increase for up to 10–12 cycles[20]. However, clomiphene is only licensed for 6 months use in the UK, and so we would advise careful counseling of patients if clomiphene citrate therapy is continued beyond 6 months.

The therapeutic options for patients with anovulatory infertility who are resistant to anti-estrogens are either parenteral gonadotropin therapy or laparoscopic ovarian diathermy. Because the polycystic ovary is very sensitive to stimulation by exogenous hormones, it is very important to start with very low doses of gonadotropins and follicular development must be carefully monitored by ultrasound scans. The advent of transvaginal ultrasonography has enabled the multiple pregnancy rate to be reduced to approximately 7% because of its higher resolution and clearer view of the developing follicles. Cumulative conception and livebirth rates after 6 months may be 62% and 54%, respectively, and after 12 months 73% and 62%, respectively[3]. Close monitoring should enable treatment to be suspended if three or more mature follicles develop, as the risk of multiple pregnancy obviously increases.

Women with PCOS are also at increased risk of developing the ovarian hyperstimulation syndrome (OHSS). This occurs if too many follicles (> 10 mm) are stimulated and results in abdominal distension, discomfort, nausea, vomiting and sometimes difficulty in breathing. The mechanism for OHSS is thought to be secondary to activation of the ovarian renin–angiotensin pathway and excessive secretion of vascular epidermal growth factor (VEGF). The ascites, pleural and pericardial effusions exacerbate this serious condition and the resultant hemoconcentration can lead to thromboembolism. The situation worsens if a pregnancy has resulted from the treatment as human chorionic gonadotropin from the placenta further stimulates the ovaries. Hospitalization is sometimes necessary in order for intravenous fluids and heparin to be given to prevent dehydration and thromboembolism. Although the OHSS is rare it is potentially fatal and should be avoidable with appropriate monitoring of gonadotropin therapy.

Ovarian diathermy is free of the risks of multiple pregnancy and ovarian hyperstimulation and does not require intensive ultrasound monitoring. Laparoscopic ovarian diathermy has taken the place of wedge resection of the ovaries (which resulted in extensive peri-ovarian and tubal adhesions), and it appears to be as effective as routine gonadotropin therapy in the treatment of clomiphene-insensitive PCOS[21].

Hyperandrogenism and hirsutism

The bioavailability of testosterone is affected by the serum concentration of SHBG. High levels of insulin lower the production of SHBG and so increase the free fraction of androgen. Elevated serum androgen concentrations stimulate peripheral androgen receptors, resulting in an increase in 5α-reductase activity directly increasing the conversion of testosterone to the more potent metabolite, dihydrotestosterone. Symptoms of hyperandrogenism include hirsutism, which is a distressing condition. Hirsutism is characterized by terminal hair growth in a male pattern of distribution, including chin, upper lip, chest, upper and lower back, upper and lower abdomen, upper arm, thigh and buttocks. A standardized scoring system, such as the modified Ferriman and Gallwey score should be used to evaluate the degree of hirsutism before and during treatments.

Treatment options include cosmetic and medical therapies. As drug therapies may take 6–9 months or longer before any improvement of hirsutism is perceived, physical treatments including electrolysis, waxing and bleaching may be helpful whilst waiting for medical treatments to work. For many years, the most 'permanent' physical treatment for unwanted hair has been electrolysis. It is time-consuming, painful and expensive and should be performed by an expert practitioner. Regrowth is not uncommon and there is no really permanent cosmetic treatment, but the last few years have seen much development in the use of laser and photothermolysis techniques. There are many different types of laser in production and each requires evaluation of dose intensity, effectiveness and safety. The technique is promising, being faster and more effective than shaving, waxing or chemical depilation. Repeated treatments are required for a near permanent effect because only hair follicles in the growing phase are obliterated at each treatment. Hair growth occurs in three cycles so 6–9 months of regular treatments are typical. Patients should be appropriately selected (dark hair on fair skin is best), and warned that complete hair removal cannot be guaranteed and some scarring may occur. At present it is not widely available and is still an expensive option.

Medical regimens should stop further progression of hirsutism and decrease the rate of hair growth. Adequate contraception is important in women of reproductive age as transplacental passage of anti-androgens may disturb the genital development of a male fetus. The best pharmacological treatment of proven effectiveness is a combination of the synthetic progestogen cyproterone acetate (50–100 mg), which is anti-gonadotropic and anti-androgenic, with ethinylestradiol (alone or as a combined oral contraceptive pill (COC)). Estrogens lower circulating androgens by a combination of a slight inhibition of gonadotropin secretion and gonadotropin-sensitive ovarian steroid production, and by an increase in hepatic production of SHBG resulting in lower free testosterone. The cyproterone is taken for the first 10 days of a cycle (the 'reversed sequential' method) and the estrogen for the first 21 days. After a gap of exactly 7 days, during which menstruation usually occurs, the regimen is repeated. As an easier and equally effective alternative, the preparation Dianette contains ethinylestradiol in combination with cyproterone, although at a lower dose (2 mg)[18]. The effect on acne and seborrhea is usually evident within a couple of months. Cyproterone acetate can rarely cause liver damage and liver function should be checked regularly (after 6 months and then annually). It is generally advised that a switch should be made to a lower-dose COC once symptom control has been achieved – usually after 6–12 months of therapy with Dianette.

Spironolactone is a weak diuretic with anti-androgenic properties and may be used in women in whom the COC is contra-indicated at a daily dose of 25–100 mg. Drosperinone is a derivative of spironolactone and contained in the new COC, Yasmin, which we are currently evaluating in women with PCOS.

Other anti-androgens such as ketoconazole, finasteride and flutamide have been tried, but are not widely used in the UK for the treatment of hirsutism in women due to their adverse side-effects. Furthermore, they are no more effective than cyproterone acetate.

Insulin-sensitizing agents and metformin

A number of pharmacological agents have been used to amplify the physiological effect of weight loss, notably metformin. This biguanide inhibits the production of hepatic glucose and enhances the sensitivity of peripheral tissue to insulin, thereby decreasing insulin secretion. It has been shown that metformin ameliorates hyperandrogenism and abnormalities of gonadotropin secretion in women with PCOS and can restore menstrual cyclicity and fertility[22]. Metformin may also enhance the efficacy of clomiphene citrate and gonadotropin therapy. The insulin-sensitizing agent troglitazone also appears to significantly improve the metabolic and reproductive abnormalities in PCOS, although this product has been withdrawn because of reports of deaths from hepatotoxicity and the introduction of newer thiazolinediones (rosiglitazone and pyoglitazone are currently being evaluated).

Metformin is the most promising and safe sensitizer to insulin available in the UK at the present time and may have benefits for short- and long-term health, by improving hyperandrogenism, fertility, insulin sensitivity and lipid profile. There has been much publicity about its use and, as usual, inadequate scientifically sound data. Further research is required with adequately powered clinical studies. The current evidence suggests significant benefit of metformin on reproductive function but not, despite earlier claims, on the ability to achieve weight loss[22].

CONCLUSIONS

In summary, PCOS is a heterogeneous condition and the commonest cause of irregular menstrual cycles. Ovarian dysfunction leads to the main signs and symptoms, and the ovary is influenced by external factors in particular the gonadotropins, insulin and other growth factors, which are dependent upon both genetic and environmental influences. There are long-term risks of developing diabetes and possibly cardiovascular disease. Therapy to date has been symptomatic but, by our improved understanding of the pathogenesis, treatment options are becoming available that strike more at the heart of the syndrome, such as the use of insulin-sensitizing agents.

PRACTICE POINTS

- Polycystic ovary syndrome is the commonest endocrine disorder in women (prevalence 15–20%)
- Polycystic ovary syndrome is a heterogeneous condition. Diagnosis is made by the ultrasound detection of polycystic ovaries and one or more of a combination of symptoms and signs (hyperandrogenism (acne, hirsutism, alopecia), obesity, menstrual cycle disturbance (oligoo/amenorrhea)) and biochemical abnormalities (hypersecretion of testosterone, luteinizing hormone and insulin)
- Management is symptom orientated
- If obese, weight loss improves symptoms and endocrinology and should be encouraged. A glucose tolerance test should be performed if the BMI is $> 30 \, \text{kg/m}^2$, or $25 \, \text{kg/m}^2$ in Asian women
- Menstrual cycle control is achieved by cyclical oral contraceptives, progestogen therapy or metformin
- Ovulation induction may be difficult and require progression through various treatments that should be monitored carefully to prevent multiple pregnancy
- Hyperandrogenism is usually managed with Dianette, containing ethinylestradiol in combination with cyproterone acetate.

A new combined oral contraceptive pill, Yasmin, may also be of benefit. Alternatives include spironolactone. Reliable contraception is required

- Insulin-sensitizing agents (e.g. metformin) are showing early promise but require further long-term evaluation and should only be prescribed by endocrinologists/reproductive endocrinologists

tumors, late-onset congenital adrenal hyperplasia, Cushing's syndrome)
- Infertility
- Rapid-onset hirsutism (to exclude androgen-secreting tumors)
- Glucose intolerance/diabetes
- Amenorrhea of more than 6 months – for pelvic ultrasound scan to exclude endometrial hyperplasia
- Refractory symptoms

INDICATIONS FOR REFERRAL TO A REPRODUCTIVE MEDICINE SPECIALIST

- Serum testosterone > 5 nmol/l (to exclude other causes of androgen excess, e.g.

REFERENCES

1. Fauser B, Tarlatziz B, Chang J, et al., the Rotterdam ESHRE/ASRM-sponsored PCOS Consensus Workshop Group. Revised 2003 consensus on diagnostic criteria amd long-term health risks related to polycystic ovary syndrome (PCOS). Hum Reprod 2004; 19: 41–7 and Fertil Steril 2004; 81: 19–25

2. Balen AH, Laven JS, Tan SL, Dewailly D. Ultrasound assessment of the polycystic ovary: international consensus definitions. Hum Reprod Update 2003; 9: 505–14

3. Balen AH, Conway GS, Kaltsas G, et al. Polycystic ovary syndrome: the spectrum of the disorder in 1741 patients. Hum Reprod 1995; 10: 2705–12

4. Clark AM, Ledger W, Galletly C, et al. Weight loss results in significant improvement in pregnancy and ovulation rates in anovulatory obese women. Hum Reprod 1995; 10: 2705–12

5. Polson DW, Adams J, Wadsworth J, Franks S. Polycystic ovaries – a common finding in normal women. Lancet 1988; 1: 870–2

6. Michelmore KF, Balen AH, Dunger DB, Vessey MP. Polycystic ovaries and associated clinical and biochemical features in young women. Clin Endocrinol (Oxf) 1999; 51: 779–86

7. Adams J, Polson DW, Franks S. Prevalence of polycystic ovaries in women with anovulation and idiopathic hirsutism. Br Med J (Clin Res Ed) 1986; 293: 355–9

8. Kyei-Mensah A, Maconochie N, Zaidi J, et al. Transvaginal three-dimensional ultrasound: reproducibility of ovarian and endometrial volume measurements. Fertil Steril 1996; 66: 718–22

9. Rodin DA, Bano G, Bland JM, et al. Polycystic ovaries and associated metabolic abnormalities

in Indian subcontinent Asian women. Clin Endocrinol (Oxf) 1998; 49: 91–9

10. Wijeyaratne CN, Balen AH, Barth J, Belchetz PE. Clinical manifestations and insulin resistance (IR) in polycystic ovary syndrome (PCOS) among South Asians and Caucasians: is there a difference? Clin Endocrinol (Oxf) 2002; 57: 343–50

11. Dahlgren E, Johansson S, Lindstedt G, et al. Women with polycystic ovary syndrome wedge resected in 1956 to 1965: a long-term follow-up focusing on natural history and circulating hormones. Fertil Steril 1992; 57: 505–13

12. Gjonnaess H. The course and outcome of pregnancy after ovarian electrocautery in women with polycystic ovarian syndrome: the influence of body weight. Br J Obstet Gynaecol 1989; 96: 714–19

13. Rajkhowa M, Glass MR, Rutherford AJ, et al. Polycystic ovary syndrome: a risk factor for cardiovascular disease? Br J Obstet Gynaecol 2000; 107: 11–18

14. Pierpoint T, McKeigue PM, Isaacs AJ, et al. Mortality of women with polycystic ovary syndrome at long-term follow-up. J Clin Epidemiol 1998; 51: 581–6

15. Norman RJ, Masters L, Milner CR, et al. Relative risk of conversion from normogly-caemia to impaired glucose tolerance or non-insulin dependent diabetes mellitus in polycystic ovary syndrome. Hum Reprod 2001; 16: 1995–8

16. Elwood JM, Cole P, Rothman KJ, Kaplan SD. Epidemiology of endometrial cancer. J Natl Cancer Inst 1977; 59: 1055–60

17. Coulam CB, Annegers JF, Kranz JS. Chronic anovulation syndrome and associated neoplasia. Obstet Gynecol 1983; 61: 403–7

18. Barth JH, Cherry CA, Wojnarowska F, Dawber RPR. Cyproterone acetate for severe hirsutism: results of a double-blind dose-ranging study. Clin Endocrinol 1991; 35: 5–10

19. RCOG. Guidelines on the initial investigation and management of infertility. London: RCOG Press, 1998

20. Kousta E, White DM, Franks S. Modern use of clomiphene citrate in induction of ovulation. Hum Reprod Update 1997; 3: 359–65

21. Farquhar C, Vandekerckhove P, Lilford R. Laparoscopic 'drilling' by diathermy or laser for ovulation induction in anovulatory polycystic ovary syndrome (Cochrane Review). In The Cochrane Library, Issue 4. Oxford: Update Software, 2002

22. Lord J, Flight I, Norman R. Insulin-sensitising drugs: a meta-analysis. Cochrane Review, 2003

Premature ovarian failure 8

D. Tucker

DEFINITION AND INCIDENCE

The reported median age of the menopause is 51 years[1]. Premature ovarian failure (POF) is a condition leading to amenorrhea, hypoestrogenism and elevated gonadotropins before the age of 40 years. The use of age 40 as a cut-off to define POF is largely empirical. An alternative definition proposed is to use two standard deviations from the expected age of menopause, or age 45 years[2]; however, the use of age 40 persists in the context of published research.

As early as the 1930s the presence of raised urinary gonadotropins was noted in patients with 'premature menopause'. Atria[3] in 1950 examined 20 patients with 'precocious menopause' and detailed typical clinical characteristics of POF.

The condition is not uncommon and may be under-reported by women who do not consider the cessation of the monthly menstrual cycle to be a medical problem. Overall, POF is responsible for 4–18% of cases of secondary amenorrhea and 10–28% of primary amenorrhea[4]. It is estimated to affect 1% of women under 40 years of age and 0.1% under 30.

ETIOLOGY

In the majority of women diagnosed with POF, the specific etiology and underlying pathophysiology remain elusive. Traditional texts have concentrated on describing ovarian failure as being associated with either a deficient number of primordial follicles from the onset of menarche, accelerated follicle atresia or follicles resistant to gonadotropin stimulation (idiopathic POF)[5].

Considering the developmental stages of the ovary, germ cells migrate from the dorsal wall of the developing gut and reach the gonadal ridges at approximately 5 weeks of gestation. Here the oogonia undergo mitotic activity, resulting in around 6–8 million primary oocytes by 20 weeks of gestational age[6]. Two-thirds of these germ cells have entered and arrested in the prophase of the first meiotic division. From 20 weeks of intrauterine life, there is gradual attrition of the primary oocytes and at birth each ovary contains around 200 000 germ cells. A further 100 000 oocytes will be lost before menarche, and ultimately only 400–500 follicles will develop fully and be released through the process of ovulation during the reproductive years.

By the time of the normal menopausal transition there is a significant reduction in the number of remaining oocytes and at menopause there will be very few remaining[7]. This is in contrast to patients with POF, where residual oocytes exist, albeit in reduced number. It is for this reason that use of the term premature menopause is inappropriate. Although it is impossible to predict likelihood of spontaneous ovulation, up to 20% of patients may ovulate in the 6 months following diagnosis[5].

Follicular versus afollicular POF

When considering the etiology of POF, dividing the condition into follicular or afollicular subgroups suggests that knowing an individual's status is either important or useful. In the absence of a non-invasive test to differentiate between follicular depletion or dysfunction, the only alternative is laparoscopic ovarian biopsy. The validity of single biopsies has not been established, indeed pregnancies have occurred despite histological lack of follicles after biopsy, suggesting sampling errors[5]. In any case, laparoscopy is not without risk and the clinical management of both types of POF is similar. A summary of the etiology of POF is listed in Table 1.

Table 1 Etiology of premature ovarian failure. Adapted from reference 6

Genetic

Enzyme deficiencies: galactosemia, 17α-hydroxylase, 17, 20-desmolase, cholesterol desmolase

X-linked

Polymorphism involving inhibin B or the FSH receptor

BEPS type I syndrome

Non-genetic

Iatrogenic: pelvic surgery, radiotherapy or chemotherapy

Autoimmune disease

Oophoritis

Idiopathic

FSH, follicle stimulating hormone; BEPS, blepharophimosis/ptosis/epicanthus

Enzyme deficiencies

A number of enzyme deficiencies have been found to be associated with an increased risk of POF. The most common of these is the autosomal recessive condition of galactosemia, that occurs due to a deficiency in the enzyme galactose-1-phosphate uridyltransferase. Accumulation of galactose results in damage to the liver, eyes and kidneys. The risk of POF has been found to be as high as 81% in affected females[8] and the cause appears to be a galactose-induced reduction in total germ cell development during oogenesis[9]. Other proposed mechanisms include accelerated follicular atresia and biologically inactive isoforms of follicle stimulating hormone (FSH)[10]. Other enzyme abnormalities associated with POF include deficiencies of 17α-hydroxylase, 17,20-desmolase and cholesterol desmolase. Patients with cholesterol desmolase are not able to produce biologically active steroids and rarely survive to adulthood. The remaining enzyme disorders are similarly rare and may be associated with concomitant adrenal insufficiency.

X-linked POF

As early as 1966 the requirement for two intact X chromosomes for normal follicular development was identified[11]. The complete absence of one X chromosome, as in Turner syndrome, results in ovarian dysgenesis and primary ovarian failure. Fragile X syndrome has been identified as placing women at higher risk of premature ovarian failure. Fragile X mutations occur at least ten times more frequently in women with POF than the general population. Following the screening of 132 women for fragile X permutations, it was found that 13% of those with familial POF and 3% with the sporadic form had fragile X permutations, compared with an expected prevalence of 1:590[12].

A critical region on the X chromosome (POF1) ranging from Xq13 to Xq26 has been identified relating to normal ovarian function in addition to a second gene of paternal origin (POF2), located at Xq13.3-q21.1[13]. Idiopathic POF can be familial or sporadic, and the familial pattern of inheritance is compatible either with X-linked (with incomplete penetrance) or with an autosomal dominant mode of inheritence[14].

FSH receptor gene polymorphism and inhibin B mutation

As might be expected, resistance to the action of gonadotropins can lead to the clinical features of POF and this has been demonstrated in a cohort of Finnish families[15]. This does, however, appear to be a very rare cause of POF. More recently an analysis of 43 patients with POF demonstrated a mutation in the inhibin gene (INHα) at a frequency ten-fold higher than control patients (7% vs. 0.7%). These patients experienced ovarian failure at an early age, frequently prior to the second decade of life[16].

Blepharophimosis/ptosis/epicanthus (BEPS) syndrome

This rare autosomal dominant condition leads to congenital abnormalities of the eye including blepharophimosis, ptosis and epicanthus inversis. In BEPS type I, eyelid malformation co-segregates with premature ovarian failure, and has been mapped to chromosome 3q[17].

Iatrogenic ovarian failure

The likelihood of ovarian failure after chemotherapy or radiotherapy depends upon the agent used, dosage levels, interval between treatments and in particular the age of the patient. The prepubertal ovary is relatively resistant to the effects of chemotherapeutic alkylating agents. Attempts to suppress ovarian activity of reproductive aged women using oral contraceptives or gonodotropin releasing hormone (GnRH) analogs in order to mimic this protection have produced conflicting results[18].

Radiation-induced ovarian failure with a total dose greater than 6 Gy usually results in sterility[19]. However, as with chemotherapy, prepubertal girls are more resistant to irradiation. Normal menstruation following treatment does not necessarily mean that the ovaries are unaffected and incipient POF may occur at a later date. Surgical transposition of the ovaries beyond the direct field of treatment has been described[20].

Autoimmune disease

POF is frequently associated with autoimmune disorders, particularly hypothyroidism[21]. Other co-existing conditions may include Crohn's disease, vitiligo, pernicious anemia, systemic lupus erythematosus or rheumatoid arthritis. Addison's disease is associated with around 3% of patients with POF and may be present as part of a polyglandular failure syndrome[5]. The type I syndrome is associated with adrenal failure, hypoparathyroidism and chronic muco-cutaneous candidiasis and mainly occurs in children, associated with primary ovarian failure. The type II syndrome may present much later with hypothyroidism and is less consistently associated with POF. Hypothyroidism affects around 25% of patients with POF and diabetes mellitus affects a further 2.5%[22].

The prevalence of antibodies directed against the ovary has been the subject of significant research. Circulating anti-ovarian antibodies have been found in 10–69% of women with POF, and importantly in a significant number of controls[23]. There is little correlation between presence of antibodies and severity or progression of disease. Antigonadotropin receptor antibodies have been isolated but their significance remains unclear. The use of antibodies directed against steroid-producing cells has proven most promising in terms of predicting patients who may develop ovarian failure as part of the polyglandular syndrome. These individuals, however, represent a minority of those affected by POF[24].

In summary, there is little evidence of involvement of autoimmunity in the etiology of POF in the absence of other manifestations of autoimmune disease. The link between the polyglandular failure syndromes and POF is well established.

Oophoritis

Rebar and Connolly reported a retrospective case review of a series of patients with POF finding 3.5% of patients had a previous infection, including malaria, varicella, or shigella[25]. Mumps orchitis is well recognized in males and a similar histological phenomenon has been described in the ovary. The exact role of viral infections in the etiology of POF, however, is unclear. Lymphocytic oophoritis was found in 11% of 215 POF patients undergoing ovarian biopsy, most of whom had steroid cell antibodies and associated adrenal disease[26].

Demographic features

The contribution of environmental factors to the development of POF has been examined in several case studies. No consistent and reliable contribution has been demonstrated with regards to education level, socioeconomic status, oral contraceptive use, smoking habit or anthropometric characteristics[27]. Nulliparity and lifelong irregular menstrual cycles are associated with an increased risk of POF[28].

PRESENTATION

There is no consistent pattern to the presentation of POF. The most common presenting symptom in POF is secondary amenorrhea in a woman under the age of 40 years. This may be preceded by irregular menses or sudden cessation of menstruation. Widespread use of combined contraceptives results in a proportion of cases presenting as persistent post-pill amenorrhea. Hot flushes may be present at the outset or develop subsequently, along with other symptoms of hypoestrogenism, including vaginal dryness or urinary symptoms.

Medical history

The important points to consider in the medical history are listed in Table 2. It is important to detect co-existing disease, in particular hypothyroidism and diabetes mellitus, the conditions most commonly associated with POF.

Table 2 History points in premature ovarian failure (POF)

Menstrual history
Duration of oligo-amenorrhea and associated symptoms

Symptoms of estrogen deficiency
Oligo-amenorrhea
Vasomotor symptoms
Vaginitis/dyspareunia
Urinary symptoms
Subfertility

Previous medical history
Previous ovarian surgery, chemotherapy or radiotherapy
Mumps
Addison's disease, thyroid disorders, diabetes mellitus, SLE, rheumatoid arthritis, vitiligo, Crohn's disease

Additional risk factors for osteoporosis
Previous low trauma fractures, smoking, excess alcohol intake, diet low in calcium, glucocorticoid therapy

Family history
POF or autoimmune disease
Family history of low trauma fractures

Systemic review
Weight loss, anorexia, fatigue, increased skin pigmentation (Addison's)
Symptoms of thyroid disease or diabetes mellitus
Headache (pituitary tumor)

SLE, systemic lupus erythematosus

Physical examination

The most important cause of POF to exclude in patients with primary amenorrhea is Turner syndrome. Typical clinical features include short stature with an increased carrying angle (cubitus valgus). Pigmented nevi or keloid scarring may be present and there is an absence of secondary sexual characteristics.

In view of the association with autoimmune diseases, physical signs of these should be sought. Graves' disease or thyroiditis may result in goiter in addition to the physical signs of hypothyroidism. Adrenal failure results in weight loss, brown hyperpigmentation of extensor surfaces and sparse axillary and pubic hair. Signs related to rare disorders such as the ophthalmic abnormalities associated with BEPS type I should be excluded. Although bitemporal hemianopia is the classical abnormality associated with pituitary tumors, any bilateral or unilateral field abnormality may occur.

Pelvic examination may reveal atrophic vaginitis due to estrogen deficiency and the ovaries may be tender on bimanual examination due to the oophoritis associated with steroid cell autoimmune POF. A neurological examination should be completed to exclude a central space-occupying lesion.

INVESTIGATIONS

Anasti[5] has suggested the diagnosis of POF may be made when the following criteria are met: 4 months of amenorrhea and two serum FSH values of $>40\,IU/l$ obtained more than 1 month apart in a women under 40 years of age. Further investigations are listed in Table 3.

Chromosomal analysis is recommended for all patients with confirmed POF due to the implications that genetic abnormalities may have for other family members. Referral for genetic counseling where appropriate is advisable. If karyotype reveals the presence of Y-chromosome material, the ovaries should be removed to prevent the development of gonadoblastoma.

Kim and colleagues examined the results of a prospective screening program in 119 patients with POF[22]. The following tests were carried out: free thyroxine, thyroid stimulating hormone

Table 3 Investigation of premature ovarian failure

Serum FSH estimation x 2 one month apart (> 40 IU/l)

Chromosome analysis

Thyroid stimulating hormone

Full blood count

Urinalysis

Fasting glucose

Autoimmune screen

+/- DXA bone mineral density estimation

+/- ACTH stimulation test

FSH, follicle stimulating hormone; DXA, dual energy X-ray absorptiometry; ACTH, adrenocorticotropic hormone

(TSH), fasting glucose, calcium, phosphate, vitamin B_{12}, electrolytes, cosyntropin stimulation test, and autoimmune screening. They reported no new diagnoses of adrenal failure, pernicious anemia or hypoparathyroidism. Twelve new cases of thyroid disease and two new cases of diabetes mellitus were discovered.

A full blood count, urinalysis and autoimmune screen may detect associated autoimmune disease. If the clinical history or examination suggests the presence of organ-specific autoimmune conditions then appropriate investigations should be carried out. Gonadotropin-producing pituitary tumors are a rare differential diagnosis of POF, but raised serum gonadotropins associated with headache and visual field defects should be investigated with magnetic resonance imaging.

Although ovarian biopsy has been considered, the diagnostic usefulness of this investigation has yet to be proven outside the context of a research setting.

CONSEQUENCES OF ESTROGEN LACK

Osteoporosis

Hypoestrogenic states are associated with the development of osteoporosis. Peak bone mass is achieved at about 30 years of age for the spine and 20 years for the proximal femur. Therefore, if POF occurs during adolescence or young adult life, peak bone mass will be impaired. If it occurs after age 30, bone loss will start early. After removal of estrogen, the rate of loss is around 2.5–6% per year from the spine, with varying rates in so-called fast or slow bone losers[29].

It is possible that the underlying cause of POF is a determinant of the rate of bone loss. This may be less rapid with spontaneous POF or that induced by cancer treatments. Howell and associates discovered no significant reduction in bone mineral density (BMD) at the lumbar spine, hip or forearm in a cohort of POF patients at a mean of 49 months amenorrhea after treatment for hematological malignancy[30]. In contrast, surgically-induced menopause may result in more rapid loss[31]. It has been suggested that this may be due to residual ovarian activity and low levels of estrogen – or their metabolites – having a persisting influence on bone density[32].

Assessment of BMD via dual energy X-ray absorptiometry (DXA) is not normally necessary, especially if the patient presents soon after onset of amenorrhea and starts estrogen replacement. If the POF was surgically induced more than 12 months previously and no estrogen replacement received, the argument for formal assessment of baseline BMD is stronger. BMD assessment is also useful in planning a long-term strategy for skeletal conservation. For every one standard deviation decrease in BMD, there is a two- to three-fold increase in risk of fracture.

Cardiovascular disease

Endogenous estrogen has an atheroprotective effect on serum lipids as well as being a systemic vasodilator. Postmenopausal loss of estrogen is associated with an increased susceptibility to cardiovascular risk factors such as hypertension, hyperlipidemia and glucose intolerance, resulting in increased cardiovascular morbidity and mortality[33,34]. Premature ovarian failure increases this risk further, with an overall seven-fold increased risk of myocardial infarction for women undergoing bilateral salpingo–oophorectomy at age 35 and not receiving estrogen replacement. Each year of prolonged endogenous estrogen exposure was found to be associated with a 2% reduction in cardiovascular mortality risk.

MANAGEMENT

A summary of the management of POF is listed in Table 4.

Table 4 Management of premature ovarian failure

Counseling about the condition and associated disorders
Estrogen replacement
Contraception if appropriate
Donor oocyte IVF if pregnancy desired
Annual review including screening for diabetes and thyroid disease

IVF, in vitro fertilization

Counseling

It is important to provide patients with adequate information about POF in an appropriate format. Some women will blame their own actions for the disease, for example long-term use of oral contraceptives. Addressing these misconceptions early can alleviate unnecessary guilt. National self-support groups for POF exist, such as The Daisy Network in the UK (http://www.daisynetwork.org.uk/), and for many these provide helpful psychological support. Women need to be aware that ovulation may again occur, often intermittently, and either cyclical menstrual bleeding or even pregnancy can result. It is important that patients with POF are aware of the symptoms of associated diseases and understand the importance of reporting these to their primary care provider.

Estrogen replacement

The mainstay of treatment for women with POF is estrogen replacement therapy, recommended until the average age of natural menopause, i.e. 51 years. This view is endorsed by regulatory bodies such as the Committee on Safety of Medicines in the UK. A commonly adopted form of treatment is the combined oral contraceptive pill (COC). This is usually provided for reasons of convenience, efficacy and minimal side-effect profile, as well as the psychological benefit of taking a therapy used by many of the patient's peer group. In women with an intact uterus, estrogen and progestogen are necessary either as sequential or continuous combined therapy. Some women may prefer sequential therapy leading to regular withdrawal bleeds rather than continuous combined therapy leading to amenorrhea. Breakthrough bleeding with either regimen may suggest return of spontaneous ovulation. If the patient has undergone hysterectomy, estrogen only is required. Women with POF may need a higher dose of estrogen than women in their 50s to control vasomotor symptoms.

There is a deficiency of controlled trial data on which to base treatment decisions. The only direct comparison of hormone replacement therapy (HRT) and ethinylestradiol and conjugated equine estrogen is a study of 17 women with Turner syndrome[35]. In this short study, there was no difference between the two estrogens with respect to effect on the endometrium, hyperinsulinemia or lipid profiles. Ethinylestradiol had a more potent effect on markers of bone turnover and suppression of gonadotropins. Estrogen replacement in normal postmenopausal women results in a decrease in the rate of bone turnover by approximately 50%, resulting in fracture reduction of 30–50% at the spine, hip and other sites[36].

Oral versus parenteral route

Whether estrogen therapy should be taken orally or parenterally is currently unresolved. Serum C-reactive protein increases with oral estrogens and this inflammatory marker is known to be a risk factor for cardiovascular events[37]. In addition, oral therapy results in increases in circulating estrone levels two to three times higher than estradiol. Transdermal estradiol is known to have less effect on coagulation and C-reactive protein levels than oral preparations, and therefore may not carry excess cardiovascular risk[38]. Avoidance of first-pass metabolism reduces the effect on hepatic

production of insulin–like growth factor and results in physiological patterns of circulating estradiol and estrone.

In view of the possibility of intermittent return of ovarian function, patients not wishing to fall pregnant should be offered the COC.

Some patients report persistent tiredness, lack of energy, reduced libido or sexual function despite apparently adequate doses of estrogen replacement. This may be more common in women who have had their ovaries removed, and consideration should be given to additional testosterone therapy. Testosterone implants may be provided along with subdermal estrogen, if this form of replacement has been chosen. When available for female use, testosterone patches provide an alternative[39].

The effect of long-term estrogen replacement by HRT or the COC in the management of POF has not been specifically addressed in clinical trials. The overall long-term safety of COC use in healthy women is reassuring, however, and although this form of estrogen replacement is probably appropriate, further research in this area is warranted.

Monitoring of treatment

Patients with POF are normally reviewed annually to ensure symptoms are adequately controlled and associated diseases are not missed. The importance of a thorough history and physical examination in the follow-up of these patients has been highlighted, without the need for extensive routine laboratory testing[5]. If there is clinical suspicion then appropriate tests are carried out. Annual screening for thyroid disease and diabetes has been suggested via serum TSH and fasting blood glucose estimations.

FERTILITY ISSUES

It has been estimated that the lifetime chance of spontaneous conception in women with karyotypically normal POF is 5–15%[5,40], the age of the patient at the time of diagnosis being an important determinant.

Empiric therapy

The published literature contains many reports of apparent successes with a variety of treatments directed at improving the chance of spontaneous pregnancy. Interventions have included gonadotropins, estrogens, GnRH agonists, growth hormone releasing hormones, corticosteroids and danazol. No evidence of effect has been proven and pregnancy is no more likely than with spontaneous conceptions[41].

Spontaneous POF

Donor oocyte in vitro fertilization (IVF) is the treatment of choice for women with both primary and secondary POF. Women with spontaneous, karyotypically normal POF have similar success rates to conventional IVF[42]. Patients can be reassured that there is no urgency for treatment following a diagnosis of POF. It is the age of the oocyte rather than the age of the recipient that determines the chance of success. Use of a sibling's oocyte has been found to decrease the pregnancy rate[43].

Turner syndrome

Oocyte donation is also an option for women with Turner syndrome and in observational studies pregnancy rates are similar to oocyte donation for other indications[44]. The risk of miscarriage is greater, however, resulting in overall significantly lower delivery rates. Cardiovascular and other complications such as hypertension and pre-eclampsia occur more frequently and it has been suggested that embryo transfer is limited to a single embryo to avoid additional complications due to multiple pregnancy. Pretreatment screening to detect previously undiagnosed maternal congenital cardiac abnormalities is essential.

POF following chemotherapy or radiotherapy

There are very few options available for preventative therapy prior to these anticancer treatments. Mature oocytes cannot be cryopreserved easily; however, oocyte survival and even successful pregnancies have been achieved[45]. The collection of mature oocytes requires ovarian stimulation, which may not be advisable in estrogen-dependent malignancies. In addition this technique is not suitable for prepubertal patients. Efforts directed at ovarian tissue cryopreservation may overcome these drawbacks, but currently remain experimental[46].

Embryo cryopreservation may be possible prior to treatment if time allows and fertility drugs are not contraindicated. Oocyte donation IVF is reported to have a lower pregnancy rate in patients with chemotherapy or radiation-induced POF than donor IVF for other indications[44,47].

SUMMARY

POF is a condition that occurs in 1% of women under the age of 40. The consequences of estrogen deficiency in a young woman include osteoporosis and cardiovascular disease, and clinicians must consider the diagnosis in all patients of reproductive age presenting with oligo-amenorrhea or symptoms of estrogen deficit. It is important to exclude co-existing autoimmune conditions with appropriate investigations. The mainstay of treatment is with hormone replacement therapy in the form of traditional HRT or the combined contraceptive pill. Oocyte donation IVF provides the greatest chance of success if fertility is desired. Annual review will ensure adequate response to estrogen replacement and provide an opportunity to screen for associated diseases.

PRACTICE POINTS

- It is important to consider the diagnosis of POF in non-pregnant women presenting with secondary amenorrhea
- Premature ovarian failure is not a benign condition and requires thorough evaluation, counseling and treatment
- Hormone replacement therapy is required to prevent short- and long-term consequences of estrogen deficiency
- Patients desiring pregnancy should be referred to local infertility services to explore the availability of ovum donation
- Local and national patient groups can provide useful information and support
- The lifetime chance of pregnancy for women with karyotypically normal premature ovarian failure is 5–15%, so contraception must be discussed with women not desiring pregnancy

REFERENCES

1. McKinlay SM, Brambilla DJ, Posner JG. The normal menopause transition. Maturitas 1992; 14: 103–15

2. Hoek A, Schoemaker J, Drexhage HA. Premature ovarian failure and ovarian auto-immunity. Endocr Rev 1997; 18: 107–34

3. Atria A. La menopausia precoz y tratamiento hormonal. Rev Med Chil 1950; 78: 373–7

4. Coulam CB, Adamson SC, Annegers JF. Incidence of premature ovarian failure. Obstet Gynecol 1986; 67: 604–6

5. Anasti JN. Premature ovarian failure: an update. Fertil Steril 1998; 70: 1–15

6. Pal L, Santoro N. Premature ovarian failure (POF): discordance between somatic and reproductive aging. Ageing Res Rev 2002; 1: 413–23

7. Richardson SJ, Senkias V, Nelson JF. Follicular depletion during menopausal transition: evidence for accelerated loss and ultimate exhaustion. J Clin Endocrinol Metab 1987; 65: 1231–7

8. Waggoner DD, Buist NR, Donnell GN. Long-term prognosis in galactosaemia: results of a survey of 350 cases. J Inherit Metab Dis 1990; 13: 802–18

9. Chen YT, Mattison DR, Feigenbaum I, et al. Reduction in oocyte number following prenatal exposure to a diet high in galactose. Science 1981; 214: 1145–7

10. Prestoz LL, Couto AS, Shin YS, Petry KG. Altered follicle stimulating hormone isoforms in female galactosaemia patients. Eur J Pediatr 1997; 156: 116–20

11. Singh RP, Carr DH. The anatomy and histology of XO human embryos and fetuses. Anat Rec 1966; 155: 369–83

12. Conway GS, Payne NN, Webb J, et al. Fragile X permutation screening in women with premature ovarian failure. Hum Reprod 1998; 13: 1184–7

13. Powell CM, Taggart RT, Drumheller TC, et al. Molecular and cytogenetic studies of an X;autosome translocation in a patient with premature ovarian failure and review of the literature. Am J Med Genet 1994; 52: 19–26

14. Van Kasteren YM, Hundscheid RD, Smits AP, et al. Familial idiopathic premature ovarian failure: an overrated and underestimated genetic disease? Hum Reprod 1999; 14: 2455–9

15. Aittomaki K, Lucena JLD, Pakarinen P, et al. Mutation in the follicle-stimulating hormone receptor gene causes hereditary hypergonadotrophic ovarian failure. Cell 1996; 82: 959–68

16. Shelling AN, Burton KA, Chand AL, et al. Inhibin: a candidate gene for premature ovarian failure. Hum Reprod 2000; 15: 2644–9

17. Amati P, Gasparini P, Zlotogora J, et al. A gene for premature ovarian failure associated with eyelid malformation maps to chromosome 3q22-q23. Am J Hum Gen 1996; 58: 1089–92

18. Morris ID, Shalet SM. Protection of gonadal function from cytotoxic chemotherapy and irradiation. Baillieres Clin Endocrinol Metab 1990; 4: 97–118

19. Howell S, Shalet S. Gonadal damage from chemotherapy and radiotherapy. Endocrinol Metab Clin North Am 1998; 27: 927–43

20. Schulz-Lobmeyr I, Schratter-Sehn A, Huber J, et al. Laparoscopic lateral ovarian transposition before pelvic irradiation for a non-Hodgkin lymphoma. Acta Obstet Gynecol Scand 1990; 78: 350–2

21. La Barbera AR, Miller MM, Rebar RW. Autoimmune etiology in premature ovarian failure. Am J Reprod Immunol 1998; 16: 115–22

22. Kim TJ, Anasti JN, Flack MR, et al. Routine endocrine screening for patients with karyotypically normal spontaneous premature ovarian failure. Obstet Gynecol 1997; 89: 777–9

23. Kim JG, Anderson BE, Rebar RW, et al. A biotin-streptavidin enzyme immunoassay for detection of antibodies to porcine granulosa cell antigens. J Immunoassay 1991; 12: 447–64

24. Ahonen P, Miettinen A, Perheentupa J. Adrenal and steroidal cell antibodies in patients with autoimmune polyglandular disease type I and risk of adrenocortical and ovarian failure. J Clin Endocrinol Metab 1987; 64: 494–500

25. Rebar RW, Connolly HV. Clinical features of young women with hypergonadotropic amenorrhea. Fertil Steril 1990; 53: 804–10

26. Hoek A, Schoemaker J, Drexhage HA. Premature ovarian failure and ovarian autoimmunity. Endocr Rev 1997; 18: 107–34

27. Testa G, Chiaffarino F, Vegetti W, et al. Case-control study on risk factors for premature ovarian failure. Gynecol Obstet Invest 2001; 51: 40–3

28. Progetto Menopausa Italia Study Group. Premature ovarian failure: frequency and risk factors among women attending a network of

menopause clinics in Italy. Br J Obstet Gynaecol 2003; 110: 59–63

29. Pouilles JM, Tremollieres F, Ribot C. Vertebral bone loss in perimenopause. Results of a 7-year longitudinal study. Presse Med 1996; 25: 277–80

30. Howell SJ, Berger G, Adams JE, et al. Bone mineral density in women with cytotoxic-induced ovarian failure. Clin Endocrinol 1998; 49: 397–402

31. Yildiz A, Sahin I, Gol K, et al. Bone loss rate in the lumbar spine: a comparison between natural and surgically induced menopause. Int J Gynaecol Obstet 1996; 55: 153–9

32. Howell SJ, Shalet SM. Etiology-specific effect of premature ovarian failure – is residual ovarian function important? Clin Endocrinol 1999; 51: 531–4

33. van der Schouw YT, van der Graaf Y, Steyerberg EW, et al. Age at menopause as a risk factor for cardiovascular mortality. Lancet 1996; 347: 714–18

34. Rosenberg L, Hennekens CH, Rosner B, et al. Early menopause and the risk of myocardial infarction. Am J Obstet Gynecol 1981; 139: 47–51

35. Guttman H, Weiner Z, Nikolski E, et al. Choosing an estrogen replacement therapy in young adult women with Turner syndrome. Clin Endocrinol 2001; 54: 159–64

36. Rossouw JE, Anderson GL, Prentice RL, et al. Risks and benefits of estrogen plus progestin in healthy postmenopausal women: principal results from the Women's Health Initiative randomized controlled trial. JAMA 2002; 288: 321–33

37. Ridker P, Hennekens C, Rifai N. Hormone replacement therapy and increased plasma concentration of C-reactive protein. Circulation 1999; 100: 713–16

38. Lindoff C, Peterson F, Lecander I, et al. Transdermal estrogen replacement therapy: beneficial effects on haemostatic risk factors for cardiovascular disease. Maturitas 1996; 24: 43–50

39. Shifren J, Braunstein GD, Simon JA, et al. Transdermal testosterone treatment in women with impaired sexual function after oophorectomy. N Engl J Med 2000; 343: 682–8

40. O'Herlihy C, Peperell RC, Evans JH. The significance of FSH elevation in young women with disorders of ovulation. Br Med J 1980; 218: 1447–50

41. van Kasteren YM, Schoemaker J. Premature ovarian failure: a systematic review on therapeutic interventions to restore ovarian function and achieve pregnancy. Hum Reprod Update 1999; 5: 483–92

42. Lydic ML, Liu JH, Rebar RW, et al. Success of donor oocyte in *in vitro* fertilization–embryo transfer in recipients with and without premature ovarian failure. Fertil Steril 1996; 65: 98–102

43. Sung L, Bustillo M, Mukherjee T, et al. Sisters of women with premature ovarian failure may not be ideal ovum donors. Fertil Steril 1997; 67: 912–16

44. National Collaborating Centre for Women's and Children's Health. Fertility: Assessment and Treatment for People with Fertility Problems. London: RCOG Press, 2004: 126–7

45. Porcu E, Fabbri R, Seracchioli R, et al. Birth of healthy female after intracytoplasmic sperm injection of cryopreserved oocytes. Fertil Steril 1997; 68: 724–6

46. Poirot C, Vacher-Lavenu M-C, Helardot P, et al. Human ovarian tissue cryopreservation: indications and feasibility. Hum Reprod 2002; 17: 1447–52

47. Pados G, Camus M, Van Waesberghe L, et al. Oocyte and embryo donation: evaluation of 412 consecutive trials. Hum Reprod 1992; 7: 1111–17

Mood and the menstrual cycle 9

F. Blake

INTRODUCTION

Gynecological experiences are closely linked with a woman's mood[1]. Disturbances of her reproductive function can upset her sense of well-being, her feelings about her sexuality, her femininity, and her self-esteem. Symptoms may affect her intimate relationships and bring greater distress than symptoms in other systems. Women presenting with gynecological problems often appear tense and anxious just because of the nature of the intimate questions and examination which they anticipate with some apprehension. Some come distressed and tearful. They may feel shame and disgust about their symptoms or because of the reaction of others. Many find the whole consultation an ordeal. The examination can remind a woman of previous threatening situations such as rape or childhood sexual abuse, or past experience of painful or demeaning examinations by previous clinicians.

Certain conditions have overtones of moral judgment such as termination of pregnancy or sexually transmitted disease. In these cases anxiety and apprehension may be considerable. Some women are suffering with problems that disturb their mood but are not primarily gynecological rather psychological or social. Gynecological complaints are presented instead because there is stigma associated with mental health problems, and social and relationship problems may seem less appropriate to present to the doctor. This chapter considers the relationship between mood and menstrual cycle problems and models of care that enable effective management whatever the cause of the distress.

MOOD AND MENSTRUAL PROBLEMS IN THE CONSULTATION

There are several patterns of presentation of mood disturbances and menstrual complaint:

(1) Distress secondary to a menstrual disorder (e.g. menorrhagia);

(2) Mood disorder presenting under the guise of menstrual complaint (e.g. depressive illness presenting as premenstrual syndrome);

(3) Mood disorder and gynecological disorder (which may or may not have a common etiology) (e.g. oligomenorrhea and anxiety disorder);

(4) Intolerance of certain gynecological events in the setting of particular social and relationship stressors (e.g. complaint of menorrhagia after stopping the oral contraceptive pill following marital breakdown) (Table 1).

Women with problems look for an explanation of their difficulties that may yield some solution or at least exemption from excessive demands. They recognize that the doctor is willing and able to listen to them and to help by diagnosing medical disorders, clarifying the role of non-medical factors where possible and reassuring them if there is no serious pathology. Gynecological problems are mysterious and abnormalities difficult to judge by women themselves. Menstrual disturbances are particularly ambiguous. Every woman has a slightly different pattern of experience, some have no pattern. Pain, mood changes, heaviness of flow are all difficult to evaluate, and pathology is hidden, requiring invasive examination. Therefore women present when their normal pattern has changed, when there is new or more intense pain or when they are worried about themselves or the impact of their symptoms on others. They may also appear following media or internet disclosure of some new way to manage a problem that they recognize in themselves. The overlap between menstrual cycle problems and psychological problems is considerable. Women need the assistance of the informed clinician to help them differentiate between the various factors that produce the symptoms and plan effective strategies.

Mood disorders and gender differences

Mood disorders in psychiatry are usually referred to under the general title of 'affective disorder' to denote a range of disturbances that are related to mood but which include anxiety disorders and depressive illness. Symptoms that range from worry to agitation, sleep problems to delusions (Table 2).

Table 1 Patterns of presentation of mood and menstrual problems

Menstrual disorder plus mood disorder
Psychological reaction to a menstrual disorder
Mood disorder presented as menstrual disorder
External stress making normal menstrual events intolerable

Table 2 Symptoms of depressive illness/disorder

Low mood
Self-blame/guilt
Suicidal thoughts
Lack of pleasure
Hopelessness
Anxiety
Plus, if there is no physical reason to explain them
Poor sleep
Poor appetite
Fatigue
Poor concentration

Surveys and interview studies show that women experience more mood problems than men particularly during their reproductive years. The difference in prevalence emerges at adolescence. By adulthood 8–12% of women at any one time have anxiety or depressive illness, twice the rate in men (Table 3). Marriage and pregnancy increase the risk, which is not explained by postnatal depression.

Psychosocial factors contribute to this excess and may predominate. Women are frequently under stress because of low social status, economic dependency, low wages, multiple roles, vulnerability to sexual and domestic violence, and being responsible for other vulnerable members of society, particularly children and the elderly. However,

Table 3 Epidemiological pattern of mood disorder in women

Increase of mood disorder at adolescence to 8–12% of female population

Female : male ratio of 2 : 1

Higher in parous women

Rate similar to that of men after 50 years of age

Excess not explained by postnatal depression

Excess not explained by help-seeking behavior

Table 4 Role of estrogen

Relieves vasomotor symptoms of the menopause

Enhances well-being in women after oophorectomy

Relieves low mood in PMS and at the menopause

Little evidence that it relieves depressive illness

PMS, premenstrual syndrome

Table 5 Role of progesterone

Popular for distress of PMS

No evidence for efficacy in PMS over placebo

Unsuitable orally so progestogens used

Progestogens may cause PMS-like symptoms

Considered safe and natural

PMS, premenstrual syndrome

this does not fully explain the difference in morbidity and it is likely that reproductive hormones make some contribution. Gonadal hormones are psychoactive but it is not clear exactly how they influence women's emotional disorders. Estrogen has antidopaminergic properties and this is most evident in the genesis of puerperal psychosis. It is also enhances the serotonin mechanisms so may have a role in mood regulation. Progesterone modulates gamma aminobutyric acid, the neurotransmitter involved in emotional control (Tables 4 and 5).

In addition women present to doctors more readily than men with both physical and psychological problems[2]. Many present psychological problems as physical symptoms and are looking for a physical explanation. This may be in the form of gynecological complaints. A woman with psychological problems is less able to tolerate premenstrual syndrome (PMS), heavy bleeding or menopausal symptoms and therefore will present to the doctor. Attention to both physical and psychological aspects of the problem is likely to offer a greater chance of appropriate management.

SPECIFIC MENSTRUAL DISTURBANCES

There are many disorders and disturbances of the menstrual cycle and all can affect mood, either directly by the impact on hormones or neurotransmitters, or by upsetting lifestyle, relationships and self-esteem, sometimes both. PMS and symptoms of the menopause are the classic examples of menstrual disorders where mood disturbances are central to most women's complaints. Other problems including menorrhagia, dysmenorrhea, polycystic ovary syndrome, subfertility, sensitivity to the oral contraceptive pill, hysterectomy, miscarriage, cancer, etc. have a psychological dimension but the mood problem is usually considered to be secondary to the evident physiological abnormality. Situations in which the mood problem is a reaction to distressing symptoms, are considered below as are those where the psychological reactions are being denied in favor of gynecological explanations but without evidence of pathology (somatization).

Premenstrual syndrome

From earliest times men have written about women's changing moods and behavior and attributed them to their female anatomy and their menstrual cycle. In the 20th century Frank[3] coined the term premenstrual tension (PMT). He perceived a link between symptoms in the latter half of the menstrual cycle and the fluctuations of the reproductive hormones. From the 1950s there was increasing recognition and treatment of such symptoms and the concept was widened and called premenstrual syndrome. Though many symptoms are associated with PMS, mood symptoms are often the most troublesome of the presenting problems. Since then PMS has received much publicity, in both the lay and medical press. Debate continues about the syndrome's definition, etiology, and treatment (Table 6). It is a complex topic that raises many questions about the interactions between hormones and physiological changes and life events and stress. A range of possible treatments has now been evaluated though only a few have an adequate evidence base.

Many women notice change in their emotional and physical feelings during the menstrual cycle. These disturbances are very variable. Different women have different symptoms and these may vary from month to

Table 6 Problems with definition of premenstrual syndrome

Many symptoms, none specific
Symptoms vary between cycles
Temporal link with the menstrual cycle crucial
Requires prospective symptom ratings
No biological markers
May be a heterogeneous group of syndromes

month in both type and severity. There are no biochemical or other physical markers for the condition and PMS may represent several heterogeneous syndromes.

While for the majority such changes are acceptable, for others they are distressing. Premenstrual changes that are distressing are now incorporated in the term 'premenstrual syndrome' rather than 'premenstrual tension', in recognition of the variable nature of the symptoms which may not always include tension. The definition of PMS has been fraught with problems, since the type of symptoms and their severity can vary enormously both between women and between cycles for individual women. There are a number of definitions of PMS available. O'Brien[4] gives a widely accepted example:

'...a disorder of non-specific somatic, psychological or behavioral symptoms recurring in the premenstrual phase of the menstrual cycle. Symptoms must resolve completely by the end of menstruation leaving a symptom-free week. The symptoms should be of sufficient severity to produce social, family or occupational disruption. Symptoms must have occurred in at least four of the six previous menstrual cycles'.

The symptoms vary but the commonest ones include: low mood, irritability, feeling out of control, anxiety, tension, clumsiness, poor memory, food craving, sleep disturbance, bloating, breast tenderness, abdominal pain, back ache, weight gain, fatigue. Some women notice only mood changes, others only physical symptoms, but it is more common for both to be experienced together. There are no specific symptom clusters but most of the women looking for help have a predominance of psychological symptoms because these interfere most with relationships in everyday life[5].

Distressing changes may start up to 14 days before menstruation, although it is more common for the symptoms to last for up to a week, and disappear at or shortly after the start of menstrual bleeding. Many women say that the severity varies from cycle to cycle. Until the timing in relation to menstruation is established, PMS can be confused with more general problems such as anxiety or depression, and may be misdiagnosed or mistreated. External stressors or events (such as Christmas, moving house) may obscure the pattern of symptoms and women appear to recall these selectively as being associated with the premenstruum and

forget or explain away symptoms at other times. Hence, the first step in diagnosis is careful and regular symptom recording to establish the nature and timing of the problems. Women should be asked to complete menstrual charts, recording their moods and other symptoms for at least two cycles. Various menstrual diaries are available (see Appendix A), or a simple practical alternative is to customize a diary for the individual based on the predominant symptoms (see Appendix B).

Three patterns emerge: 'pure' PMS, premenstrual magnification of another problem (such as anxiety), or a problem not linked to the menstrual cycle (such as depressive illness or relationship stress) (Figure 1).

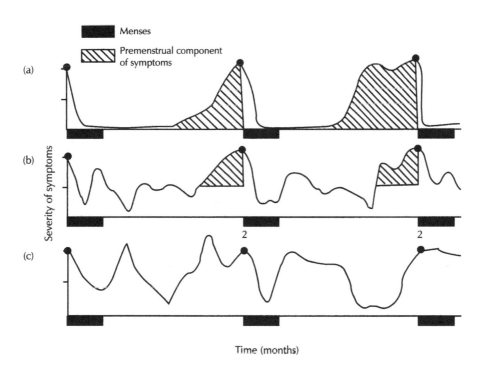

Figure 1 Patterns of symptoms presenting as premenstrual syndrome (PMS). (a) 'Pure' PMS; (b) premenstrual exacerbation of an underlying disorder; (c) symptoms that are non-cyclical (and may be part of another disorder, e.g. depression). Adapted from Sampson G.A. Premenstrual syndrome. Baillieres Clin Obstet Gynaecol 1989; 3: 687–704 with permission

Premenstrual dysphoric disorder

The most disabling form of PMS involves mood and other psychological symptoms. In research, especially in the USA, a subset of PMS sufferers has been identified using strict criteria. These criteria describe a condition called premenstrual dysphoric disorder (PMDD) that picks out the women with severe affective symptoms related to the menstrual cycle that are disabling and enduring. It must be confirmed by prospective diary evidence. Only 3–5% of women meet such criteria. This disorder is included in the American Psychiatric Association's *Diagnostic and Statistical Manual of Mental Disorders*[6], a classification for psychiatric problems (Table 7).

Etiology

There have been many hypotheses about the etiology of PMS, each associated with particular treatments, some contradicting each other. The gonadal hormones have always been at the center of investigations with nutritional deficiencies also popular. Some interest has been taken in psychopharmacological etiologies especially as so many women who complain have mood problems. With the advent of fluoxetine and the other selective serotonin re-uptake inhibitors (SSRIs) this has become a focus of research as these drugs offer realistic treatment with acceptably few side-effects (Tables 8 and 9). The link between PMS and affective disorder is strong especially among those with PMDD[7]. Many sufferers have a history of affective disorder, and many have had affective disorders associated with reproduction. Women who have suffered from depression often report exacerbation of depressed mood premenstrually. This has led to researchers considering PMDD as an intermittent affective disorder[8].

Psychosocial factors are also important. This is evident from the response of symptoms to stress, especially relationship difficulties and the large placebo response associated with PMS treatments.

Management

Most women complaining of PMS are unclear about what they themselves mean by PMS or what doctors mean by it. They have often been influenced by comments in the media or from friends who may have advocated a specific

Table 7 DSM-4 criteria for premenstrual dysphoric disorder

In most menstrual cycles during the past year, five (or more) of the following symptoms were present for most of the time during the last week of the luteal phase, began to remit during menses and were absent in the week post menses: low mood, hopelessness, self-deprecating thoughts; anxiety, tension, edginess; lability of mood; anger, irritability, loss of interest; poor concentration; lethargy, fatigue; overeating or cravings; hypersomnia or insomnia; feeling overwhelmed, out of control; physical symptoms, e.g. breast tenderness, bloating, headaches, joint aches, weight gain

The syndrome markedly disturbs work or school and relationships

Disturbance is not an exacerbation of another disorder

Criteria above must be confirmed by prospective daily symptom ratings for at least 2 consecutive months

---

Table 8 Treatment for premenstrual syndrome

Psychosocial: lifestyle adjustment, relaxation training, cognitive behavioral therapy

Hormones: estrogen, progesterone, progestogens

Special treatments: danazol, gonadotropin releasing hormone agonists

Symptomatic treatments: diuretics, mefenamic acid, evening primrose oil

Nutritional supplements: evening primrose oil, pyridoxine, magnesium, zinc, *Vitex agnus castus* fruit, special diets

Antidepressants: SSRIs

SSRIs, selective serotonin re-uptake inhibitors

Table 9 Selective serotonin re-uptake inhibitors (SSRIs) and premenstrual syndrome (PMS)

SSRIs are superior to placebo for PMS

Confirmed by several randomized controlled trials

Trials have usually been for PMDD

Non-SSRI antidepressants are not as effective

Intermittent treatment is as effective as continuous

A link between estrogen and serotonin neurotransmitters has been suggested

PMDD, premenstrual dysphoric disorder

treatment. Women may also have information from the Internet.

As always the history of the symptoms, their duration, the timing and associated events will help guide the discussion. It is important to enquire why the sufferer has chosen to present now, and to consider the social and relationship context. Often there will have been a crisis, an outburst or other life event. The usual examination and investigations will be required to explore likely pathology. Exploration of what the woman has heard or read about the problem and what she has tried so far, may prove useful.

Education, understanding and support are the cornerstones of management. The woman

needs to feel that you have listened, taken her seriously and that you have shed some light on her distress. Simple explanations and encouragement to problem solve may be enough to enable her to recover her equilibrium. If further help is required then some effort should be made to persuade her to keep a simple daily symptom diary. Diary keeping is difficult and many women simply cannot manage it, but for those who do, there are benefits beyond establishing the diagnosis. The diary can give a woman a sense of control, validation for her experiences and assist in clarifying which problems can be solved. It can also be used to demonstrate the effectiveness of any prescribed intervention.

Most pharmacological interventions are associated with a large placebo response (up to 94%!)[9]. Thus it may take 3–4 months to establish whether a new treatment has been effective. Treatments offered should be as simple as possible, be suitable for long-term use, and be compatible with the woman's other needs.

Hormones

Randomized controlled trials (RCTs) have shown that estrogen patches at high dose (100 μg twice weekly) are effective[10]. There is less evidence for oral estrogen preparations. Progesterone has not been shown to be better than placebo in RCTs[11].

More potent drugs such as danazol or gonadotropin releasing hormone agonists are used when symptoms are severe and unresponsive to other treatments. These produce a reversible medical menopause and establish whether the PMS can be relieved by removing the cycle altogether. This can be a preliminary to the most drastic measure of all – hysterectomy and oophorectomy[12].

Nutritional supplements

Nutritional supplements are still under review as evidence so far is inadequate. They are prescribed readily because they are acceptable and relatively safe. Megadose preparations should be avoided. Oil of evening primrose oil is helpful for breast tenderness and may help other symptoms. It is likely that pyridoxine (vitamin B_6) helps in mild PMS[13]. A recent RCT has found that extract of *Vitex agnus castus* fruit helps PMS symptoms[14].

Serotonin re-uptake inhibitors

For women with mainly psychological symptoms, antidepressants such as fluoxetine can help[15]. Fluoxetine is a serotonin re-uptake inhibitor. It can be used continuously or intermittently on symptomatic days[16]. Other drugs in this group include citalopram, paroxetine, setraline and clomipramine[17,18]. Other antidepressants are less effective.

Symptomatic treatment

Symptomatic relief can be offered. Mefenamic acid helps pain and fatigue. Diuretics, particularly spironolactone, relieve bloating. Oil of evening primrose helps breast tenderness[19].

Psychological strategies can enhance the education and support that are offered to all women. Exercise and improving lifestyle can help. There is evidence to show that cognitive behavioral therapy can be effective in relieving symptoms by giving women new perspectives

on themselves, their symptoms and others around them. This enhances their ability to identify solvable problems and succeed in managing their lives better. Such a treatment resource is scarce, but for badly affected women who are unable to tolerate, or keen to avoid, pharmaceutical strategies it may be appropriate[20].

MENOPAUSE

Definition

Menopause is the cessation of the menstrual cycle associated with the failure of the ovaries to produce sufficient estrogen to sustain ovulation and formation of a corpus luteum. The menopause is established when periods have been absent for 1 year.

About 20% of women will complain of symptoms that they associate with the menopause. On average the menopause occurs at about age 50 but, for several years before the cessation of periods, there is a decline in the production of reproductive hormones. This period of hormone decline is known as the climacteric and is associated with the development of menopausal symptoms and an increase in psychological symptoms[21].

Symptoms

Symptoms that are clearly linked to hormone decline are sweats, flushes and vaginal dryness. These are the symptoms that respond most consistently to hormone replacement therapy (HRT). Other symptoms common at this time include depressed mood, insomnia, fatigue, anxiety, joint pain, memory and concentration difficulty. These are less readily explained by hormonal decline but may be linked to the secondary effect of insomnia and fatigue due to night sweats, relationship difficulties secondary to dyspareunia or anxiety due to embarrassing flushing[22].

Psychological aspects

Psychosocial pressures appear to be more significant than hormonal changes in women with these other symptoms, and it is clear in many cases that the women have been under considerable pressure emotionally and physically for years, but it is as they get older that they simply have less resilience to cope. They often come in the hope of 'a boost' to flagging energy[23].

Some women feel that the menopause heralds old age and marks the end of their usefulness, their youth and desirability. This may be the result of media coverage that suggests that HRT is the elixir of youth! On the other hand, there may be reluctance to accept hormones for relief of vasomotor symptoms because of fears of long-term side-effects such as breast cancer. This anxiety will add to the stress of physical symptoms, and needs careful discussion and exploration to enable the woman to make an informed choice and minimize risks to herself. There will be women who present with menopausal symptoms whose main problem is depressive illness. Depressive illness is not actually more common at the menopause, but it occurs in at least 10% of women at this time and such women may present more readily because they also have menopausal symptoms. Both issues need attention. Affective disorder should always be considered if psychological symptoms are prominent or if HRT is ineffective. Women with a psychiatric history should be actively treated for their mental disorder but they also need appropriate help when they present with symptoms that denote estrogen decline (Tables 10 and 11).

OTHER MENSTRUAL CONDITIONS ASSOCIATED WITH MOOD PROBLEMS

Use of hormonal contraceptives

Women use the combined oral contraceptive pill (COC) mainly for fertility control, but many clinicians also recommend it for cycle regulation and to limit menorrhagia. The estrogen suppresses ovulation, and the bleeding is not due to the failing corpus luteum but a with-

Table 10 Menopause and other reproductive mood disturbances

Menopause clinic attenders with mood symptoms have frequently reported a past history of:
Oral contraceptive pill dysphoria
Premenstrual syndrome
Postnatal depression
Family history of reproductive mood disturbance

Table 11 Menopause and mood disorder

There is no evidence of 'involutional melancholia'
There is no excess of menopausal depressive disorder
There is a higher rate of minor psychological symptoms in the 5 years premenopause
More of the distress is due to life stresses than mental illness
A subset of women may have depression triggered by estrogen decline

drawal bleed when hormones stop during the pill-free week. Some women cannot tolerate the COC because they feel low in mood while taking it. The mechanism for this is not entirely clear but it is thought that excess progestogens or relative lack of estrogen, may be a factor. So a preparation with a different progestogen, or one higher in estrogen may improve this symptom. The COC is not associated with any increase in depressive illness. Women who have mood disturbance at the menopause are more likely to have had a history of similar problems while on oral contraceptives.

MOOD PROBLEMS AS REACTIONS TO MENSTRUAL EVENTS

Miscarriage, termination and infertility

Most couples expect to be able to enjoy the pleasure and responsibilities of parenthood. They also look for a level of control over their fertility unimaginable a hundred years ago. Technology now appears to allow a woman to choose when and whether to have children and families and friends collude with this, putting pressure on couples as though they can simply switch on a pregnancy.

Miscarriage

A proportion of pregnancies miscarry. This is not uncommon in the first trimester. Some women regard an early miscarriage as no more than a late period and have not made an emotional bond with the potential child. Others find the miscarriage demanding physically, especially if it is accompanied by pain or is prolonged. Quite a few women grieve for the unborn baby no matter how early the miscarriage and take some time to regain a normal mood. These days fewer babies are lost later in pregnancy and therefore a loss at this stage is less expected. A woman feels the loss more if it occurred later in the pregnancy and if she has already made a relationship with the baby or if the baby is longed for and the pregnancy has been achieved with difficulty. This does not amount to a depressive illness but can be quite intense.

Ambivalence towards the pregnancy can also bring mood disturbance. Low mood can be accompanied by guilt if the woman loses a baby that she had considered aborting anyway.

Termination

Pregnancy is not always planned, predicted or welcome. Termination of pregnancy is usually a hurried and pragmatic resolution to a threat to lifestyle, career, relationship or well-being. It is loaded with moral importance and is frequently conducted in secret and associated with guilt. Nevertheless it is not associated with high levels of psychiatric morbidity afterwards and most people come to terms with their decision. A minority, however, pursue such a course of action with great ambivalence. In such cases it can be helpful to talk things through with a counselor who can support the woman as she makes her decision. Few women have long-term regrets though these can emerge if there is difficulty conceiving in the future. Counseling can also be important if the woman needs help to come to terms with feelings of guilt, anger and remorse and to accept the positive and negative consequences of her choice[24].

Infertility

As many as one in six couples seek help with conception. This number is likely to grow, as couples become more intolerant of advice to wait and see, especially when they have chosen to defer childbearing until late in the woman's reproductive life. Also, couples' expectations are high as technology offers more procedures to overcome childlessness. Unless the process of investigation and treatment is relatively brief and with a good outcome, the issue becomes a major stress in the lives of such couples. Fertility treatment can be a roller coaster of hope and disappointment. Sexual activity becomes linked with failure, menstruation is accompanied by disappointment and distress, and life plans revolve around treatment cycles. Often the couple are hesitant to share their dilemmas and can feel isolated among their peers who are reproducing with apparent ease. The desire for a child can become an obsession and the couple may not agree on its importance. Treatment is stressful but it can be equally hard to stop, and deciding to cease treatment is a demanding decision which may be accompanied by a grief process for the baby that will never be. Even achieving the much-wanted pregnancy can bring alarming dysphoria when the baby turns out to be exhausting and motherhood overwhelming after years of imagined parental bliss.

Menorrhagia and menstrual irregularities

Heavy periods are difficult for women practically and emotionally. This is made worse if the loss is sufficient to cause anemia and therefore physical debility, or if accompanied by dysmenorrhea or other pelvic pain. Women vary in their tolerance of the inconvenience and discomfort of menstruation and it is difficult to evaluate the actual complaint of any particular woman. Once the history has been established investigations will be recommended to investigate pathology.

If no pathology emerges the problem is often addressed by use of non-steroidal anti-inflammatory drugs (such as mefenamic acid or naproxen) or antifibrinolytics (tranexamic acid) or by modifying the cycle with the combined oral contraceptive pill or progestogens. This makes the cycle more predictable as well as more bearable. Some women do not respond to these measures. This often results in surgery; hysterectomy or endometrial ablation. Hysterectomy used to be thought to be associated with a high rate of depressive illness afterwards. Epidemiological research then found that even more women were depressed before the operation[25]! In some women the depression was caused by the symptoms of menorrhagia, in others the depression was comorbid with the menstrual issue that prompted the operation. Further it may be that for some women their distress was not due to excessive bleeding but to their inability to tolerate menstruation when depressed. Perhaps surgeons were too ready to believe that a woman would be better off without her womb whatever her distress!

Dysmenorrhea

Women frequently experience pain associated with menstruation. Most find ways of managing this within their lifestyle, or with the help of hormonal (oral contraceptive pill) or pain-relieving medication (non-steroidal anti-inflammatory drugs). A few have pain that is chronic and difficult to treat and may have been evaluated by a gastroenterologist as well as a gynecologist. The gynecologist looks for endometriosis and often finds it. Curiously, although undoubtedly endometriosis causes pain in many sufferers, the degree of endometriosis found is not in proportion to the severity of pain.

Once the main treatment strategies have been tried it can be frustrating for both patient and doctor that the problem continues. In primary care it is important to maintain a positive stance but to resist the temptation (or the pressure from the patient) to continue to investigate or try unorthodox treatments, as this tends to foster the hope that somewhere, someday a 'cure' will be found. It is better to encourage coping, improving general lifestyle and making the most of support and resources already available. Adopting the sick role and seeking evermore exotic and sometimes dangerous procedures can lead to the illness giving meaning and importance to the woman's life that can be difficult to give up especially if family and social support have been lacking in the past.

CONCLUSION

Menstruation is associated with many issues that affect mood. These are not just about gynecological pathology, but about normality, well-being and femininity. Having problems with reproductive function and sexuality can cause anxiety and have negative effects on mood which disorders in other systems do not generate. In some the mood is primary and a result of reproductive hormones interacting with neurotransmitter systems controlling mood. In others the low mood is a reaction to the underlying gynecological condition. In many women both their mood and menstrual disorder are affected by social and relationship factors that govern why and when the woman presents to her doctor. These factors are important for outcome and patient satisfaction, as correct diagnosis and effective treatment rely on judging the balance of several contributing factors and on helping the woman manage them appropriately. As research continues the role of psychological treatments and psychiatric medication is becoming established, which acknowledges that mood and menstruation are linked.

REFERENCES

1. Byrne P. Psychiatric morbidity in a gynaecological clinic: an epidemiological study. Br J Psychiatry 1984; 144: 28–34

2. Piccinelli M, Wilkinson G. Gender differences in depression. Br J Psychiatry 2000; 177: 486–92

3. Frank RT. The hormonal causes of premenstrual tension. Arch Neurol Psychiatry 1931; 26: 1053–7

4. O'Brien PM. The premenstrual syndrome. Br J Fam Plann 1990; 15 (Suppl): 13–18

5. Connelly M. Premenstrual syndrome: an update on definitions, diagnosis and management. Adv Psychiatr Treat 2001; 7: 469–77

6. American Psychiatric Association. Diagnostic and Statistical Manual of Mental Disorders, 4th

edn. Washington, DC: American Psychiatric Association, 1994

7. Fava M, Pedrazzi F, Guaraldi GP, et al. Comorbid anxiety and depression among patients with late luteal dysphonic disorder. J Anx Disord 1992; 6: 325–35

8. Roy-Byrne PP, Hoban MC, Rubinoiw DR. The relationship of menstrually related mood disorder to psychiatric disorders. Clin Obstet Gynecol 1987; 30: 386–95

9. Magos AL, Brincat M, Studd JW. Treatment of the premenstrual syndrome by subcutaneous estradiol implants and cyclical oral norethisterone: placebo controlled study. BMJ 1986; 292: 1629–33

10. Smith RN, Studd JW, Zamblera D, Holland EF. A randomised comparison over 6 months of 100 mg and 200 mg twice-weekly doses of transdermal oestradiol in the treatment of severe premenstrual syndrome. Br J Obstet Gynaecol 1995; 102: 475–84

11. Wyatt KM, Dimmock PW, Jones PW, O'Brien PM. Progesterone therapy: a systematic review of its efficacy in the premenstrual syndrome. Neuropsychopharmacology 2000; 23: S2

12. Muse K, Cetel N, Futterman L, et al. The premenstrual syndrome: effects of medical ovariectomy. N Engl J Med 1984; 311: 1345–9

13. Wyatt KM, Dimmock PW, O'Brien PM. Vitamin B6 therapy: a systematic review of its efficacy in the premenstrual syndrome. BMJ 1999; 318: 1375–81

14. Schellenberg GR. Treatment of the premenstrual syndrome with Agnus Castus fruit extract: a prospective, randomised, placebo controlled study. BMJ 2001; 322: 134–8

15. Steiner M. Fluoxetine in the treatment of LLPDD: a multicentre, placebo-controlled, double-blind trial. Int J Gynaecol Obstet 1994; 46: 122

16. Pearlstein MD, Stone AB. Long-term fluoxetine treatment of late luteal phase dysphoric disorder. J Clin Psychiatry 1994; 55: 332–5

17. Eriksson E. Serotonin reuptake inhibitors for the treatment of premenstrual dysphoria. Int Clin Psychopharmacol 1999; 14: S2, S27–S33

18. Dimmock PW, Wyatt KM, Jones PW, O'Brien PM. Efficacy of selective serotonin reuptake inhibitors in premenstrual syndrome: a systematic review. Lancet 2000; 136: 1131–6

19. Budeiri DJ, Li WP, Dornan JC. Is evening primrose oil of value in the treatment of the premenstrual syndrome? Controlled Clin Trials 1996; 17: 60–8

20. Blake F, Gath D, Salkovskis P, et al. Cognitive therapy for the premenstrual syndrome: a controlled trial. J Psychosom Res 1998; 45: 307–18

21. Greene JG. The Social and Psychological Origins of the Climacteric Syndrome. Aldershot: Gower, 1984

22. Zweifel JE, O'Brien WH. A meta-analysis of the effect of hormone replacement therapy upon depressed mood. Psychoneuroendocrinology 1997; 22: 189–212

23. Pearce J, Hawton K, Blake F. Psychological and sexual symptoms associated with the menopause and the effects of hormone replacement therapy. Br J Psychiatry 1995; 67: 163–73

24. Gilchrist AC, Hannaford P, Frank P, et al. Termination of pregnancy and psychiatric morbidity. Br J Psychiatry 1995; 167: 243–8

25. Gath D, Cooper P, Day A. Hysterectomy and psychiatric disorder: I. Levels of psychiatric morbidity before and after hysterectomy. Br J Psychiatry 1982; 140: 335–50

Appendix A

Daily Symptom Diary

Choose the four symptoms that trouble you most, (e.g. irritability, depression, tiredness), list them at the top of the columns. Score these symptoms each evening as follows:

None	=	0
Mild	=	1 (present but tolerable)
Moderate	=	2 (interferes with normal activities)
Severe	=	3 (incapacitating)

Add any relevant comments about what is happening in your life in the last column. Note bleeding with an M (for menstruation) in the 'Bleeding' column

Date	Bleeding	Symptom 1	Symptom 2	Symptom 3	Symptom 4	Comments

Appendix B

Premenstrual assessment chart for clinical use (based on the Prism calendar, O'Brien)

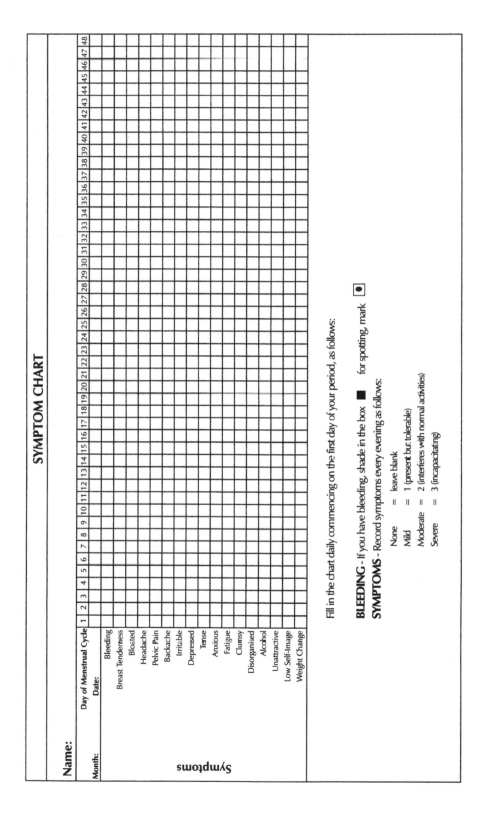

SYMPTOM CHART

Name:

Month:

Day of Menstrual Cycle	1	2	3	4	5	6	7	8	9	10	11	12	13	14	15	16	17	18	19	20	21	22	23	24	25	26	27	28	29	30	31	32	33	34	35	36	37	38	39	40	41	42	43	44	45	46	47	48
Date:																																																
Bleeding																																																
Breast Tenderness																																																
Bloated																																																
Headache																																																
Pelvic Pain																																																
Backache																																																
Irritable																																																
Depressed																																																
Tense																																																
Anxious																																																
Fatigue																																																
Clumsy																																																
Disorganised																																																
Alcohol																																																
Unattractive																																																
Low Self-Image																																																
Weight Change																																																

Symptoms

Fill in the chart daily commencing on the first day of your period, as follows:

BLEEDING - If you have bleeding, shade in the box ▪ for spotting, mark ⊡

SYMPTOMS - Record symptoms every evening as follows:

None	=	leave blank
Mild	=	1 (present but tolerable)
Moderate	=	2 (interferes with normal activities)
Severe	=	3 (incapacitating)

Surgical interventions: hysterectomy/endometrial destruction for excessive menstrual bleeding

10

D.E. Parkin

INTRODUCTION

It is little over a decade since hysteroscopic methods of endometrial destruction started to be rigorously assessed and were found to give the first effective alternative to hysterectomy as a surgical treatment for excessive or dysfunctional uterine bleeding (DUB) for 100 years (Table 1). The two initial methods were endometrial laser ablation (ELA) and transcervical resection of the endometrium (TCRE), later to be joined by rollerball endometrial ablation (REA).

These new methods were introduced at the time that assessment with suitable randomized controlled trials (RCTs) was becoming the standard. This meant that much reliable knowledge was gained not only about these new hysteroscopic methods but also about hysterectomy which was prospectively assessed with RCTs for the first time.

The hysteroscopic (first generation) methods were difficult to master with only a minority of gynecologists being able to offer these procedures. This led to the development of new (second generation) methods of endometrial ablation that do not require hysteroscopic skills and are much easier to learn (Table 2).

A choice now exists for women and gynecologists. It is vitally important, owing to the depth and breadth of evidence, that women are counseled and informed in an accurate and unbiased manner (Table 3). Unfortunately this is

Table 1 Hysterectomy versus endometrial ablation

Issues	Hysterectomy	Endometrial ablation
Fertility	offered only if no fertility goals	offered only if no fertility goals
Contraception	provided	not provided
Cervical smears	no need unless subtotal	need to continue
Hormone replacement therapy	no need for progestogen	need progestogen
Hospital stay	3–7 days	day case or outpatient
Time to recovery	8–12 weeks	2 weeks
Satisfaction	90%	80%
Amenorrhea	100%	30–50%
Further surgery at 5 years	10%	hysterectomy in 20–24%
Pelvic pain at 5 years	15%	18%

Table 2 Methods of endometrial ablation

First generation
Transcervical resection of the endometrium (TCRE)
Endometrial laser abation (ELA)
Rollerball endometrial ablation (REA)

Second generation
Thermal balloons (ThermaChoice, Cavatherm)
Microwave Endometrial Ablation (MEA)
Circulating hot saline (HydroTherm Ablator)
Cryotherapy

Table 3 Issues in patient counseling and consent

Fertility wishes
Likely satisfaction
Amenorrhea rate
Risk of further surgery
Recovery
Complications

not happening as widely as it should be. This is of vital importance as surgical treatment for DUB is such a major health burden both for women and the society that provides the health care.

WHO SHOULD BE REFERRED FOR SURGICAL TREATMENT?

All the surgical methods, hysterectomy and ablation should only be offered to women who have completed their family, because of the absolute sterility caused by hysterectomy and the relative sterility and possible risks of pregnancy following endometrial ablation.

When hysterectomy was the only surgical treatment for DUB it was traditional practice for women to have to earn their hysterectomy unless there was an obvious abnormality that demanded surgery such as very large fibroids. Otherwise hysterectomy was not offered before numerous and usually ineffective medical treatments had been tried and failed. In addition, a number of dilatations and curettages were usually carried out. As hysterectomy is a major procedure with risks, involving hospitalization and a period of recovery, this seemed reasonable. In health-care systems where waiting lists are the norm this also allowed a degree of control over the number of hysterectomies performed. There was and still is no clinical evidence, however, that this is the correct management. Observational studies suggest that 10% of women will undergo a hysterectomy for DUB[1]. No thought seems to have been given to whether women were happy with this approach. This was despite observational studies showing poor results with the commonly used progestogen therapy and a 90% satisfaction with hysterectomy[2].

When first-generation endometrial ablation was introduced the same rationale regarding delaying surgery until medical treatment had failed was used as it was seen as an alternative to hysterectomy.

The only evidence from a RCT regarding when women should be referred comes from a trial of women referred to a gynecologist with a clinical diagnosis of DUB who had completed their family. In this trial of 187 women management with potentially effective oral medical treatment was compared with immediate surgical treatment with TCRE. Results of this trial have now been published giving follow-up data after 4 months, 24 months and 5 years[3–5].

The early results at 4 months in the women randomized to initial TCRE were not surprising. The amenorrhea rate was 38%, and

78% of these women were very satisfied with the result of their surgery. In the TCRE arm there was a significant increase in hemoglobin levels especially in those who were mildly anemic pre-operatively. In the group randomized to medical treatment after 4 months of follow-up only 20% of women were happy to continue with their prescribed treatment and there was no change in hemoglobin levels. Assessment of quality-of-life measures are perhaps more important. The quality-of-life tool Short Form 36 (SF36) demonstrated that both groups were significantly disabled by their symptoms at the start of the trial. At 4 months the women in the TCRE group returned to normal values for their age while the women in the medical group did not. When these women were followed 2 years after initial treatment the same differences were still present. By this time 49% of the women randomized to medical treatment had undergone TCRE and 15% hysterectomy. Only 20% of the TCRE group required any further treatment and in this group the hysterectomy rate was 10%. The fact that there were fewer hysterectomies among those randomized to immediate TCRE is reassuring in that offering early endometrial ablation does lead to a higher ultimate hysterectomy rate. Of interest and concern was the fact that those women randomized to medical treatment who then subsequently had a TCRE never achieved the same normal SF36 score of those randomized to initial TCRE. This may be due to a dissatisfaction if acceptable improvement in symptoms is delayed by first using an ineffective medical treatment, despite the fact that there is no reason to believe that there would be any difference in the efficacy of TCRE between the two groups.

After 5 years of follow-up, of the women allocated to medical treatment only 10% were still using this treatment and nearly 90% had undergone either TCRE (77%), hysterectomy (15%) or both. Despite the high number treated surgically these women were significantly less likely to be totally satisfied or to recommend their treatment to a friend than those in the initial TCRE group. Bleeding and pain scores were similar in both groups and notably reduced in both. In the TCRE arm, significantly more women had no or very light bleeding and they had significantly fewer days' heavy bleeding. The hysterectomy rates at 5 years for the two arms were very similar (18% in the medical arm and 20% in the TCRE arm).

Not only did the TCRE group have improvement in all eight health scales of the SF36 (compared to four after medical treatment), it actually restored them to normative levels. The conclusion is that when compared with medical treatment, immediate TCRE achieved higher levels of satisfaction, better menstrual status, and a greater improvement in health-related quality of life without an increase in the hysterectomy rate[5].

If a woman is keen or willing to be treated medically in the first instance then immediate endometrial ablation would not be appropriate. However, if a woman does not wish medical management then it would be unreasonable to withhold surgical treatment with endometrial ablation, were she not satisfied with the outcome of the chosen medical management she may not ultimately achieve the same level of satisfaction. The conclusion from these papers is that patient choice must be taken into account when deciding on the management of menorrhagia.

HYSTERECTOMY

Which route?

The three choices are abdominal, vaginal or laparoscopically assisted, though through most of the developed world the abdominal route is the most common. In the British VALUE study of hysterectomy carried out between 1994 and 1995[6] this cohort comprised 37 298 hysterectomies for benign reasons, with DUB as the most common indication (46%). In this group 67% had a total abdominal hysterectomy (TAH), 30% a vaginal hysterectomy (VH) and only 3% a laparoscopically assisted hysterectomy (LAVH). Those undergoing hysterectomy for DUB had it performed abdominally, in 73%, and vaginally, 20%.

The laparoscopic route has received great publicity over recent years but the above figures suggest that it has not been widely incorporated into practice in the UK. A RCT from Scotland compared TAH with LAVH in a trial of 200 women needing a hysterectomy for benign disease[7]. In the LAVH group 8% needed conversion to an open procedure though there were fewer complications with this method (8%) than with TAH (14%). The operating time was significantly longer for LAVH (81 min compared with 47 min) but the postoperative hospital stay was reduced. Perhaps disappointingly there was no difference in recovery time or satisfaction at 4 weeks between the two groups.

A larger RCT, the EVALUATE study, has been completed which compares LAVH with both TAH and VH. Although results have been presented this study is not yet published.

It is obvious that the vaginal route is underused, though the merits of this approach have to be put into context with the high satisfaction of TAH seen in the RCTs comparing hysterectomy with endometrial ablation.

Morbidity

The complications of hysterectomy are often underestimated. Minor pyrexial morbidity was found in 47% of women after abdominal hysterectomy in a RCT comparing hysterectomy with endometrial ablation, with 11% having a vaginal vault hematoma and 5% requiring a blood transfusion[8] (Table 4). There were also three major complications in this series.

The VALUE study in England and Wales is the most recent assessment of complications[6]. Unfortunately, only 45% of cases were reported and there is a suspicion that complication rates were higher in the unreported group (M. Maresh, personal communication).

Overall operative complications occurred in 3.5% with 9% getting a postoperative complication. A severe postoperative com-

Table 4 Hysterectomy

Risks
Pyrexia 30%
Transfusion 5%
Return to theater 1%
Visceral damage 0.75%
Death 1/3000

Sequelae
Amenorrhea
Sterility
? Bladder dysfunction
? Early menopause

plication was found in 1% and the death rate at 6 weeks after surgery was 0.38 per 1000.

Visceral damage occurred in 0.76% after TAH, 0.61% after VH and 1.13% after LAVH. Significant bleeding was found in 2.3% of TAH cases (though this included the women with large fibroids), 1.9% after VH and 4.2% after LAVH. Following LAVH 1.5% of women returned to theater compared with 0.7% after TAH or VH. It seems that the laparoscopic approach gives a higher complication rate.

In a large retrospective study from the United States of 1851 premenopausal women undergoing hysterectomy[9] the procedure was performed by the abdominal route in 1283 and vaginally in 568 women. The rate of fever after TAH was 30% and 15% needed a blood transfusion. Vaginal hysterectomy had a lower rate of febrile morbidity of 15%. Bowel injury occurred in 3/1000 women following abdominal hysterectomy and 6/1000 after vaginal hysterectomy. The urinary tract was damaged in 3/1000 after abdominal hysterectomy but 14/1000 with the vaginal route. The mortality was 1/1000. A similar rate of bowel damage has been found in another large American study where the rate of bowel damage in abdominal gynecological surgery has been reported as 8.4/1000 and 7.3/1000 for vaginal surgery[10]. Though this study advocated vaginal hysterectomy because of a 70% higher rate of complications after abdominal hysterectomy the difference was mainly caused by relatively minor febrile problems. There was, however, more damage to the bowel or urinary tract during vaginal hysterectomy.

Long-term results and sequelae

Hysterectomy is a very effective treatment for heavy menstruation. A total hysterectomy effectively guarantees amenorrhea and a subtotal hysterectomy almost does the same. It would seem logical to expect 100% satisfaction in women complaining of DUB. Observational but prospective work by Gath and colleagues in the 1980s showed that satisfaction after hysterectomy for DUB was 86%[2].

Three major RCTs comparing hysterectomy with TCRE have been published, all funded by peer-reviewed competitive grants. These were the first RCTs of hysterectomy for DUB despite a century of widespread use. They differ in their methodological soundness and also the length of follow-up. Dwyer and associates randomized 200 women to either hysterectomy or TCRE (ratio 1 : 1) at the time of the decision to offer surgical treatment for their heavy periods and follow-up was for 2 years[11]. Pinion and colleagues, randomized 204 women to either receive hysterectomy or hysteroscopic surgery (1 : 1 ratio)[8]. Follow-up is now published between 4 and 6 years postoperatively. O'Connor and co-workers published an MRC-funded multicenter study[12]. This study used a 3 : 1 randomization between TCRE and hysterectomy and had a prolonged period of recruitment with 75% of eligible women declining to enter the study. Despite the methodological differences between these studies the results are remarkably consistent.

In the Dwyer study satisfaction was 93% following hysterectomy. Pinion found after 12 months' follow-up that 89% were satisfied after hysterectomy. O'Connor found 96% satisfaction after hysterectomy at a median follow-up of 2 years though there were only 28 women in the hysterectomy group. All three studies showed significantly longer recovery time, longer hospital stay and significantly more complications after hysterectomy compared with endometrial ablation[8,11,12].

These studies confirmed the previous observational findings that hysterectomy does not lead to 100% patient satisfaction when carried out for excessive menstrual loss despite giving complete amenorrhea.

Importantly these studies were pragmatic and included women with uterine enlargement up to the size of a 10-week pregnancy and 20% had fibroids identifiable at hysteroscopy.

Long-term follow-up of the Pinion study from Aberdeen has been published[13]. The follow-up period was 4–6 years with a median of 5.1 years. There was no significant difference in satisfaction between the hysterectomy and the TCRE/ELA groups. The relative symptomatic results of the two treatment approaches are best assessed by the use of RCTs as shown above. These are large enough to give an indication of the relative frequency of common complications, but for the study of uncommon complications large prospective series are needed.

Long-term sequelae are important. The major one is the effect of surgical castration and the role of hormone replacement therapy. This is a huge topic and outside the role of this chapter.

As hysterectomy disrupts the local nerve supply, and alters the anatomical position and relation of the remaining pelvic organs, two unknowns about the long-term effects of hysterectomy are the effect on bladder and pelvic floor function and on sexual function. Because preserving the cervix may give fewer local changes the debate has now spread to the question of whether or not the cervix should be removed at the time of the hysterectomy.

Uncontrolled studies are of little or no value here as the pre-existing state is often unknown. The randomized trials comparing hysterectomy with endometrial ablation have given some data as performing an endometrial ablation should have no physical effect on either the bladder or sexual function.

In the Aberdeen trial there was no difference in sexual satisfaction between hysterectomy and endometrial ablation[14]. A follow-up urodynamic study found no difference in bladder function between the two groups[15]. This indirect and circumstantial but prospective and randomized evidence strongly suggests that hysterectomy does not adversely affect either the bladder or sexual outcome.

Recently two studies have been published that have gone a long way towards answering these questions. A prospective observational study comparing the effects of VH, TAH and subtotal abdominal hysterectomy was published in 2003[16]. This study looked at 413 women who were having a hysterectomy for benign reasons; and the gynecologist chose the type of hysterectomy. Sexual pleasure increased in all groups and the number of women with sexual problems was the same after all three types of hysterectomy.

A RCT was published in 2002 looking at a group of 279 women undergoing a hysterectomy for benign disease[17]. They were randomized in a double-blind manner to either TAH or subtotal abdominal hysterectomy. Both groups had an equal reduction in bladder symptoms at 12 months after the surgery. There was no change in either sexual function or bowel symptoms.

This evidence suggests that there is no long-term symptom benefit from the subtotal operation and that hysterectomy for benign causes does not give rise to adverse long-term sequelae apart from the hormonal problems caused by castration.

ENDOMETRIAL ABLATION

The new endometrial ablative methods (including resection) gave the promise of replacing hysterectomy with a minor, quick and safe technique. They have since been joined by the non-hysteroscopic second-generation methods of endometrial ablation which may be easier to learn and therefore be more widespread in their use. The early 1990s was a time when the concept of evidence-based medicine was becoming established. This meant that the newly introduced endometrial ablative methods were rigorously assessed with RCTs comparing them with hysterectomy, medical treatment and the differing methods of ablation. Evidence regarding all the surgical methods including hysterectomy therefore began to accrue. At the same time national audits of endometrial ablation, and recently hysterectomy, gave robust data regarding safety.

Despite the increasing acceptance of the role of randomized trials and the concept of grading evidence as used by the Scottish Intercollegiate Guidelines Network it is unfortunate that even to this day the majority of publications in this area are uncontrolled observational studies. Furthermore, only the minority of studies have used power calculations to determine the size of the population studied.

A problem with studies on surgery for DUB is the question of outcome measures. Patient satisfaction is the most useful and important measure, followed by hysterectomy rates in women treated by conservative surgical methods. Amenorrhea rates are useful when comparing one ablative method with another, but less so when comparing ablation with hysterectomy. Surrogate measures of menstrual loss are even less useful as even the pictorial blood loss assessment chart (PBLAC) score has been shown to be unreliable in women with DUB[18].

Patient selection for trials and studies is another area where bias is possible. A number of prognostic factors for the success or failure of endometrial ablation have been recognized. Success is more likely in women who are older, have genuinely heavy periods and who have less dysmenorrhea[19,20]. Studies can therefore be biased if the population is not representative. It follows that care must be taken when interpreting results of studies, especially those which are not randomized or have inclusion and exclusion criteria based on PBLAC scores.

Indications and patient selection

Whilst some selection criteria are fairly obvious, others have become clearer as the evidence has accrued. From the beginning the ablative procedures have only been offered to women whose family is complete because of the probable subfertility and the potential risks to both mother and fetus of a pregnancy following endometrial ablation. As it became obvious that pregnancies could occur after ablation, women had to continue adequate contraception after the procedure. It was also obvious that ablation would not deal with a very large fibroid uterus.

There is now evidence as to the prognostic factors for successful ablation based on randomized trials and the large audit studies.

Women whose menstrual blood loss is genuinely excessive have a better outcome after TCRE than those with normal menstrual blood loss. Gannon and colleagues showed that if menstrual blood loss was above 80 ml per cycle the subjective failure rate was 9% compared with 18% if periods were perceived to be heavy but in fact constituted normal menstrual loss[19]. Patient age may be important with younger women having a lower satisfaction than older women. A Scottish audit of hysteroscopic surgery showed a lower satisfaction in women under 40 years of age, though this was still 79% compared with 88% in women aged over 40[20].

The presence of irregular periods or menstrual dysmenorrhea is not a predictor of a poor outcome. In a large RCT comparing TCRE and ELA there was no difference in satisfaction using either of these criteria[21].

Whether endometrial ablation of the endometrium succeeds or fails is probably multifactorial, with symptom severity, both genuine and perceived, patient expectation and uterine pathology all being determinants. In addition there is the individual variation in efficacy and performance of the procedure as well as the pathological healing processes in the uterus.

One method of determining reasons for the failure of endometrial ablation is to look at the pathology of the uterus in women who have a hysterectomy for failure. The problem with this approach is that it reveals nothing about the uterus in those women who have had a successful ablation.

Davis and colleagues have studied the histopathological status of the removed uterus following hysterectomy for failure of REA to control symptoms[22]. In women still complaining of bleeding excessively they found that endometrium was present focally but not diffusely in the uterine cavity. Fibroids were found in 30% and adenomyosis in 27%. As already stated in the Pinion study, where the women had a clinical diagnosis of dysfunctional uterine bleeding, those randomized to hysterectomy were found to have endometriosis in 8%, adenomyosis in 17% and fibroids in 20%[8]. Presumably as it was a randomized study the same uterine pathology would be present in those women undergoing TCRE or ELA. Despite this the hysterectomy rate 4–6 years after treatment is only 22%[13]. It is probable that even in women with this range of pathology, many will have a satisfactory result from endometrial ablation if the indication for endometrial ablation is DUB rather than pain. The finding of fibroids, endometriosis or adenomyosis at hysterectomy in those who fail following endometrial ablation may overestimate the importance of that abnormality and shows the value of a randomized trial. Despite this knowledge we still cannot reliably predict the outcome for an individual woman following endometrial ablation.

First-generation techniques of endometrial ablation: results

A large number of uncontrolled series of TCRE and ELA have been published as well as randomized studies comparing them with each other and with medical treatment. The two uncontrolled studies that give the best estimate as to the long-term outcome are the long-term follow-up studies of TCRE and ELA. O'Connor and Magos followed up 525 women for up to 5 years, though the mean follow-up was actually 31 months and only 43 women were followed up for the full 5 years. The hysterectomy rate was only 9% and 80% avoided further surgery[23]. The Middlesbrough group reported long-term follow-up of 1000 ELA procedures, with 746 women followed up for up to 6 years. The rate of repeat surgery was 15%, but by using life-table analysis they predicted a hysterectomy rate of 21% at 6.5. years[24]. Despite the size of these studies they are less useful than the long-term follow-up of RCTs. These studies along with long-term follow-up of the Aberdeen randomized trial show that the great majority of women will avoid a hysterectomy following first-generation endometrial ablation.

TCRE has been compared with ELA in a randomized trial of 372 patients[21]. This study showed that TCRE had a shorter operating time than ELA. There was less mean fluid absorption following TCRE and fewer patients absorbed a large volume during TCRE than with ELA. There were no differences in complications between the two methods. There was no difference in outcome as measured by satisfaction (90%), amenorrhea rate (45%), or hysterectomy rate (20%) between the two methods.

Rollerball endometrial ablation (REA) is a widely used method especially outside the UK. It has never been subject to a published randomized trial compared with hysterectomy or TCRE. Uncontrolled results give this method a similar success rate to the other hysteroscopic methods.

First-generation techniques of endometrial ablation: safety

The incidence of complications following the hysteroscopic methods of TCRE and ELA has been determined firstly by a Scottish audit of hysteroscopic surgery[20] then by the MISTLETOE study in England and Wales[25] giving combined results from over 11 000 patients. In both audits it was estimated that over 90% of procedures were reported and that there was no difference in the complication rate in the unreported group. In the MISTLETOE study of over 10 000 cases the rate of bowel damage due to TCRE was 0.7/1000. The Scottish audit of hysteroscopy surgery of just under 1000 cases reported no cases of bowel damage. This gives a rate of 1/1000 for bowel damage due to TCRE[20,25]. ELA is felt to be safer than TCRE with no case of bowel damage in 1764 cases in MISTLETOE and 314 in the Scottish audit but there was a case of small bowel damage in the Aberdeen randomized study[8].

REA is felt to be a safer method than TCRE as the surface of the uterine cavity is coagulated rather than resected. No visceral damage was reported with this method in MISTLETOE, but there were only 650 cases[25]. There have been a number of case reports of large and small bowel damage after REA.

In the MISTLETOE study the rate of emergency hysterectomy was 6/1000 overall and 2/1000 in the Scottish audit. Blunt uterine perforation is reported in 15/1000 cases in the MISTLETOE and 10/1000 in the Scottish audit[20,25]. This is of little consequence if the perforation is recognized and does not involve the use of electrodiathermy or laser energy.

All the hysteroscopic methods use fluid to distend and irrigate the uterine cavity and excessive absorption of irrigation fluid is a potential risk. During TCRE using glycine, changes in electrolytes especially serum sodium can be avoided if the procedure is abandoned when absorption is noted to be reaching

Table 5 Morbidity of first-generation methods

Uterine perforation	1%
Excessive fluid absorption	1%
Emergency hysterectomy	0.6%
Visceral damage	0.1%
Death	0.027%

1500 ml[26]. In MISTLETOE there was a 1% rate of fluid absorption >2000 ml and 1% in the Scottish audit (Table 5). Both audits and a RCT comparing TCRE with ELA have shown a greater rate of fluid absorption following ELA compared with TCRE[20,21,25]. Combining the two audit studies the mortality from the hysteroscopic methods of endometrial resection and ablation was 0.27/1000.

Second-generation endometrial ablation methods

Second-generation ablative techniques represent a rapidly expanding area of medical technology. The majority use tissue heating as the method of endometrial destruction including, electrical energy (Vesta system), microwave energy (microwave endometrial ablation (MEA)), laser (endometrial laser intrauterine thermotherapy (ELITT)) or heated saline/glycine irrigating the uterus (Hydro-ThermAblator (HTA) and circulating hot saline) or heated saline/dextrose contained within a balloon device (ThermaChoice (Figure 1) and Cavatherm systems). Second-generation techniques are mostly blind in nature (no hysteroscopy) and most avoid the need for fluid distention media and its risks. They are quicker and much simpler to learn and perform than first-generation techniques, which many gynecologists failed to master. Some also offer the benefits of local anesthesia (MEA and ThermaChoice).

These new procedures all postdate the earlier national safety audits. The new techniques must prove equal efficacy but also safety before they can become widely accepted. Their efficacy should be compared in randomized trials of adequate power with the now established gold standard of TCRE. Adequate training is vital to reduce the potential for serious complications with the second-generation techniques.

Second-generation endometrial ablation methods: results

The only methods that to date have been subject to adequate assessment are Therma-Choice, MEA, the Vesta system and the HTA.

Thermal balloon has been compared in a RCT with REA, which, although a first-generation technique, has not been validated against hysterectomy and is not therefore seen as a gold standard.

A multicenter North American trial randomized 275 women to thermal uterine balloon therapy (ThermaChoice) or REA to

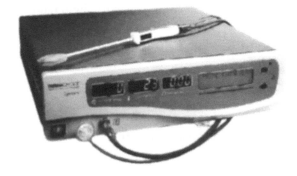

Figure 1 ThermaChoice, a second-generation endometrial ablation method

study efficacy and safety[27]. The study was powered to detect 20% less efficacy for rollerball versus balloon. The study was restricted to women with small, regular uterine cavities and with high PBLAC scores and therefore was less generalizable than the trials of first-generation methods. No pretreatment endometrial hormonal preparation was used in either arm, instead the endometrium was prepared with a 5-min suction aspiration. At 1 year both techniques significantly reduced the PBLAC score; 68.4% in the rollerball arm and 61.6% in the balloon arm had a reduction by over 90% with no significant difference in the two groups. Quality-of-life scores, satisfaction and improvement in dysmenorrhea/premenstrual syndrome were also similar. The balloon treatment was significantly quicker with no complications, compared with 3.2% of the rollerball group. The amenorrhea rate was significantly lower after ThermaChoice (15%) compared with (27%) after REA, despite the fact the amenorrhea rate after REA was considerably less than expected with a first-generation method. This study was re-analyzed at 2 and 3 years of follow-up[28]. At 2 years' follow-up it was found that in both groups 15 hysterectomies had been performed, 11 in the rollerball arm and four in the balloon arm. Of the 214 who were followed for 3 years the results of uterine balloon therapy and REA remained similar, with little difference at 3 years compared with results at 1 year. There was a suggestion of an increase in hysterectomies in the rollerball group (14) compared with the uterine balloon therapy group (8) at 3 years.

It was concluded that both methods were highly successful at avoiding hysterectomy and relieving symptoms and that patient satisfaction remained high.

MEA has been validated against the gold standard of TCRE in a RCT. The probe (Figure 2) is 8 mm in diameter and delivers microwaves of 9.2 GHz frequency to the probe tip. The Aberdeen group randomized 263 women to MEA or TCRE (the study had sufficient power to detect an 8% difference in satisfaction between the groups)[29]. The inclusion criteria were the same as for the previous studies from that group[3,8,21], specifically the uterus could be up to the size of a 10-week pregnancy and fibroids were not excluded. MEA was a significantly faster procedure (11 vs. 15 min) and had fewer operative complications. In the 2-year follow-up 95% of the subjects returned questionnaires[30]. Similar menstrual data was reported in both arms with a higher amenorrhea rate after MEA (47%) than TCRE (41%), though this was not significant. Satisfaction was significantly higher after MEA with 79% of women either completely or generally satisfied compared with 67% after TCRE. Quality of life was similarly increased in both groups. Hysterectomy rates of 12% at 2

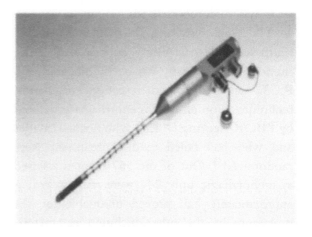

Figure 2 Microwave probe used in microwave endometrial ablation (MEA)

years were similar after both treatments. The group concluded that MEA was as effective as the TCRE.

A RCT comparing MEA under local anesthesia with that under general anesthesia has recently been published[31]. In this study of 359 women referred for MEA, 191 (59% of those eligible) agreed to randomization to general anesthesia or local anesthesia and 131 (41%) agreed to participate in the patient-preference arm of the study. Of the procedures started under local anesthesia 91% were completed under local anesthesia and 87% found local anesthesia totally or generally acceptable. Despite this only 75% of those randomized to local anesthesia would have their treatment the same way, significantly less than those randomized to general anesthesia (88%).

The safety of MEA has been reported in a prospective series of 1400 cases[32]. The data covered 13 gynecological units in the UK and Canada. Out of 1433 cases one major complication of small bowel damage occurred giving an incidence of 0.7/1000. There were few minor complications and fluid absorption is impossible. In conclusion MEA appeared safer than hysteroscopic methods.

The Vesta system, a disposable dispensable multielectrode-carrying balloon utilizing monopolar diathermy, has been compared in a RCT with combined resection/coagulation technique. Women with menorrhagia as defined by PBLAC scoring (> 150) with normal cavities and who had failed medical treatment were randomized[33]. Out of the 557 women assessed as menorrhagic only 244 were randomized, as approximately half proved unsuitable for the procedure by the other inclusion parameters. PBLACs were used in selection and definition of outcome success (a score PBLAC < 75

defined success). Success was achieved in 86.9% of the Vesta arm and 83% in TCRE at 1 year. Amenorrhea rates were 31% in the Vesta arm and 34% in the TCRE arm. No significant complications were reported. Of the Vesta procedures 87% were performed under local anesthesia ± sedation as an outpatient. Of note there were 18 (10.6%) technical failures in the Vesta arm and one Vesta procedure had to be abandoned as the device had entered a weakened cesarean scar. The benefits of avoiding fluid overload and local anesthesia are present. It was concluded that the Vesta method was equally effective and safe as TCRE. However, the Vesta system is not currently being commercially marketed.

HTA unlike the rest of the second-generation techniques requires hysteroscopy. However, no manipulation by the operator is required. The technique relies upon circulating heated saline within the endometrial cavity. The saline is heated externally prior to being introduced into the hysteroscope and achieves an intrauterine temperature of 90°C. This method seems suitable for irregular cavities unlike the balloon methods. The device is 8 mm and takes 10 min of active treatment.

A multicenter RCT study comparing HTA with REA has been published[34]. Two hundred and seventy-six patients with menorrhagia were randomized to HTA (187) or Rollerball (89). PBLAC diaries were used for inclusion criteria and follow-up. Success was defined as a PBLAC score of < 75. Success rates as defined were 77% after HTA and 82% for REA.

Amenorrhea rates were 40% HTA and 51% REA at 1 year. It was concluded that HTA was safe and effective, offering safety benefits with the associated use of hysteroscopy and the potential to be performed as an outpatient procedure.

With the exception of the trials on MEA all the above trials on second-generation methods were initiated to obtain FDA approval in the USA and were under the control of the device manufacturers. All use PBLAC as the entry criteria and reducing the PBLAC score to normal as the primary endpoint.

Other techniques exist such as photodynamic therapy, cryoablation, circulating hot saline and Novacept. None of these have enough data to make any recommendations. The ELITT device utilizes an intrauterine diode laser that scatters a laser beam around the endometrial cavity. It is a non-hysteroscopic, non-contact procedure and purports the benefit of treating irregular cavities and difficult-to-access areas (e.g. the cornua) equally well. To date, evidence is encouraging but is limited only to observational prospective series.

At present the most thoroughly evaluated second-generation technique remains MEA. Morbidity levels of second-generation techniques of endometrial ablation are shown in Table 6.

Second-generation endometrial ablation methods: applicability

The first-generation methods have shown themselves to be adaptable to a wide range of uterine cavity sizes and irregularities as shown by the fact that all the RCTs on these methods were very pragmatic[8,11,12]. None of these trials excluded fibroids and accepted an enlarged uterus up to the size of a 10-week pregnancy.

The second-generation methods show more variation. The ThermaChoice, Cavatherm and Vesta systems will only adapt to a regular normal-sized uterine cavity and the FDA trial inclusion criteria for the ThermaChoice reflected that. The HTA and MEA will both treat irregular and relatively large cavities. MEA performed as well as TCRE in the independent trial comparing these methods[29,30].

There seems to be a trade-off for some of these methods between ease of use and applicability. Only MEA and HTA seem to have the same spectrum of use as the first-generation methods.

CONCLUSION

The evidence regarding the results and problems of both hysterectomy and endometrial ablation are robust and well known. Despite this most women are still offered only hysterectomy. Though this is a successful procedure more women should be offered at least one of the proven ablative methods.

Table 6 Morbidity of second-generation methods

Uterine perforation	1%
Excessive fluid absorption	0% (except HydroThermAblator)
Emergency hysterectomy	?%
Visceral damage	?%
Death	?%

PRACTICE POINTS

- Offer choice of appropriate evidence-based treatments
- Counsel patients in an unbiased fashion
- Only perform endometrial ablation after training in that technique
- Keep to the patient-selection and treatment protocols for second-generation methods
- Audit your results

REFERENCES

1. Vessey MP, Villard-Mackintosh L, McPherson K, et al. The epidemiology of hysterectomy: findings in a large cohort study. Br J Obstet Gynaecol 1992; 99: 402–7

2. Gath D, Cooper P, Day A. Hysterectomy and psychiatric disorder. I. Levels of psychiatric morbidity before and after hysterectomy. Br J Psychiatry 1982; 140: 335–42

3. Cooper KG, Parkin DE, Garratt AM, et al. A randomized comparison of medical and hysteroscopic management in women consulting a gynecologist for treatment of heavy menstrual loss. Br J Obstet Gynaecol 1997; 104: 1360–6

4. Cooper KG, Parkin DE, Garret AM, Grant AM. Two-year follow-up of women randomized to medical management or transcervical resection of the endometrium for heavy menstrual loss; clinical and quality of life outcomes. Br J Obstet Gynaecol 1999; 106: 258–65

5. Cooper KG, Jack SA, Parkin DE, Grant AM. Five-year follow-up of women randomized to medical management or transcervical resection of the endometrium for heavy menstrual loss: clinical and quality of life outcomes. Br J Obstet Gynaecol 2001; 108:1222–8

6. Maresh MJA, Metcalfe MA, McPherson K, et al. The VALUE national hysterectomy study: description of the patients and their surgery. Br J Obstet Gynaecol 2002; 109: 302–12

7. Lumsden MA, Twaddle S, Hawthorn R, et al. A randomized comparison and economic evaluation of laparoscopic-assisted hysterectomy and abdominal hysterectomy. Br J Obstet Gynaecol 2000; 107: 1386–91

8. Pinion SB, Parkin DE, Abramovich DR, et al. Randomized trial of hysterectomy, endometrial laser ablation and transcervical resection for dysfunctional uterine bleeding. BMJ 1994; 309: 979–83

9. Krebs HB. Intestinal injury in gynecologic surgery: a ten-year experience. Am J Obstet Gynecol 1986; 155: 509–14

10. Dicker RC, Greenspan JR, Strauss LT. Complications of abdominal and vaginal hysterectomy among women of reproductive age in the United States. Am J Obstet Gynecol 1982; 144: 841–8

11. Dwyer N, Hutton J, Stirrat GM. Randomized controlled trial comparing endometrial resection with abdominal hysterectomy for the surgical treatment of menorrhagia. Br J Obstet Gynaecol 1993; 100: 237–43

12. O'Connor H, Broadbent JA, Magos AL, McPherson K. Medical Research Council randomized trial of endometrial resection versus hysterectomy in the management of menorrhagia. Lancet 1997; 349: 891–901

13. Aberdeen Endometrial Ablation Trials Group. A randomized trial of endometrial ablation versus hysterectomy for the treatment of dysfunctional uterine bleeding: outcome at four years. Br J Obstet Gynaecol 1999; 106: 360–6

14. Alexander DA, Naji. AA, Pinion SB, et al. Randomized trial comparing hysterectomy with endometrial ablation for dysfunctional uterine bleeding: psychiatric and psychological aspects. BMJ 1996; 312: 280–4

15. Bhattacharya S, Mollison J, Pinion SB, et al. A comparison of bladder and ovarian function two years following hysterectomy or endometrial ablation. Br J Obstet Gynaecol 1996; 103: 898–903

16. Roovers JP, van der Bom JG, van der Vaart CH, Heintz AP. Hysterectomy and sexual wellbeing: prospective observational study of vaginal hysterectomy, subtotal abdominal hysterectomy and total abdominal hysterectomy. BMJ 2003; 327: 774–8

17. Thakar R, Ayers S, Clarkson P, et al. Outcomes after total versus subtotal abdominal hysterectomy. N Engl J Med 2002; 347: 1318–25

18. Reid PC, Cocker A, Coltart R. Assessment of menstrual blood loss using a pictorial chart: a validation study. Br J Obstet Gynaecol 2000; 107: 320–2

19. Gannon MJ, Day P, Hammadich N, et al. A new method of measuring menstrual blood loss and its use in screening women before endometrial ablation. Br J Obstet Gynaecol 1996; 103: 1029–33

20. Scottish Hysteroscopy Audit Group. A Scottish audit of hysteroscopic surgery for menorrhagia: complications and follow up. Br J Obstet Gynaecol 1995; 102: 249–54

21. Bhattacharya S, Cameron IM, Parkin DE, et al. A pragmatic randomized comparison of transcervical resection of the endometrium with endometrial laser ablation for the treatment of menorrhagia. Br J Obstet Gynaecol 1997; 104: 601–7

22. Davis JR, Maynard KK, Brainard CP, et al. Effects of thermal endometrial ablation. Clinicopathologic correlations. Am J Clin Path 1998; 109: 96–100

23. O'Connor H, Magos A. Endometrial resection for the treatment of menorrhagia. N Engl J Med 1996; 335: 151–6

24. Phillips G, Chien PF, Garry R. Risk of hysterectomy after 1000 consecutive endometrial laser ablations. Br J Obstet Gynaecol 1998; 105: 897–903

25. Overton C, Hargreaves H, Maresh M. A national survey of the complications of endometrial destruction for menstrual disorders: the MISTLETOE study. Minimally Invasive Surgical Techniques–Laser Endo-Thermal or Endoresection. Br J Obstet Gynaecol 1997; 104: 1351–9

26. Byers GF, Pinion S, Parkin DE, et al. Fluid absorption during transcervical resection of the endometrium. Gynecol Endosc 1993; 2: 21–3

27. Meyer WR, Walsh BW, Grainger JF, et al. Thermal balloon and rollerball ablation to treat menorrhagia: a multicenter comparison. Obstet Gynecol 1998; 92: 98–103

28. Loffer FD. Three-year comparison of thermal balloon and rollerball ablation in treatment of menorrhagia. J Am Assoc Gynecol Laparosc 2001; 81: 48–54

29. Cooper KG, Bain C, Parkin DE. Comparison of microwave endometrial ablation and transcervical resection of the endometrium for treatment of heavy menstrual loss: a randomized trial. Lancet 1999; 354: 1859–63

30. Bain C, Cooper KG, Parkin DE. Microwave endometrial ablation versus endometrial resection: a randomized controlled trial. Obstet Gynecol 2002; 99: 983–7

31. Wallage S, Cooper KG, Graham W, et al. A randomised trial comparing local versus

general anaesthetic for microwave endometrial ablation. Br J Obstet Gynaecol 2003; 110:799–807

32. Parkin DE. Microwave endometrial ablation: a safe technique. Complication data from a prospective series of 1400 cases. Gynecol Endosc 2000; 9: 385–8

33. Corson SL, Brill AI, Brooks PG, et al. One-year results of the vesta system for endometrial ablation. J Am Assoc Gynecol Laparosc 2000; 7: 489–97

34. Corson SL. A multicenter evaluation of endometrial ablation by Hydro ThermAblator and rollerball for treatment of menorrhagia. J Am Assoc Gynecol Laparosc 2001; 8: 359–67

Laparoscopic surgery

11

T.J. Child

INTRODUCTION

Laparoscopy has revolutionized the investigation and management of women in gynecological practice. Though first described over 90 years ago[1] it is really only in the past two to three decades that advances in light delivery systems and camera/video technology have allowed the performance of advanced procedures. The aim of this chapter is to review the indications, procedures, and complications of laparoscopic surgery as applied to women with an abnormal menstrual cycle. Evidence-based recommendations are used where possible.

THE BASICS OF LAPAROSCOPY

Standard laparoscopy is performed under general anesthesia and involves the creation of a carbon dioxide pneumoperitoneum. The abdomen is inflated via a Veress needle inserted subumbilically. A 10-mm diameter trochar is inserted, again in the subumbilical position, and a telescope inserted through the trochar sleeve to view the internal organs (Figure 1). A uterine manipulator is passed into the cervix to allow optimal views of the pelvis. The legs are held in stirrups and the patient put into a steep Trendelenburg's (head down) position to displace bowel from the pelvis. One to three

5-mm secondary ports are placed along the 'bikini line' in the suprapubic or iliac fossae areas for the introduction of graspers, scissors, suction–irrigation or diathermy instruments. In modern laparoscopy the camera is linked to one or two video monitors to allow optimum views of the procedure for the surgeon and assistants. The operation may be recorded on videotape or digital videodisc (DVD) and kept in the department or, as in Oxford (UK), handed to the patient for safe-keeping and personal viewing. The latter approach also permits surgeons in other units to view the operative findings and procedures as the need dictates.

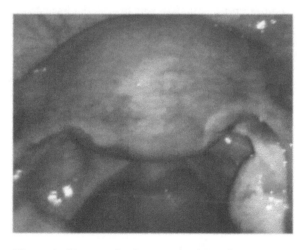

Figure 1 Photograph of a normal pelvis at laparoscopy

INDICATIONS FOR LAPAROSCOPIC SURGERY

The indications for surgery with reference to this book include pelvic pain and/or irregular or heavy menstruation. These symptoms may be due to pathology of the uterus, tube, ovary, peritoneum or adhesions between these structures and to the bowel (Table 1). Surgery may be divided into diagnostic or operative procedures. A diagnostic laparoscopy is generally performed as a day-case procedure whilst operative procedures often, but not necessarily, involve a stay of one or more nights post-surgery.

PROCEDURES

It is fair to say that just about any abdominopelvic operative procedure can be performed laparoscopically. However, just because a procedure can be done laparo-scopically, it does not follow that it necessarily should be performed this way. There are, however, a number of advantages of laparoscopy over laparotomy including reduced pain scores, time in hospital, and time to return to normal functioning[2-4]. However, operative time may be increased, equipment costs are higher, and increased surgical experience may be required[4].

DIAGNOSTIC LAPAROSCOPY

The aim of a diagnostic laparoscopy is to investigate the pathological cause of symptoms listed in Table 1. Diagnostic laparoscopies are usually performed as day-case procedures with women going home 3–4 h after surgery. If pathology is found the management options are discussed with the patient before discharge and/or at a later clinic appointment. An alternative approach is to 'see and treat'. Women with symptoms suggestive of, for instance, endometriosis may be asked to give their consent to ablation of small areas of disease and

Table 1 Pelvic pathology leading to an abnormal menstrual cycle and amenable to minimal access surgery

Structure	Pathology	Possible surgical interventions
Uterus	fibroids	myomectomy, hysterectomy
	dysfunctional uterine bleeding	hysterectomy, endometrial resection/ablation
Fallopian tubes	hydrosalpinx	salpingectomy, salpingostomy
Ovary	polycystic ovary syndrome	laparoscopic ovarian drilling
	endometrioma	drainage and ablation cystectomy, oophorectomy
	dermoid cyst	cystectomy, oophorectomy
Peritoneum	endometriosis	resection/ablation of endometriosis
Rectovaginal septum	endometriotic nodule	nodule resection
Adhesions between any of above and to bowel		adhesiolysis

still go home the same day. In general, it is probably best not to treat more than minor degrees of endometriosis or adhesions during a diagnostic laparoscopy.

Patients with abdominopelvic pain, randomized to the control arm of trials examining operative laparoscopy, appear to have some reduction in pain scores following diagnostic laparoscopy alone that may persist for at least 12 months[5,6]. The mechanism for this finding is unclear. Photographic reinforcement of normal findings in pelvic pain patients has not been shown to be better than no re-inforcement in a randomized controlled trial (RCT)[7].

OPERATIVE LAPAROSCOPY

The term operative laparoscopy encompasses a wide range of procedures from ablation of a small amount of endometriosis to resection of a large rectovaginal nodule or total laparoscopic hysterectomy. Consequently, the risks and benefits of operative laparoscopy vary with the extent, type and location of disease, the procedure planned, and the expertise of the surgical team. A prospective study of 25 764 laparoscopies performed in 72 Dutch hospitals during 1994 revealed a complication rate of 2.7/1000 for diagnostic and 17.9/1000 for operative laparoscopies[8]. A complication was defined as any unexpected or unplanned event requiring intra- or postoperative intervention. Hemorrhage of the epigastric vein and bowel injuries were the most commonly observed complications. Two deaths occurred. The laparotomy rate was 3.3/1000. Previous laparotomy and surgical experience were identified as variables associated with risk of complication.

Uterus

Hysterectomy for heavy and/or painful periods is a common procedure traditionally performed by the abdominal or vaginal route. During abdominal hysterectomy the body of the uterus is usually removed with the cervix (total abdominal hysterectomy) though sometimes the cervix is left *in situ* (subtotal abdominal hysterectomy). The ovaries may either be removed or left *in situ* depending on the age of the woman and presence of ovarian pathology. During vaginal hysterectomy the cervix is removed and the ovaries normally left *in situ* since access is generally limited. Women wishing to preserve fertility who have fibroids may undergo myomectomy. For those with multiple or large fibroids not desirous of fertility an abdominal hysterectomy is normally indicated. For menstrual dysfunction alternative treatments to hysterectomy include oral medications, a levonorgestrel uterine device (Mirena; Schering) or endometrial ablation/resection (see Chapters 3, 5 and 10). For fibroids an alternative treatment to myomectomy or hysterectomy is uterine artery embolization (see Chapter 6).

Hysterectomy

The ideal minimal access approach to removal of the uterus is vaginal hysterectomy since the operation is fast, has been in use for many years, has no abdominal incisions and is associated with a generally rapid recovery. Laparoscopic hysterectomy should be considered as an alternative to abdominal hysterectomy for cases in which there are absolute or relative contraindications to the vaginal approach. Such contraindications may include minimal uterine descent, a large uterus, ovarian pathology necessitating oophorectomy, or pelvic adhesions due to endometriosis or previous surgery. Laparoscopic hysterectomy has been described for over 20 years. The three main types of procedure are total laparoscopic hysterectomy (TLH), subtotal laparoscopic hysterectomy (STLH), and laparoscopic assisted vaginal hysterectomy (LAVH). During TLH the complete procedure is performed 'from above' meaning that all pedicles are taken laparoscopically using diathermy and scissors, clips or sutures, the uterus is removed through the vagina, and the vaginal vault is sutured via the laparoscopic ports. In a STLH the pedicles down to the uterine arteries are taken laparoscopically at which point the uterine body is separated from the cervix and removed from the abdomen using a laparoscopic morcellator. During a LAVH some pedicles (usually down to and including the uterine arteries) are taken from above whilst the rest are secured vaginally. The procedure is completed as per a standard vaginal hysterectomy.

Though a number of RCTs have been described comparing laparoscopic hysterectomy against vaginal or abdominal approaches these have in general been small, underpowered studies from single centers of laparoscopic excellence. This would tend to bias the results towards the laparoscopic approach.

Recently, however, two large parallel, multicenter $(n = 30)$, randomized trials have been reported comparing: (1) laparoscopic with abdominal hysterectomy, and (2) laparoscopic with vaginal hysterectomy[4] along with cost analyses in 1380 women[9]. These are important trials, with some shortcomings, so will be discussed in detail. Gynecologists entered patients for randomization into either the

abdominal or vaginal trial on clinical grounds. Following randomization to the laparoscopic arm of the trial the particular procedure performed, TLH, STLH or LAVH, was chosen by the surgeon. All surgeons had performed at least 25 of each procedure before participating in the trial. Exclusion criteria included second – or third-degree uterine prolapse or a uterine size > 12 weeks. The primary endpoint was the occurrence of at least one major complication which included outcomes such as bowel, bladder and ureteric injuries, hemorrhage requiring transfusion, and, somewhat contentiously, intraoperative conversion to laparotomy.

In the abdominal trial laparoscopic hysterectomy took about 30 min longer to complete and was associated with a significantly higher incidence of major complications (11.1%) compared with abdominal hysterectomy (6.2%) (Table 2). Intraoperative conversion to laparotomy accounted for 23 of the 65 major complications reported in the laparoscopic group. It could be argued that conversion of a planned laparoscopic hysterectomy to an abdominal procedure should not be considered a 'major complication', in the absence of additional problems such as hemorrhage or bowel damage, by women who, in the end, still achieve their aim of hysterectomy. A potentially severe complication during hysterectomy by any route is damage to the ureter as it runs close to the cervix below the uterine artery or bladder as it is dissected from the anterior cervix. In the abdominal trial 3% of patients undergoing laparoscopic hysterectomy had damage to the urinary tract compared with 1% of those undergoing abdominal hysterectomy.

Compared with abdominal hysterectomy, women undergoing laparoscopy had significantly less pain, a quicker recovery, and improved quality-of-life indicators in the short term though by 4 months' post-surgery there was no difference in physical or mental wellbeing scores between the two groups. Patients undergoing laparoscopy spent 1 day less in hospital though the difference was not subjected to statistical analysis. Cost-effectiveness analysis demonstrated no significant difference between the abdominal and laparoscopic approach, since the former cost more in terms of time in hospital and the latter had higher theater costs due to duration of surgery and use of non-reusable instruments[9].

In the vaginal trial laparoscopic hysterectomy took twice as long as vaginal hysterectomy though the major complication rate was 9–10% for both groups (Table 2)[4]. Laparoscopic hysterectomy cost an average of £401 (at year 2000 prices) more than vaginal hysterectomy[9]. These findings would confirm the opinion that, when vaginal hysterectomy is possible, laparoscopic surgery does not offer any advantage and in fact costs more.

Table 2 Summary of outcomes of hysterectomy trials from reference 4. Values are numbers (percentages) of participants unless indicated

	Abdominal trial		Vaginal trial	
	Abdominal hysterectomy (n = 292)	Laparoscopic hysterectomy (n = 584)	Vaginal hysterectomy (n = 168)	Laparoscopic hysterectomy (n = 336)
Major complications (a patient may have had more than one)				
Ureteric injury	0	5 (0.9)	0	1 (0.3)
Bladder injury	3 (1)	12 (2.1)	2 (1.2)	3 (0.9)
Hemorrhage	7 (2.4)	27 (4.6)	5 (2.9)	17 (5.1)
Bowel injury	3 (1)	1 (0.2)	0	0
Pulmonary embolus	2 (0.7)	1 (0.2)	0	2 (0.6)
Anesthetic problems	0	5 (0.9)	0	2 (0.6)
Unintended laparotomy				
intraoperative conversion	1 (0.3)	23 (3.9)	7 (4.2)	9 (2.7)
return to theater	1 (0.3)	3 (0.5)	0	1 (0.3)
Wound dehiscence	1 (0.3)	1 (0.2)	0	1 (0.3)
Hematoma	2 (0.7)	4 (0.7)	2 (1.2)	7 (2:1)
Other complications	0	0	1 (0.6)	0
At least one major complication	18 (6.2)	65 (11.1)	16 (9.5)	33 (9.8)
Length of surgery (min) median (range)	50 (19–155)	84 (10–325)	39 (14–168)	72 (21–220)
Length of hospital stay (days) median (range)	4 (1–36)	3 (1–36)	3 (1–16)	3 (1–19)

Following trial publication a number of criticisms were made. Many felt that, due to the higher complication rate in the laparoscopic arm, the trial showed laparoscopic hysterectomy in an unfair light. Some felt that the inclusion of intraoperative conversion to laparotomy as a major complication was incorrect[10]. The study authors admitted that some within the trial steering group agreed with this view. Others felt that the high complication rate was in part due to surgeons' inexperience since other groups report better statistics[11]. The study authors countered that their findings reflect surgery in the real world, not that from single centers of international excellence. In summary these two trials demonstrate that: (1) laparoscopic hysterectomy has no advantages over vaginal hysterectomy, and (2) laparoscopic hysterectomy has advantages over abdominal hysterectomy in terms of length of stay in hospital and postoperative pain and quality-of-life scores, though laparoscopy is associated with a significantly longer surgical time and a 3.9% chance of intraoperative conversion to laparotomy. The rates of other complications were similar between laparoscopic and abdominal hysterectomy[4].

Myomectomy

The surgical and medical treatment of fibroids has been reviewed elsewhere in this volume. Laparoscopic myomectomy, briefly discussed here, can be performed for intramural, subserosal or pedunculated fibroids. A disadvantage of laparoscopic myomectomy is the time taken to remove large fibroids from the abdomen through the small 10-mm ports. Fibroid extraction from the abdomen can potentially take longer than removal of the myoma from the uterus. Though the fibroid could be cut into small pieces within the abdomen for removal through the ports a morcellator is generally used. This is a 10–15-mm diameter tubular device inserted through the abdominal wall. Grasping forceps pass down the center of the morcellator to hold and pull the free myoma up to the circular lower serrated edge of the instrument. An electric motor then rotates the serrated sleeve resulting in coring of the myoma, bit by bit, until all tissue is removed. Morcellators are potentially very dangerous instruments since the serrated teeth will cut through any tissue, such as bowel or blood vessels, inadvertently placed in the way and fatalities have been reported[12]. With myomectomy by any route intra- and postoperative hemorrhage is a major concern. The vascular bed of the myoma must be secured with intra- or extracorporeal sutures in two to three layers. Good approximation of uterine muscle is also vital to minimize the risk of uterine rupture in any subsequent pregnancy. Elective cesarean section may be the safest approach following the removal of large myomas. Depending on surgical experience and available equipment, the maximum diameter of fibroids appropriate for laparoscopic myomectomy is probably 7–9 cm.

An RCT ($n = 109$) comparing abdominal and laparoscopic myomectomy found no difference in pregnancy rate or miscarriage rates[13]. There was a significantly higher incidence of postoperative fever and a drop in hemoglobin and hospital stay in the group following abdominal myomectomy. A further RCT ($n = 40$) demonstrated reduced pain scores and duration of hospital stay with laparoscopic myomectomy[2]. The recurrence rate of fibroids is similar following laparoscopic or abdominal myomectomy[14].

Fallopian tubes

Large hydrosalpinges may be associated with pelvic pain. Laparoscopic treatment options include salpingectomy in which the tube is removed or alternatively salpingostomy in which the tube is opened and drained. With salpingostomy the hydrosalpinx may potentially re-form if the hole closes. The presence of hydrosalpinges is known to reduce the chance of livebirth significantly during *in vitro* fertilization (IVF) treatment probably through leakage of tubal fluid via the cornu into the uterine cavity. A systematic review of three RCTs showed that salpingectomy for hydrosalpinx before IVF increases the odds ratio of livebirth by 2.13 (95% confidence interval (CI) 1.24–3.65)[15].

Ovary

Abnormal menstrual cycles may be due to pathology involving the ovaries such as polycystic ovary syndrome (PCOS) or cysts including endometriomas or dermoids. PCOS is the commonest cause of oligoamenorrhea in women of reproductive age and has been covered in detail elsewhere. Here, the surgical management of PCOS will be described in terms of laparoscopic ovarian diathermy (LOD) for anovulation. The laparoscopic treatment of ovarian cysts by either cystectomy or oophorectomy will then be described.

Polycystic ovary syndrome

It has been recognized for many years that surgical damage to the quiescent polycystic ovary can result in resumption of spontaneous ovulatory cycles. Originally this was achieved through a 'wedge resection'[16] but the association of this procedure with severe periovarian adhesions and loss of ovarian tissue meant its fall from use by the early 1980s. Subsequently medical ovulation induction using oral clomiphene citrate or injected gonadotropins became standard treatment. However, ovulation induction is associated with the dual risks of multiple pregnancy and ovarian hyperstimulation syndrome. More recently the technique of LOD has gained prominence in the management of anovulatory PCOS. During LOD a shielded monopolar diathermy electrode is inserted through the ovarian capsule and into the stroma to a depth of about 8 mm. Current is applied for a few seconds before the electrode is withdrawn and the procedure repeated at 4–15 points in each ovary. The mechanism through which LOD achieves ovulation is not entirely clear but probably involves partial destruction of the androgen-producing ovarian stroma, a fall in serum androgen and luteinizing hormone levels[17], and a general restoration of the normal hormonal milieu[18].

Ovulation rates of between 50–80% by 6 months after surgery have been reported[18]. A retrospective analysis of LOD in 112 women with clomiphene citrate-resistant anovulatory infertility demonstrated a cumulative conception rate of around 70% by 24 months after surgery (Figure 2)[17]. Fifteen women who had not conceived by 12 months after LOD underwent a second-look laparoscopy. Four of these patients were found to have flimsy periovarian adhesions. In a few trials anovulatory PCOS patients have been randomized to receive either LOD or a course of gonadotropin ovulation induction treatment. A meta-analysis demonstrated no significant difference in cumulative ongoing pregnancy rate at 12 months

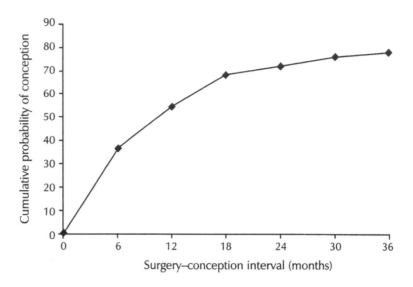

Figure 2 Cumulative probability of conception following laparoscopic ovarian diathermy in 112 clomiphene citrate-resistant anovulatory women with polycystic ovary syndrome. Reproduced from reference 17 with permission from American Society for Reproductive Medicine

follow-up (equivalent to up to six cycles of gonadotropin ovulation induction)[18]. Importantly, however, the multiple pregnancy rate was significantly lower in the LOD group (odds ratio (OR) 0.16; 95% CI 0.03–0.98). Data suggest that the benefits of LOD can persist for a number of years after surgery[19]. The cost per live birth achieved is around one-third cheaper with LOD compared with gonadotropins[20].

LOD can be performed as a day-case procedure and is often scheduled at the same time as confirmation of tubal patency with transcervical dye insufflation. The risks of LOD, on top of those of any laparoscopic procedure, include the formation of periovarian adhesions at the diathermy site[17,21] and damage to bowel with the monopolar electrode or heat from the ovarian capsule. The risk of bowel damage should be absolutely minimal if, as usual during surgery, the electrode tip is watched constantly when in the abdomen and only activated when in the correct position. Saline flushing over the ovary immediately after diathermy results in cooling and further risk reduction. As an alternative to electrodiathermy the use of laser has been reported. Results appear to be similar[18].

Ovarian cysts

Ovarian cysts encountered in women of reproductive age and possibly causative of pain include endometriomas, dermoids and large simple cysts. The possibility of ovarian malignancy must always be considered. For any cysts other than those that are obviously identified as endometriomas or simple cysts on preoperative ultrasound it is prudent to measure the serum CA-125. If ultrasound features of the cyst are suspicious or the CA-125 raised then discussion with a gynecological oncologist as to the most appropriate treatment is advisable.

Rupture of the capsule during laparoscopic cystectomy is not uncommon, which, in the case of malignancy, can alter the staging.

Treatment options for benign ovarian cysts include either oophorectomy or cystectomy. The decision will depend on the size of the cyst, amount of viable ovarian tissue remaining, fertility aspirations of the woman and surgical expertise. In general the rule should be to conserve ovarian tissue apart perhaps from women in their 40s. Oophorectomy has the obvious advantage of preventing cyst recurrence on that side. At the start of laparoscopy the pelvis, abdomen, liver and diaphragm should be carefully evaluated to exclude sinister pathology.

Oophorectomy Oophorectomy is performed by mobilizing the ovary and securing and ligating the suspensory and infundibulopelvic ligaments and vessels. To avoid cyst rupture and spillage the ovary can be nestled in a laparoscopic bag during oophorectomy and then withdrawn safely from the abdomen.

Cystectomy for endometrioma Ovarian endometriotic cysts appear to form from the invagination of endometriotic deposits on the ovarian surface. A pseudocapsule forms within which is found altered blood with the appearance and consistency of melted chocolate, hence the term 'chocolate cyst'. Endometriomas can give rise to symptoms as detailed in Chapter 2. The medical management of ovarian endometriosis is recognized to be relatively unsuccessful, leaving surgery as the treatment of choice.

Laparoscopically there are two approaches to treatment. The first is to open the cyst, drain the contents, and then ablate the cyst wall with diathermy or laser. The second is to strip the cyst wall after drainage from the ovarian cortex and stroma (Figures 3 and 4). Debate continues

regarding the most appropriate method. As the cyst wall is firmly stuck to the cortex and stroma the concern with stripping is that ovarian tissue, containing oocytes, is also likely to be removed. Furthermore, large cysts are likely to be hypervascular at the hilum risking heavy

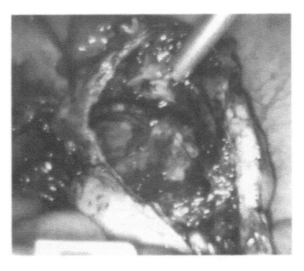

Figure 3 Photograph of cavity of endometrioma ready for stripping of cyst wall

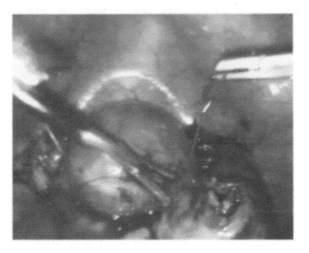

Figure 4 Suturing of ovarian capsule following cyst wall stripping

bleeding, occasionally requiring oophorectomy for hemostasis. However, there are advantages of cyst stripping: tissue is sent for histology since occasionally cysts thought to be benign are not, and, in addition, there is a lower recurrence rate in stripped compared with ablated cysts[22]. Furthermore, the cumulative conception rate is significantly higher following stripping compared with ablation[22].

Dermoid cysts (benign teratomas) Dermoid cysts, often discovered incidentally during pelvic imaging, may cause discomfort due to pressure or twisting effects if large. Contents generally include hair and sebum, and often teeth, epithelium, cartilage and nervous tissue revealing their germ cell origin. A concern with large dermoid cysts is the chance of torsion or spontaneous rupture and the possibility of a chemical peritonitis. Rupture is said to be more common during pregnancy. Cystectomy may be performed by laparoscopy or laparotomy. Both these routes were compared in a recent RCT involving 40 women with unilateral dermoid cysts < 10 cm diameter[3]. Patients were followed up every 6 months for 5 years. A higher proportion of women had milder pain, reduced stay in hospital and duration of convalescence following laparoscopy than laparotomy. There was no recurrence of teratoma in either arm of the study[3].

At surgery the aim is to shell out the capsule without cyst rupture. If rupture does occur then copious suction–irrigation with at least 3 litres of saline is required to remove noxious tissue and reduce/eliminate the risk of a sterile peritonitis. Alternatively, before commencing cystectomy the ovary can be nestled within a laparoscopic bag so that if rupture does occur the contents are contained.

Simple cysts The capsule of simple cysts may be very thin and inseparable from the ovarian cortex and stroma. Consequently, the simplest technique may be to drain the cyst using a laparoscopic needle, sending the fluid for cytology, and excising the redundant thin ovarian/cyst wall tissue. If simply drained and left the cyst is likely to recur.

Risks of ovarian surgery Whenever ovarian surgery is performed, particularly cystectomy, there is always the possibility of hemorrhage. Generally bleeding can be controlled with use of bipolar diathermy or laparoscopic suturing though occasionally the only way to stem the flow is to perform oophorectomy, obviously a last resort if fertility is an issue.

If the ovary is stuck in the ovarian fossa due to adhesions and/or endometriosis it should be mobilized prior to cystectomy. The ureter runs along the base of the ovarian fossa and is at risk of mechanical or heat trauma during mobilization or diathermy to raw peritoneal areas. More proximally the ureter enters the pelvis near the base of the infundibulopelvic ligaments and vessels and may be damaged during oophorectomy.

Non-ovarian endometriosis

Peritoneal implants of endometriosis causing pain may be treated through medical or surgical means. Medical treatments are based on ovulation suppression, and therefore suppression of endometrial tissue, and whilst potentially successful in pain resolution are not curative since the endometriosis still exists. Furthermore, conception cannot occur during medical treatment and so is not beneficial if fertility is a concern. In this case surgery should be considered.

Peritoneal endometriosis can be resected or ablated using diathermy or laser. An advantage of resection is that tissue is gained for histology. The majority of studies examining the role of surgery in pain treatment are non-randomized and uncontrolled[23]. Fortunately, a prospective, double-blind, RCT comparing laparoscopic laser treatment of minimal to moderate stages of endometriosis against no treatment for women with pelvic pain has been reported[5]. Seventy-four women were randomized. Six months after surgery, 62.5% of treated women, compared with 22.6% untreated, reported improvement or resolution of symptoms. The results were poorest for stage I and best for stage III disease (although only six women had moderate endometriosis). The median visual analog pain scores plotted against time are reproduced from

the original article in Figure 5[5]. The difference was statistically significant at 6 months ($p = 0.01$). Note that the y-axis begins at a score of four not zero, which does have the effect of over-emphasizing the reduction in pain scores (the median decrease in pain score from baseline in the laser group was 2.85). Unfortunately, the surgical intervention included laser vaporization of deposits and laparoscopic uterine nerve ablation (LUNA) as required. Consequently, it is not clear what the relative contribution of either of these laser techniques to the pain reduction was.

The Cochrane group has completed a systematic review of the surgical interruption of pelvic nerve pathways for dysmenorrhea (including dysmenorrhea due to endometriosis)[24]. Interventions included LUNA and also presacral neurectomy (PSN). Uterine nerve ablation involves transection of the uterosacral ligaments at their insertion into the cervix, whereas PSN involves total removal of the presacral nerves lying within the bounds of the interiliac triangle. These procedures both interrupt the majority of the cevical sensory nerve fibers, thus diminishing uterine pain. One small sequentially randomized study was identified comparing LUNA ($n = 10$) against diagnostic laparoscopy alone ($n = 11$) for women with primary dysmenorrhea[25]. LUNA resulted in significant pain relief at 6 and 12 months' follow-up though the effect decreased with time[25]. However, the small size of the study suggests that further research is required before LUNA can be considered a proven treatment option. Two studies were identified comparing LUNA with routine endometriosis deposit ablation versus deposit ablation alone for secondary dysmenorrhea[24]. Combined treatment was no more effective in reducing pain

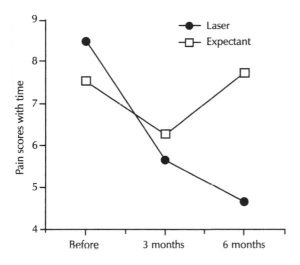

Figure 5 Median visual analog pain scores (with time) in 63 women with minimal to moderate endometriosis randomized to laser surgery or diagnostic laparoscopy. Reproduced from reference 5 with permission from American Society for Reproductive Medicine

than deposit ablation alone and, therefore, cannot be recommended. Uterine nerve ablation is not without risk, as blood vessels and ureters run very close to the ligaments, and deaths have been reported. In comparative studies PSN was as effective as LUNA in treating primary dysmenorrhea in the short term and significantly more effective in the long term. For secondary dysmenorrhea, PSN plus endometriosis deposit ablation was no more effective than deposit ablation alone[24]. PSN is a significantly more difficult procedure to perform than LUNA and the vascular nature of the presacral area raises the risks. A high proportion of women undergoing PSN developed constipation[24]. The Cochrane group concluded that there is insufficient evidence to recommend the use of nerve interruption in the management of dysmenorrhea, regardless of cause. They recommended that future RCTs be undertaken[24].

Deeply infiltrating endometriosis can be associated with severe pain and difficult surgical excision. Again, no RCTs have been reported but large observational series suggest a cure rate for pelvic pain of 70% and a recurrence rate of 5% at 5 years[26].

Rectovaginal disease may be associated with the usual pain symptoms of endometriosis plus cyclical dyschezia (pain on opening bowels) and/or rectal bleeding. Surgery to remove rectovaginal nodules is difficult and carries a number of risks secondary to the possibility of bowel perforation. Approaches include performing an anterior resection followed by reanastomosis, generally by laparotomy but possible laparoscopically, or via a disc resection of the diseased tissue with suturing of the bowel defect laparoscopically.

Adhesions and adhesiolysis

The relationship between adhesions and pain is unclear. A retrospective review of 100 consecutive laparoscopies for chronic pelvic pain and 88 for infertility did not find a significant difference in the density or the location of adhesions between the groups[27]. Again, studies examining the role of treatment are in general retrospective or observational rather than randomized and controlled. Observational, uncontrolled studies suggest an improvement rate of 67–84% in pain after adhesiolysis[28]. Adhesion reformation has been observed in 97.1% of patients and at 66% of the sites of the original adhesiolysis[29].

However, a suitably powered multicenter RCT examining the role of adhesiolysis in treating chronic abdominal pain in patients at risk for adhesions has recently been reported[6]. Recruited patients were those undergoing a diagnostic laparoscopy for chronic abdominal pain attributed to adhesions following the exclusion of other causes for their pain; 87% of patients were women. Adhesions were attributable to previous gynecological surgery in about a half of all patients and appendicectomy in one-quarter. If adhesions were found patients were randomly assigned at the time of surgery to either laparoscopic adhesiolysis or diagnostic laparoscopy alone. Patients and assessors were unaware of treatment allocation. Pain was assessed for 1 year by visual analog score (VAS; scale 0–100), pain change score, use of analgesics, and quality-of-life score.

Fifty-two patients underwent laparoscopic adhesiolysis and 48 received no treatment. Both groups reported substantial pain relief and a significantly improved quality of life which persisted to 12 months of follow-up. There was no statistical difference in outcome between the experimental and control groups. The authors conclude that although laparoscopic adhesiolysis relieves chronic abdominal pain, it is not more beneficial than diagnostic laparoscopy alone[6]. Importantly, five (10%) of the adhesiolysis patients had six complications including two small bowel perforations, one hemorrhage, one abdominal abscess, one rectovaginal fistula, and protracted paralytic ileus after surgery compared with no complications in the control group. A later subgroup analysis including only the women who had adhesions secondary to previous gynecological surgery also confirmed no benefit of adhesiolysis over diagnostic laparoscopy alone[6].

The additional risks of adhesiolysis over and above the general laparoscopy risks are those of causing damage to structures joined by the adhesions, particularly bowel. The exact risk will of course depend on the extent and density of adhesions, and the proximity to bowel or other delicate organs.

There is increasing recognition of the need to prevent adhesion formation post-surgery. Surgical adhesions account for a proportion of patient re-admissions in the years following open gynecological surgery with procedures on the ovaries and tubes being particularly adhesiogenic[30]. Laparoscopic surgery is generally considered to be less adhesiogenic than open procedures mainly due to reduced tissue handling. However, more recent data suggest that the overall risk of re-admission for adhesion-related problems is similar following either laparoscopic or open surgery[31]. Adhesions form between damaged peritoneal surfaces and can be reduced by minimizing tissue handling, drying and bleeding[31]. In addition to these peroperative techniques workers have examined the role of agents left in the pelvis at the end of surgery to minimize adhesions[32]. These are either gels or films applied directly over the incision site, for instance the serosal myometrial incision following myomectomy, with the aim of separating areas of damaged peritoneum, or flotation agents that are left in the abdomen and absorbed over 5–6 days. The true value of gels, films or fluid agents in preventing adhesions remains to be fully established in adequately powered RCTs utilizing second-look laparoscopies to assess the change in adhesion score[31].

CONCLUSION

Most gynecological operations can now be performed laparoscopically. However, relatively few suitably powered and methodologically sound RCTs have been reported in which the efficacy of operative laparoscopy is compared against treatment alternatives including diagnostic laparoscopy, open surgery or medical management. Some notable exceptions are discussed above. More of these large scale, expensive trials will need to be performed if we are to continue with our aim of practicing evidence-based surgery.

REFERENCES

1. Steptoe P. Laparoscopy in Gynecology. London: Livingstone, 1967

2. Mais V, Ajossa S, Guerriero S, et al. Laparoscopic versus abdominal myomectomy: a prospective, randomized trial to evaluate benefits in early outcome. Am J Obstet Gynecol 1996; 174: 654–8

3. Mais V, Ajossa S, Mallarini G, et al. No recurrence of mature ovarian teratomas after laparoscopic cystectomy. Br J Obstet Gynaecol 2003; 110: 624–6

4. Garry R, Fountain J, Mason S, et al. The eVALuate study: two parallel randomised trials, one comparing laparoscopic with abdominal hysterectomy, the other comparing laparoscopic with vaginal hysterectomy. BMJ 2004; 328: 129

5. Sutton CJ, Ewen SP, Whitelaw N, et al. Prospective, randomized, double-blind, controlled trial of laser laparoscopy in the treatment of pelvic pain associated with minimal, mild, and moderate endometriosis. Fertil Steril 1994; 62: 696–700

6. Swank DJ, Swank-Bordewijk SC, Hop WC, et al. Laparoscopic adhesiolysis in patients with chronic abdominal pain: a blinded randomised controlled multi-centre trial. Lancet 2003; 361: 1247–51

7. Onwude JL, Thornton JG, Morley S, et al. A randomised trial of photographic reinforcement during postoperative counselling after diagnostic laparoscopy for pelvic pain. Eur J Obstet Gynecol Reprod Biol 2004; 112: 89–94

8. Jansen FW, Kapiteyn K, Trimbos-Kemper T, et al. Complications of laparoscopy: a prospective multicentre observational study. Br J Obstet Gynaecol 1997; 104: 595–600

9. Sculpher M, Manca A, Abbott J, et al. Cost effectiveness analysis of laparoscopic hysterectomy compared with standard hysterectomy: results from a randomised trial. BMJ 2004; 328: 134

10. Atkinson SW. Results of eVALuate study of hysterectomy techniques: conversion to open surgery should not be regarded as major complication. BMJ 2004; 328: 642

11. Donnez J, Squifflet J, Jadoul P, Smets M. Results of eVALuate study of hysterectomy techniques: high rate of complications needs explanation. BMJ 2004; 328: 643

12. Milad MP, Sokol E. Laparoscopic morcellator-related injuries. J Am Assoc Gynecol Laparosc 2003; 10: 383–5

13. Seracchioli R, Rossi S, Govoni F, et al. Fertility and obstetric outcome after laparoscopic myomectomy of large myomata: a randomized comparison with abdominal myomectomy. Hum Reprod 2000; 15: 2663–8

14. Rossetti A, Sizzi O, Soranna L, et al. Long-term results of laparoscopic myomectomy: recurrence rate in comparison with abdominal myomectomy. Hum Reprod 2001; 16: 770–4

15. Johnson NP, Mak W, Sowter MC. Surgical treatment for tubal disease in women due to undergo in vitro fertilisation (Cochrane review). In the Cochrane Library. Chichester, U.K: John Wiley & Sons, Ltd., 2004

16. Stein IF, Cohen MR. Surgical treatment of bilateral polycystic ovaries. Am J Obstet Gynecol 1939; 38: 465–73

17. Felemban A, Tan SL, Tulandi T. Laparoscopic treatment of polycystic ovaries with insulated needle cautery: a reappraisal. Fertil Steril 2000; 73: 266–9

18 Farquhar C, Vandekerckhove P, Lilford R. Laparoscopic 'drilling' by diathermy or laser for ovulation induction in anovulatory polycystic ovary syndrome. In the Cochrane Library. Chichester, UK: John Wiley & Sons, Ltd., 2004

19. Amer SA, Gopalan V, Li TC, et al. Long-term follow-up of patients with polycystic ovarian syndrome after laparoscopic ovarian drilling: clinical outcome. Hum Reprod 2002; 17: 2035–42

20. Farquhar CM, Williamson K, Brown PM, Garland J. An economic evaluation of laparoscopic ovarian diathermy versus gonadotrophin therapy for women with clomiphene citrate resistant polycystic ovary syndrome. Hum Reprod 2004; 19: 1110–15

21. Greenblatt EM, Casper RF. Adhesion formation after laparoscopic ovarian cautery for polycystic ovarian syndrome: lack of correlation with pregnancy rate. Fertil Steril 1993; 60: 766–70

22. Beretta P, Franchi M, Ghezzi F, et al. Randomized clinical trial of two laparoscopic treatments of endometriomas: cystectomy versus drainage and coagulation. Fertil Steril 1998; 70: 1176–80

23. Child TJ, Tan SL. Endometriosis: aetiology, pathogenesis and treatment. Drugs 2001; 61: 1735–50

24. Proctor ML, Farquhar CM, Sinclair OJ, et al. Surgical interruption of pelvic nerve pathways for primary and secondary dysmenorrhoea. In the Cochrane Library. Chichester, UK: John Wiley & Sons, Ltd., 2004

25. Lichten EM, Bombard J. Surgical treatment of primary dysmenorrhea with laparoscopic uterine nerve ablation. J Reprod Med 1987; 32: 37–41

26. Koninckx PR, Martin D. Treatment of deeply infiltrating endometriosis. Curr Opin Obstet Gynecol 1994; 6: 231–41

27. Rapkin AJ. Adhesions and pelvic pain: a retrospective study. Obstet Gynecol 1986; 68: 13–15

28. Sutton C, MacDonald R. Laser laparoscopic adhesiolysis. J Gynecol Surg 1990; 6: 155–9

29. Operative Laparoscopy Study Group. Post-operative adhesion development following operative laparoscopy: evaluation at early second-look procedures. Fertil Steril 1991; 55: 700–4

30. Lower AM, Hawthorn RJ, Ellis H, et al. The impact of adhesions on hospital readmissions over ten years after 8849 open gynecological operations: an assessment from the Surgical and Clinical Adhesions Research Study. Br J Obstet Gynaecol 2000; 107: 855–62

31. Trew G. Consensus in adhesion reduction management. Obstet Gynecol 2004; 6 (2 Suppl)

32. Al-Jaroudi D, Tulandi T. Adhesion prevention in gynecologic surgery. Obstet Gynecol Surv 2004; 59: 360–7

Alternative medicines 12

K. Reddy

INTRODUCTION

Many women feel that alternative and complementary therapies (ACTs) are safer and more 'natural' than orthodox medicines. Currently, there is continuous and intense publicity regarding ACTs and it is not surprising that a growing proportion of women consider such therapies for prevention or treatment of a wide range of medical conditions, including disorders of the menstrual cycle.

Studies of use of ACTs are relatively limited. A UK population survey of lifetime use in the past 12 months for acupuncture, chiropractic, homeopathy, hypnotherapy, medical herbalism and osteopathy showed that 10.6% of the general population in the UK visited an alternative practitioner in a 12-month period[1]. If all therapies and remedies purchased over the counter were included, the estimated proportion rose to 28.3% (95% confidence interval (CI) 26.6–30) for use in the last 12 months and 46.6% (95% CI 44.6–48.5) for lifetime use. A study of 300 women in New York found that more than half had used an alternative treatment or remedy, and 40% had visited an alternative practitioner[2]. In 2001, it was estimated that one in two practices in England offered their patients some access to ACTs (95% CI 46–52)[3].

The evidence regarding the various strategies are reviewed in this chapter. Most studies relate to dysmenorrhea but there are some data for menorrhagia, amenorrhea and premenstrual syndrome. The evidence from randomized trials suggesting that complementary and alternative therapies improve abnormal menstrual symptoms or have the same benefit as medical therapy is poor, but this does not deter women from trying them.

HERBALISM

Interest in the physiological role of bioactive compounds present in plants has increased dramatically over the past decade. Herbal and dietary therapies number among the more popular complementary medicines for the treatment of primary and secondary dysmenorrhea. In the USA, herbs and other phytomedicinal products have been legally classified as dietary supplements since 1994.

Sweet fennel (*Foeniculum vulgaredulce*)

In one cohort study for the treatment of dysmenorrhea, essence of fennel fruit (2%; 25 drops 4 hourly) was compared with mefenamic acid (250 mg 6 hourly). It was concluded to be a safe and effective herbal drug; however, the dosages used may have been of a lower potency then mefenamic acid and the bad fennel odor resulted in discontinuation in 16%[4].

Fresh maritime pine bark extract (Pycnogenol® (PYC))

Maritime pine bark extract appears to have a wide spectrum of favorable pharmacological properties. Chemically it is composed primarily of procyanidins and phenolic acids. Procyanidins are biopolymers of catechin and epicatechin subunits that are recognized as important constituents in human nutrition. The phenolic acids are derivatives of benzoic and cinnamic acids. PYC has been shown to relieve pre-menstrual symptoms, including menstrual pain, and this action may be associated with the spasmolytic action of the phenolic acids constituents[5].

Japanese herbal combination (Toki-shakuyaku-san (TSS))

Kampo (Japanese traditional herbal medicine) remedies are often used for the treatment of gynecological complaints. The herbal remedy TSS is one of the most important prescriptions, and has been used empirically as a remedy for amenorrhea, luteal phase dysfunction and dysmenorrhea[6]. TSS is a combination of six medicinal plants: toki, senkyu, shakuyaku, sojutsu, takusha and bukuryo. In a recent trial by Kotani and associates[7], the herbal remedy TSS was compared with placebo and was found to be significantly more effective in reducing pain after 2 months of treatment in women with complex symptoms.

Oil of evening primrose

This is a very popular remedy used for a variety of gynecological complaints in particular pre-menstrual syndrome (PMS). However, studies are sparse and meta-analysis suggests that it is of little value[8–10]. Further larger studies are required to unveil any small effects since there is a noticeable placebo response in studies evaluating treatment for PMS.

Traditional Chinese medicine

Chinese medicinal therapy, considered a feasible alternative medicine, comprises decoctions of mixtures of up to 20 herbs that are customized for each individual patient. Traditional Chinese medicine (TCM) represents one aspect of Chinese medical philosophy that is characterized by its emphasis on maintaining and restoring balance[11]. One *in vitro* study examining the effectiveness of Wen-Jing Tang on uterine contractility in rats had encouraging results; however, proper randomized studies in humans are lacking[12].

Rubidatum, another traditional Chinese medicine, was proven to be safe and effective in decreasing and shortening abnormal menstrual loss in women who used an intrauterine contraceptive device[13].

In a study of 30 perimenopausal women presenting with leiomyomas, menstrual flow and pain were improved by using the Chinese herbal medicines Keishi-bukuryo-gan and Shakuyaku kanzo[14].

VITAMINS AND MINERALS

Magnesium

Results from small trials[15,16] suggest that magnesium is a promising treatment for dysmenorrhea, but the required dosage or treatment regimen are unclear and, therefore, no strong recommendation can be made until further evaluation has been carried out. A large trial by Seifert and co-workers[17] yielding data on the levels of prostaglandin $F_{2\alpha}$ ($PGF_{2\alpha}$) in menstrual blood, found that women who underwent magnesium therapy had substantially lower levels of $PGF_{2\alpha}$ in their menstrual blood than those on placebo ($p < 0.05$), which mirrored the therapeutic decrease in pain experienced by the participants. This highlights the possible biological rationale behind magnesium therapy for dysmenorrhea.

Magnesium has been noted to fluctuate across the menstrual cycle and is involved in PMS[18]. The clinical evidence, however, on magnesium supplementation, while promising, remains limited. A double-blind, randomized study in 1991 examined the effect of magnesium (360 mg/day) for two cycles compared with placebo[19]. Magnesium was administered during the luteal phase of the menstrual cycle until the onset of menstruation. Although magnesium was found to reduce total symptom scores and the negative-effect group of symptoms, baseline symptom scores between treatment groups were significantly different and the expected placebo effect was lacking in this trial. Walker and colleagues[20] also investigated the benefit of magnesium supplementation in PMS in a double-blind crossover trial over four menstrual cycles. A daily supplement of 200 mg of magnesium was provided to 41 women with PMS for two cycles. Of the six categories of symptoms investigated (anxiety, craving, depression, hydration, other and total symptoms) the hydration (bloating) group was significantly affected compared with placebo.

Calcium

Three trials have demonstrated the efficacy of calcium treatment for PMS. In 1989, a randomized, double-blind crossover trial was conducted to assess the effectiveness of 1000 mg calcium daily in 33 women with PMS[21]. At the end of the 3-month trial, 73% of the women treated with calcium cited global improvement of symptomatology compared with placebo. In 1993, Penland and co-workers[22] conducted a metabolic study of calcium and manganese nutrition in ten women with premenstrual and menstrual distress symptomatology. Women were assigned in a double-blind manner to one of four dietary periods of either 587 mg or 1336 mg of calcium with 1 mg or 5.6 mg of manganese per day. The high dietary calcium intake of 1336 mg per day was found to benefit mood and behavior, and improve pain and water retention symptoms significantly during the menstrual cycle. In 1998, a prospective, randomized, double-blind, placebo-controlled, parallel group, multicenter clinical trial was conducted in women with moderate to severe PMS to determine the efficacy of calcium in symptom reduction[23]. Four hundred and ninety-seven women were randomly assigned to receive 1200 mg of elemental calcium per day in the form of calcium carbonate or placebo for three menstrual cycles. By the third treatment cycle, calcium effectively resulted in an overall 48%

reduction in total symptom scores. Calcium was found to be effective for the four core symptom factors of PMS (negative effect, water retention, food cravings and pain) as well as for 15 of the 17 individual symptoms.

Vitamin B$_6$

Vitamin B$_6$ has become a popular remedy for treating PMS. Unfortunately, clinical studies have failed to support any significant benefit[24]. Diegoli and colleagues[25] indicated that placebo was as likely to relieve symptoms of PMS as vitamin B$_6$. In addition, vitamin B$_6$ toxicity has been seen in increasing numbers of women who take it for PMS. One review indicated that neuropathy was present in 23 of 58 women taking daily vitamin B$_6$ supplements for PMS whose blood levels of B$_6$ were above normal[26]. There is thus no convincing scientific evidence to support recommending vitamin B$_6$ supplements for PMS.

Vitamin B$_1$

Vitamin B$_1$ plays an important role in metabolism, and deficiency can be characterized by fatigue, muscle cramps and reduced tolerance to pain, all factors that could be associated with dysmenorrhea. One randomized, double-blind, placebo-controlled study was carried out on 556 girls aged 12–26 years. Thiamine hydrochloride was given in a dose of 100 mg orally, daily for 90 days. The combined final results of both the 'active treatment first' group and the 'placebo first' group, after 90 days were 87% completely cured, 8% relieved (pain reduced or almost nil) and 5% with no effect whatsoever[27].

Vitamin E

It has been suggested that vitamin E has analgesic and anti-inflammatory properties. A randomized trial of vitamin E for rheumatoid arthritis has shown significant reduction in pain parameters, which lends further support to this theory[28]. However, large randomized trials are needed to prove its efficacy in the treatment of dysmenorrhea.

PHYTOESTROGENS

Phytoestrogens are bioactive compounds found predominantly in soybeans and red clover. They are structurally similar in chemical structure to the mammalian estrogen, estradiol, and thus are viewed as possible selective estrogen receptor modulators. This is based on recent data of their conformational binding to selective estrogen receptors and stronger relative binding affinity to estrogen receptor-β[29]. The two major classes of dietary phytoestrogens are the isoflavones and lignans. The isoflavones are probably the most extensively studied of the phytoestrogen class; however, their occurrence in foods is limited largely to soybeans and a few other legumes[29]. Lignans, are widely distributed but they have been studied relatively little. Although isoflavones have estrogenic activity 100–1000 times weaker than estradiol, some foods and dietary supplements contain comparatively high amounts of these compounds. Where this is the case, plasma levels may exceed endogenous estrogen levels by several orders of magnitude and therefore these compounds have the potential to exert biological effects *in vivo*[29]. Studies of phytoestrogens in menstrual disorders are limited, with most research concentrating on use in menopausal women. There is some evidence that phytoestrogen supplements may alter menstrual cycle length but the results are conflicting[30,31].

DIETARY INTERVENTIONS – OMEGA-3 FATTY ACIDS (FISH OIL)

Levels of polyunsaturated fatty acids (PUFAs) are correlated with menstrual pain, with higher levels of the omega-3 fatty acids associated with milder menstrual symptoms[32]. PUFAs are metabolized into specific prostaglandins associated with dysmenorrhea and it appears that the ratio of omega-3 to omega-6 fatty acids is associated with menstrual symptoms; therefore, a diet higher in omega-3 fatty acids is possibly associated with less dysmenorrhea. One small trial [33] showed fish oil to be more effective than placebo for pain relief, but the trial was of short duration, only 2 months, which may not be enough to assess properly the effect of dietary intervention. Thus, large studies are needed to assess its clinical efficacy.

TRANSDERMAL PROGESTERONE AND WILD YAM CREAMS

Topical, 'natural' progesterone cream has, been extensively marketed through the internet and lay media as a reputedly effective treatment for PMS and other gynecological complaints[34]. Unfortunately, evidence of efficacy is scant and progesterone is absorbed poorly through the skin[35]. Wild yam cream is popular, and claims have been made that steroids such as diosgenin in yams (*Dioscorea villosa*) are converted in the body to progesterone. However, this is biochemically impossible in humans.

MECHANICAL

Transcutaneous electrical nerve stimulation

The technique of transcutaneous electrical nerve stimulation (TENS) has been shown to be effective for pain relief in a variety of conditions. In dysmenorrhea, TENS is thought to work by alteration of the body's ability to receive or perceive pain signals rather than by exertion of a direct effect on uterine contractions. Proctor and associates[36] concluded high-frequency TENS to be effective, but the trials to support this are small[37–42]. Furthermore, there is insufficient evidence to determine the effectiveness of low-frequency TENS in reducing dysmenorrhea.

Acupuncture and acupressure

Acupuncture is the stimulation of special points on the body, usually by the insertion of fine needles, and originated in the Far East about 2000 years ago. It is thought to excite receptors or nerve fibers through a complicated interaction with mediators such as serotonin and endorphins to block pain impulses.

In its original form acupuncture was based on the principles of traditional Chinese medicine. According to these principles, the workings of the human body are controlled by a vital force or energy called 'Qi' (pronounced 'chee'), that circulates between the organs along channels called meridians[43].

There are 12 main meridians, and these correspond to 12 major functions or 'organs' of the body. Qi energy must flow in the correct strength and quality though each of these meridians and organs for health to be maintained. The acupuncture points are located along the meridians and provide one means of altering the flow of Qi. Acupuncture has long been used in the treatment of pain, although proof of its effects are uncertain. There is insufficient evidence to determine the effectiveness of these therapies in reducing dysmenorrhea; however, a single, small, but methodologically sound trial suggests benefit for this modality[36,44].

Spinal manipulation

One popular treatment modality is spinal manipulation therapy. Several hypotheses support the use of musculoskeletal manipulation to treat dysmenorrhea. One is that mechanical dysfunction in the spinal vertebrae can cause spinal mobility. This could affect sympathetic nerve supply to the blood vessels supplying pelvic viscera, leading to dysmenorrhea as a result of vasoconstriction. Another is that dysmenorrhea is referred pain arising from musculoskeletal structures that share the same pelvic nerve pathways.

Results from randomized controlled trials suggest that the spinal manipulation technique was no more effective than sham manipulation used in controls[45–49]. Overall, there is no evidence to suggest spinal manipulation is effective treatment for dysmenorrhea. However, the risk of adverse effects with spinal manipulation is no higher than that of sham manipulation.

Chiropractic manipulation

A systematic review of the available clinical trials reveals that the evidence for or against the effectiveness of chiropractic manipulation in non-spinal conditions like dysmenorrhea is not based on rigorous clinical trials[50].

Esogetic Colorpuncture™ Therapy

A review of recent research studies[51] was conducted in Europe to evaluate the efficacy of Peter Mandel's Esogetic Colorpuncture Therapy (ECT) – a holistic aculight system. This is a powerful new method of holistic healing and is utilized as a treatment for various health problems including uterine bleeding. Croke and colleagues[51] concluded that ECT led to a dramatic improvement of symptoms and that it could offer fast, economical, non-invasive and non-toxic methods for treating selected health problems. However, limitations in research design and sample size imply that these studies be viewed as pilot or preliminary research.

CONCLUSION

Beneficial effects of the most common supplements and mechanical methods available for the treatment of menstrual complaints are limited, as are the clinical data regarding their efficacy. However, as alternative and complementary therapies are one of the fastest expanding areas in the consumer markets throughout the world, the requirement for large randomized studies is great.

PRACTICE POINTS

- There is insufficient evidence to recommend
  any of the herbal and dietary therapies for the management of abnormal menstrual bleeding and dysmenorrhea

- Chinese medicinal therapy is being considered as a feasible alternative medicine. However, randomized studies are lacking
- Trials suggest that vitamins and minerals like magnesium are a promising treatment for dysmenorrhea, but no strong recommendation can be made until further evaluation on the dose or regimen of treatment is carried out
- Calcium has been found to be effective in the treatment of premenstrual syndrome
- There is no convincing evidence to support recommending vitamin B_6 supplements for premenstrual syndrome
- Studies of phytoestrogens in menstrual disorders are limited. There is some evidence that they may alter menstrual cycle length, but the results are conflicting
- There is insufficient evidence to suggest that mechanical methods such as transcutaneous electrical nerve stimulation, acupuncture, spinal manipulation, chiropractic manipulation and Esogetic Colorpuncture Therapy are effective in the treatment of dysmenorrhea

ACKNOWLEDGMENT

Many thanks to Ms Denise Tiran, at Expectancy Ltd (www.expectancy.co.uk), for providing information on complementary therapies.

REFERENCES

1. Thomas KJ, Nicholl JP, Coleman P. Use and expenditure on complementary medicine in England: a population based survey. Complement Ther Med 2001; 9: 2–11

2. Factor-Litvak P, Cushman LF, Kronenberg F, et al. Use of complementary and alternative medicine among women in New York City: a pilot study. J Altern Complement Med 2001; 7: 659–66

3. Thomas KJ, Coleman P, Nicholl JP. Trends in access to complementary or alternative medicines via primary care in England: 1995–2001 results from a follow-up national survey. Fam Pract 2003; 20: 575–7

4. Namavar Jahromi B, Tartifizadeh A, Khabnadideh S. Comparison of fennel and mefenamic acid for treatment of primary dysmenorrhea. Int J Gynaecol Obstet 2003; 80: 153–7

5. Rohdewald P. A review of French maritime pine bark extract (Pycnogenol), a herbal medication with a diverse clinical pharmacology. Int J Clin Pharmacol Ther 2002; 40: 158–68

6. Terasawa K. Kampo Japanese–Oriental Medicine: Insights from Clinical Cases. Tokyo, Japan: KK Standard McIntyre, 1993

7. Kotani N, Oyama T, Sakai I, et al. Analgesic effect of a herbal medicine for treatment of primary dysmenorrheal – a double-blind study. Am J Chi Med 1997; 25: 205–12

8. Budeiri D, Li Wan Po A, Dornan JC. Is evening primrose oil of value in the treatment of premenstrual syndrome? Control Clin Trials 1996; 17: 60–8

9. Khoo SK, Munro C, Battistutta D. Evening primrose oil and treatment of premenstrual syndrome. Med J Aust 1990; 153: 189–92

10. Collins A, Cerin A, Coleman G, Landgren BM. Essential fatty acids in the treatment of premenstrual syndrome. Obstet Gynecol 1993; 81: 93–8

11. Yuan R, Lin Y. Traditional Chinese medicine: an approach to scientific proof and clinical validation. Pharmacol Ther 2000; 86: 191–8

12. Hsu CS, Yang JK, Yang LL. Effect of a dysmenorrhea Chinese medicinal prescription on uterine contractility *in vitro*. Phytother Res 2003; 17: 778–83

13. Wu XZ. Evaluation of rubidatum treatment of abnormal uterine bleeding after IUD insertion: analysis of 255 cases. Shengzhi Yu Biyun 1992; 12: 33–6

14. Sakamoto S, Mitamura T, Iwasawa M, et al. Conservative management of perimenopausal women with uterine leiomyomas using Chinese herbal medicines and synthetic analogs of gonadotropin-releasing hormone. In Vivo 1998; 12: 333–7

15. Davis LS. Stress, vitamin B6 and magnesium in women with and without dysmenorrhea: a comparison and intervention study. Dissertation, University of Texas at Austin, 1988

16. Fontana-Klaiber H, Hogg B. Therapeutic effects of magnesium in dysmenorrhea. Schweiz Rundsch Med Prax 1990; 79: 491–4

17. Seifert B, Wagler P, Dartsch S, et al. Magnesium – a new therapeutic alternative in primary dysmenorrhea. Zentralbl Gynakol 1989; 111: 755–60

18. Thys-Jacobs S. Micronutrients and the premenstrual syndrome: the case for calcium. J Am Coll Nutr 2000; 19: 220–7

19. Facchinetti F, Borella P, Sances G, et al. Oral magnesium successfully relieves premenstrual mood changes. Obstet Gynecol 1991; 78: 177–81

20. Walker AF, De Souza MC, Vickers MF, et al. Magnesium supplementation alleviates premenstrual symptoms of fluid retention. J Womens Health 1998; 7: 1157–65

21. Thys-Jacobs S, Ceccarelli S, Bierman A, et al. Calcium supplementation in premenstrual syndrome: a randomized crossover trial. J Gen Intern Med 1989; 4: 183–9

22. Penland JG, Johnson PE. Dietary calcium and manganese effects on menstrual cycle symptoms. Am J Obstet Gynecol 1993; 168: 1417–23

23. Thys-Jacobs S, Starkey P, Bernstein D, Tian J. Calcium carbonate and the premenstrual syndrome: effects on premenstrual and menstrual symptoms. Premenstrual Syndrome Study Group. Am J Obstet Gynecol 1998; 179: 444–52

24. Johnson SR. Premenstrual syndrome therapy. Clin Obstet Gynecol 1998; 41: 405–21

25. Diegoli MS, da Fonseca AM, Diegoli CA, Pinotti JA. A double-blind trial of four medications to treat severe premenstrual syndrome. Int J Gynaecol Obstet 1998; 62: 63–7

26. Dalton K. Pyridoxine overdose in premenstrual syndrome. Lancet 1985; 1: 1168–9

27. Gokhale LB. Curative treatment of primary (spasmodic) dysmenorrhea. Indian J Med Res 1996; 103: 227–31

28. Edmonds SE, Winyard PG, Guo R, et al. Putative analgesic activity of repeated oral doses of vitamin E in the treatment of rheumatoid arthritis. Results of a prospective placebo controlled double blind trial. Ann Rheum Dis 1997; 56: 649–55

29. Setchell KD, Cassidy A. Dietary isoflavones: biological effects and relevance to human health. J Nutr 1999; 129: 758S–67S

30. Cassidy A, Bingham S, Setchell KD. Biological effects of a diet of soy protein rich in isoflavones on the menstrual cycle of

premenopausal women. Am J Clin Nutr 1994; 60: 333–40

31. Maskarinec G, Williams AE, Inouye JS, et al. A randomized isoflavone intervention among premenopausal women. Cancer Epidemiol Biomarkers Prev 2002; 11: 195–201

32. Deutch B. Menstrual pain in Danish women correlated with low n-3 polyunsaturated fatty acid intake. Eur J Clin Nutr 1995; 49: 508–16

33. Harel Z, Biro FM, Kottenhahn RK, Rosenthal SL. Supplementation with omega-3 polyunsaturated fatty acids in the management of dysmenorrhoea in adolescents. Am J Obstet Gynecol 1996; 174: 1335–8

34. Lee LR. Natural progesterone. The multiple role of a remarkable hormone. Sebastopol, CA: BLL Publishing, 1995

35. Wren BG, McFarland K, Edwards L, et al. Effect of sequential transdermal progesterone cream on endometrium, bleeding pattern, and plasma progesterone and salivary progesterone levels in postmenopausal women. Climacteric 2000; 3: 155–60

36. Proctor ML, Smith CA, Farquhar CM, Stones RW. Transcutaneous electrical nerve stimulation and acupuncture for primary dysmenorrhoea. Cochrane Database Syst Rev 2002; 1: CD002123

37. Dawood MY, Ramos J. Transcutaneous electrical nerve stimulation (TENS) for the treatment of primary dysmenorrhea: a randomized crossover comparison with placebo TENS and ibuprofen. Obstet Gynecol 1990; 75: 656–60

38. Lewers D, Clelland JA, Jacksin VR, et al. Transcutaneous electrical nerve stimulation in the relief of primary dysmenorrhea. Phys Ther 1989; 69: 3–9

39. Lundeberg T, Bondesson L, Lundstrom V. Relief of primary dysmenorrhea by transcutaneous electrical nerve stimulation. Acta Obstet Gynecol Scand 1985; 64: 491–7

40. Mannheimer JS, Whalen EC. The efficacy of transcutaneous electrical nerve stimulation in dysmenorrhoea. Clin J Pain 1985; 1: 75–83

41. Milsom I, Hedner N, Mannheimer C. A comparative study of the effect of high-intensity transcutaneous nerve stimulation and oral naproxen on intrauterine pressure and menstrual pain in patients with primary dysmenorrhea. Am J Obstet Gynecol 1994; 170: 123–9

42. Neighbors LE, Burnham TL, George KL, et al. Transcutaneous electrical nerve stimulation for pain relief in primary dysmenorrhoea. Clin J Pain 1987; 3: 17–22

43. Vickers A, Zollman C. ABC of complementary medicine. Acupuncture. BMJ 1999; 319: 973–6

44. Helms JM. Acupuncture for the management of primary dysmenorrhea. Obstet Gynecol 1987; 69: 51–6

45. Boesler D, Warner M, Alpers A, et al. Efficacy of high-velocity low-amplitude manipulative technique in subjects with low-back pain during menstrual cramping. J Am Osteopathic Assoc 1993; 93: 203–14

46. Hondros MA, Long CR, Brennan PC. Spinal manipulation therapy versus a low force mimic maneuver for women with primary dysmenorrhoea: a randomized, observer-blinded clinical trial. Pain 1999; 81: 105–14

47. Kokjohn K, Schmid DM, Triano JJ, Brennan PC. The effect of spinal manipulation on pain and prostaglandin levels in women with primary dysmenorrhea. J Manipulative Physiol Ther 1992; 15: 279–85

48. Snyder BJ, Sanders GE. Evaluation of the Toftness system of chiropractic adjusting for subjects with chronic back pain, chronic tension headache or primary dysmenorrhoea. Chiropract Tech 1996; 8: 3–9

49. Thomason PR, Fisher BL, Carpenter PA, Fike GL. Effectiveness of spinal manipulative therapy in treatment of primary dys-

menorrhoea: a pilot study. J Manipulative Physiol Ther 1979; 2: 140–5

50. Ernst E. Chiropractic manipulation for non-spinal pain – a systematic review. NZ Med J 2003; 116: U539

51. Croke M, Bourne RD. A review of recent research studies on the efficacy of Esogetic Colorpuncture Therapy – a holistic acu-light system. Am J Acupunct 1999; 27: 85–94

Contraceptive preparations and the abnormal menstrual cycle

13

I.R. Pirwany and T.C. Rowe

INTRODUCTION

Contraceptive preparations play an important role in the management of menstrual disorders. Since their discovery in the 1960s, hormonal contraceptives have held great promise as an answer to menstrual disturbances. The therapeutic use of estrogens and progestins is widespread, and, although used primarily to prevent pregnancy, they also have significant health benefits beyond contraception. Their popularity in part stems from their widespread availability, acceptance, and familiarity of use.

In recent years, however, the use of hormonal contraceptives has been tempered by the realization of their side-effect profile as well as by their limitations. Notably, some contraceptive preparations may paradoxically cause menstrual disturbances. For example, low-dose combined oral contraceptive preparations, although effective, may not be as efficacious in regulating menstrual cycles as their higher-dose counterparts. Similarly, parenteral medroxyprogesterone, and subdermal and intrauterine levonorgestrel preparations, although effective agents in the management of some menstrual abnormalities may themselves cause irregular vaginal bleeding. A paucity of reliable data is one of the reasons for the uncertainty surrounding the use of contraceptives in the management of the abnormal menstrual cycle. Despite four decades of widespread clinical use for fertility regulation, surprisingly few studies have examined the effect of contraceptive preparations on menstrual cyclicity exclusively.

When dealing with abnormalities of the menstrual cycle, therefore, it is important for the practitioner to be aware not only of the choices available, but also of the relative merits and demerits of the various agents in order to effectively manage women with abnormal menstrual cycles. This chapter explores the role of various contraceptive preparations in the management of the abnormal menstrual cycle, with a particular emphasis on the role of hormonal contraceptive preparations.

Contraceptives may be broadly classified into reversible and irreversible methods, and hormonal or non-hormonal preparations. Sterilization is the most effective, non-reversible method of contraception. The perception of increased menstrual loss following the procedure is a commonly held misconception. Although change in follicular phase of the cycle[1] has been suggested as a possible cause of abnormal menstrual function following surgery, the discontinuation of oral contraception and the resulting derangement in menstrual cyclicity is the most likely cause of the perceived menorrhagia after surgery[2].

AMENORRHEA

Amenorrhea is traditionally categorized as either primary (no history of menstruation) or secondary (cessation of menses after a variable time). The causes of primary amenorrhea are diverse. Although the classification of amenorrhea can be useful for identifying the mechanism of disease and differential diagnosis, it is important to appreciate that some disorders can initially present with either primary or secondary amenorrhea. For example, although polycystic ovary syndrome (PCOS) usually presents as oligomenorrhea, it may also present with primary amenorrhea. Where possible the treatment should be directed to the primary cause of the disorder.

Gonadal dysgenesis is an important cause of primary amenorrhea. Although most women with this disorder present with primary amenorrhea, some patients may have residual follicles, may menstruate and indeed may ovulate[3]. These events may be followed by complete cessation of periods. Management of these patients involves the use of hormonal contraception to develop and maintain secondary sexual characteristics. It is advantageous to commence with a higher-dose combined oral contraceptive formulation (COC), and to titrate the dosage in relation to the appearance of side-effects[4].

Secondary amenorrhea is most often due to chronic anovulation. The causes of secondary amenorrhea can be broadly categorized as listed in Table 1.

Establishing any association of secondary amenorrhea with various life events is extremely useful. For example, an unusual dietary history, supported by evidence of estrogen deficiency and low circulating levels of gonadotropins, is suggestive of bulimia or anorexia nervosa. In fact, approximately half of all adolescents with bulimia nervosa will also exhibit hypothalamic dysfunction and oligomenorrhea[5]. There is no clearly defined threshold between infertility and normal reproductive health and, despite suboptimal weight, many women do become pregnant[6]. Although most affected women have normal pregnancies and healthy babies[6], there appears to be a higher incidence of pregnancy-related complications. In particular, these patients are at a higher risk of miscarriage (38% compared with 16% in controls)[7], preterm premature rupture of membranes (PPROM)[8], and preterm delivery than women of normal weight[9]. As expected, women with anorexia nervosa are at a higher risk of hyperemesis gravidarum and postpartum depression than controls. As with hypothalamic amenorrhea the COC provides effective contraception and exerts a protective effect on bone density (see below). It may also allow an opportunity to delay pregnancy permitting the body weight to stabilize at $\geq 45 \, \text{kg}$.

A derangement in the pulsatile secretion of luteinizing hormone releasing hormone (LHRH) has been suggested as the underlying etiological factor in functional (or hypothalamic) amenorrhea. If anovulation persists for more than 6 months, or if reversal of the primary cause is not practical (e.g. professional

Table 1 Causes of secondary amenorrhea

Hypothalamic dysfunction (functional amenorrhea)

Ovarian failure

Pituitary origin (hyperprolactinemia)

Androgen excess

Primary uterine disease (intrauterine adhesions, e.g. after a postpartum curettage)

Chronic illness

athletes, ballerinas), the long-term adverse effect of hypoestrogenism on bone metabolism must be considered. Associated insulin-like growth factor I deficiency, hypercortisolism, or nutritional factors may all exacerbate bone loss in these patients[10,11]. Estrogen replacement therapy in the form of a low-dose OC offers the best treatment option in these groups of patients[12]. Given the documented, albeit transient, association of injectable progesterone contraceptives with reduced bone density, it is prudent to avoid these in this group of patients for fear of worsening bone mineral density.

Premature ovarian failure (POF) may occur as an isolated autoimmune disorder or in association with hypothyroidism, diabetes mellitus, hypoadrenalism, hypoparathyroidism, or systemic lupus erythematosus, or as part of a polyendocrinopathy[13] (see Chapter 8). The management of POF depends upon the desire for pregnancy, and has been discussed elsewhere. It is important to note that ovulation may occur, often intermittently, and pregnancy can result. If pregnancy is not desired, a low-dose OC is the treatment of choice and confers a protective effect on bone density. Clinical studies have indicated that an OC containing 20–35 μg/day of ethinylestradiol in combination with the progestin norethindrone produces the optimal bone-sparing effect in premenopausal women[14]. This should be the treatment of choice in non-smoking women with no risk factors for venous thromboembolism[15].

The single most common cause of secondary amenorrhea of pituitary origin is hyperprolactinemia resulting from a prolactinoma (18% of cases)[16]. Other pituitary causes of secondary amenorrhea, e.g. empty sella syndrome, Sheehan's syndrome, and Cushing's disease, are rare (1% of cases). Currently, the most effective form of treatment is the use of dopamine agonists, bromocriptine and cabergoline[17]. Tumor shrinkage is achieved in most cases with a reduction in prolactin levels, resolution of headaches and galactorrhea, and the resumption of menses and fertility. Oral contraceptives were believed to be contraindicated in women with pituitary adenomas for fear of causing tumor enlargement or growth promotion of the lesion[18]. Reassuringly, however, preliminary evidence from case–control studies indicates that use of the OC does not result in documented radiological tumor enlargement over 2 years of administration[19], supporting the use of the OC in this clinical setting.

For primary uterine abnormalities as a cause of secondary amenorrhea, particularly uterine adhesions, hysteroscopic lysis of the intrauterine adhesions followed by long-term estrogen therapy is the treatment of choice. Although the role of hormonal contraception in the management of these patients has not been studied extensively, it would appear that the increase in endometrial thickness and volume that may result from their use may hasten endometrial regeneration[20]. In cases of recurrence, insertion of an intrauterine contraceptive device provides additional protection against re-adherence of the uterine walls. The use of exogenous estrogen in combination with the levonorgestrel releasing intrauterine system (LNG-IUS; Mirena®, Schering, Germany) may not only impede uterine wall apposition, but, in combination with exogenous estrogen, may provide further protection against uterine re-adherence. However, this has not been studied in the context of a randomized study. The risk of abnormal placentation and the possibility of placenta accreta should be borne in mind if these patients become pregnant[21].

OLIGOMENORRHEA

The most prevalent cause of oligomenorrhea is PCOS, a heterogeneous disorder that is present in 6–10% of women of reproductive age[22] and is discussed in detail in Chapter 7.

Low-dose OCs containing 30 µg or less of ethinlyestradiol in combination with a third-generation progestin should be the treatment of choice in non-smoking patients with PCOS who desire contraception, and who do not have any risk factors for venous thromboembolism. In addition to providing adequate contraception and endometrial protection, this combination is effective in suppression of circulating androgen levels[23]. Used alone, low-dose OCs are effective in controlling mild hirsutism which is the most frequent hyperandrogenic manifestation of the syndrome[24]. In part, this effect is secondary to increased hepatic sex hormone binding globulin (SHBG) production resulting in lower free circulating testosterone levels[25]. Additionally, the progestogen in the COC can lead to an antagonism of 5α-reductase and the androgen receptor, and a further decrease in SHBG concentrations[26]. It is advisable to select an OC containing a progestin with low androgenic activity. Predictable withdrawal bleeding in response to oral contraceptive treatment is reassuring evidence against the development of endometrial hyperplasia, rendering frequent endometrial assessments unnecessary[27].

The LNG-IUS may also be used to obviate the effect of unopposed estrogen on the endometrium. Limited data from small case series suggest that this may be an excellent treatment for endometrial hyperplasia[28]; however, corroboratory evidence from results of long-term studies is lacking.

A concern regarding possible insulin desensitizing effects of oral contraceptives has been raised[29]. Although older, higher-dose oral contraceptives worsen insulin sensitivity, long-term follow-up studies have failed to detect any increase in the incidence of diabetes mellitus in past or current users of high-dose pills[30]. Furthermore, the effect of the OC on insulin metabolism appears to be dose related[31], thus it is advisable to use the newer generation of low-dose contraceptive preparations. These preparations containing ethinylestradiol 30 µg or less and desogestrel, norgestimate, or gestodene as the progestin component do not appear to worsen lipid and lipoprotein profile or adversely affect the surrogate biochemical markers of cardiovascular disease[32]. Neither do they appear to have a deleterious effect on insulin sensitivity in women with PCOS[33].

Cyproterone acetate in conjunction with ethinlyestradiol is superior to the combined estrogen progestin pill alone in the management of the hyperandrogenic manifestations of the disorder, particularly hirsutism[34]. Cyproterone acetate is a 17-hydroxyprogesterone acetate derivative with strong progestogenic properties. The drug mainly acts as an anti-androgen by competing with dihydrotestosterone (DHT) and testosterone for binding to the androgen receptor. There is also some evidence that cyproterone acetate and ethinylestradiol in combination can inhibit 5α-reductase activity in the skin[35]. Treatment in a reverse sequential manner (using 50 mg of cyproterone in the early follicular phase of the cycle, with the addition of ethinlyestradiol 50 µg from day 5 to 25) is now seldom used. Smaller doses (2 mg) in daily combination with 35 µg of ethinylestradiol (Dianette®, Schering Health Care, West Sussex, UK) administered daily is a popular contraceptive preparation for hyperandrogenic women with PCOS, and is an effective treatment for hirsutism. However, disturbingly, a four-fold higher risk of venous thromboembolism (VTE) is associated with its use compared with levonorgestrel in a large case–control study[36]. Other studies however, have not been able to confirm this association[37,38]. Clearly more studies are needed to clarify the association between cyproterone acetate and VTE. Pending better elaboration of its safety profile, cyproterone should be used after due counseling and after considering the potential benefits of this treatment. More severe forms of hirsutism may warrant alternative strategies. Discussion of these is beyond the scope of this chapter.

MENORRHAGIA

Menorrhagia is defined as blood loss greater than 80 ml per cycle and/or menstrual periods or a complaint of regular excessive menstrual bleeding over several consecutive cycles (see Chapter 2). The complaint accounts for 12% of all gynecological referrals for menstrual dysfunction to gynecologists in the UK[39].

Combined contraceptives

Contraceptive preparations are often tried as first-line treatments, and various delivery systems are available. These include oral, transdermal and vaginal routes.

Combined oral contraceptives

COCs are frequently used in the primary management of menorrhagia especially when contraception is needed. COCs, may act by several mechanisms to decrease the menstrual blood loss (MBL)[32]. They act primarily by suppressing the estrogen-induced mid-cycle surge of gonadotropin secretion, and thus inhibition of ovulation. Combination of regular shedding of the thin endometrium and anovulation results in endometrial atrophy[23,40]. In the absence of contraindications, pills containing at least 30 μg of ethinylestradiol should be prescribed. Although clinically the combined COC is an effective treatment for menorrhagia, most studies on its use are limited by methodological shortcomings and inadequate patient numbers[41], as well as by the dissimilar dose of ethinylestradiol employed in the various studies. Notwithstanding these inadequacies, evidence from these controlled observational studies[42], and meta-analysis[43] points to a modest, but significant benefit of the COC in reducing menstrual blood loss compared to baseline measurements. This benefit appears to be greater in studies that have employed higher dose of estrogen than the 30–35 mg of preparations currently in use. The effectiveness of lower-dose pills in reducing MBL is unclear. Indeed, lower-dose combination pills may paradoxically cause irregular uterine bleeding. It has been suggested that the perturbations in menstrual cyclicity with these preparations may be countered by altering the progestin dosage. It is unclear whether changing the progestin type has an appreciable beneficial effect on the MBL in patients with menorrhagia[44].

Clearly the simplicity of treatment, familiarity with its usage, and the appreciation of the non-contraceptive benefits of the pill ensure a place for the COC in the primary management of menorrhagia in women desiring contraception. The non-contraceptive benefits of the COC, include reduction in dysmenorrhea, and reduction in the incidence of ovarian and endometrial cancers[45]. The absolute contraindications for estrogen use are previous VTE event or stroke, history of an estrogen-dependent tumor, and liver disease. Undiagnosed abnormal uterine bleeding, hypertriglyceridemia, and women over age 35 years who smoke should also be regarded as contraindications to its use. Although pregnancy should be regarded as an absolute contra-indication, inadvertent COC use during early pregnancy has not been associated with an increase in risk of congenital anomalies with the possible exception of congenital urinary tract abnormalities[46]. Caution should be exercised in using COCs in women with poorly controlled hypertension, those on anticonvulsant therapy, and women with migraine, particularly those with associated focal neurological symptoms, who may be at increased risk of stroke cerebro-vascular incident[47].

Non-oral routes of administration

Non-oral routes have the advantage of better patient compliance and equal contraceptive effectiveness. For example, the transdermal contraceptive patch (Ortho Evra®, Ortho-Mcneil, Raritan, NJ, USA), which delivers 20 µg of ethinylestradiol and 150 µg of norelgestromin daily, and the contraceptive ring (NuvaRing®, Organon, Roseland, NJ, USA), which delivers 15 µg ethinylestradiol and 120 µg of etonogestrel daily intravaginally, offer highly effective contraception with few side-effects[48]. However, given the paucity of long-term studies, it is not possible to comment on their effectiveness as viable therapeutic agents in the management of women with abnormal menstrual rhythm. Pending further elucidation of its role in the symptomatic management of menorrhagia, and despite the higher incidence of irregular bleeding with these preparations, the user-friendly mode of non-oral administrations

ensures excellent patient compliance and satisfaction compared with the COC, and has a lower rate of discontinuation[49]. Thus, despite the shortcomings, these preparations may be a method of choice in women who also desire contraception.

Progesterone-only contraceptives

Oral preparations

Oral, parenteral and intrauterine methods are available; however, contraceptive efficacy is lower when compared to combined oral contraceptive pills. Limited data exist on the use of the progesterone-only contraceptive pill (POP) or the 'minipill' in women with menor-rhagia. Irregular bleeding pattern, however, is a common side-effect of all POPs, which may limit their value in patients with menorrhagia. Indeed, one-third to half of all POP users experience prolonged menstruation, and up to 70% report breakthrough bleeding or spotting in one or more cycles. These disturbances in menstrual cyclicity are consequent upon variable and unpredictable endometrial response that include irregular secretory endometrium, increased capillary fragility, alteration in endometrial vascular structure[50] and a lack of, or suppressed, endometrial proliferation[51]. Newer POPs containing desogestrel cause a more pronounced ovarian inhibition: they are more efficacious, and may have a correspondingly better bleeding pattern than levonorgestrel-containing minipills[52]. However, their use in the management of women with menstrual dysfunction has not been explored, and the data on their effect on menstrual cyclicity are limited.

Higher dose oral progesterone therapy (norethisterone or medroxyprogesterone) administered cyclically either from day 5 or 12 of the cycle may also be useful in the management of ovulatory and anovulatory dysfunctional uterine bleeding[53]. However, as the results of a recent meta-analysis have indicated, this treatment is significantly less effective than tranexamic acid or the LNG-IUS[54].

Parenteral progestogen preparations and the LNG-IUS may be particularly good choices in women with heavy menstrual loss in whom an estrogen-containing contraceptive is either contraindicated or causes additional health concerns, such as women with a history of exacerbations of migraine who take the OC and those who are prescribed anticonvulsants.

Parenteral progestogens

Depot medroxyprogesterone acetate (DPMA) acts primarily by inhibiting ovulation[55], and is a highly effective contraceptive[56]. Ideally, the first intramuscular injection of 150 mg DMPA is administered within 5 days of the onset of menses: alternative contraception is then not necessary. Women who receive the first injection after the seventh day of the cycle, however, should use a second method of contraception for 7 days. The same dose is repeated at 12-week intervals. Ovulation is suppressed for at least 14 weeks, so a delay in administering subsequent doses of up to 2 weeks should not reduce contraceptive efficacy.

Although irregular or prolonged bleeding are commonly reported early side-effects following the first injection, 50% of women report amenorrhea by 1 year[57]. Interestingly, follicular growth and maturation have been documented in those patients who continue to bleed following DPMA, indicating the need for repeat depot injection earlier than every 12 weeks[50]. If the bleeding is troublesome, various strategies may be used which include using 50 μg of ethinylestradiol for 14 days[58]. Other strategies for reducing the abnormal bleeding in these women include the use of non-steroidal anti-inflammatory agents (NSAIDS), and cyclical mifepristone (50–200 mg). While the evidence for the effectiveness of the former treatment is questionable, the latter drug, though efficacious, is not licensed for this use in the UK. The irregular bleeding is however, likely to recur after estrogen is stopped. Recurrent or persistent episodes of irregular bleeding may necessitate a reconsideration of methods. Notwithstanding the tenuous association between DPMA use and androgenic side-effects (acne, headaches, weight gain and depression), these side-effects remain the most commonly cited reasons for treatment discontinuation by 1 year in over 70% of women[59,60]. The effect of prolonged DPMA use on increased bone resorption and reduction in bone density is transient and reversible[61], and does not increase the risk of fracture or postmenopausal osteoporosis[62]. Indeed, DPMA use confers significant non-contraceptive benefits, including a reduction in the risk of endometrial cancer and pelvic inflammatory disease.

Most women have a return of fertility 6–9 months after the last injection. However, this may be delayed for up to 18 months after cessation of DMPA[55]. Thus, this mode of contraception is not suitable for women who may wish to become pregnant soon after cessation of contraception.

Noristerat® (Schering Health Care, West Sussex, UK), another injectable progestogen which contains norethisterone enanthate has a similar mode of action to DPMA. In contrast to

DPMA, however, the 200 mg injection is usually administered every 2 months. Ostensibly, the side-effects are reduced, though, in the absence of studies, it is unclear whether this is at the cost of its contraceptive efficacy.

Derangements in menstrual cyclicity following injectable progestogens have been the impetus for the development of the combined injectable methods. Monthly contraceptives comprising progestogens and estrogens have the advantage of maintaining the high efficacy of the combined methods and the added benefit of allowing withdrawal bleeding to resemble the physiologic menstrual cycles.

Medroxyprogesterone acetate (MPA)/ estradiol cypionate (E$_2$C) (Lunelle®, Pfizer Inc., NY, USA) is a combined (25 mg MPA and 5 mg E$_2$C), highly effective, injectable contraceptive available in the USA[63], that has several desirable features over DMPA such as faster resumption of fertility upon discontinuation[64], reduced incidence of irregular bleeding, and better side-effect profile[65]. However, monthly injections are required, which is less convenient than DMPA. Its effectiveness in reducing MBL is unclear.

Subdermal delivery

While subdermal levonorgestrel systems are effective contraceptives[66] and are very effective in reducing MBL, the side-effects have precluded their widespread use. An example in point is Norplant® (Leiras Oy, Finland), the six-rod subcutaneous implantable system, that has comparable efficacy to the LNG-IUS system[67], with a concomitant reduction in dysmenorrhea and irregular menstrual bleeding. However, Norplant, was withdrawn from the market because of retrieval complications. Implanon® (Organon Laboratories Ltd., Cambridge, UK), and Jadelle® (Leiras Oy, Finland), a single-rod and two-rod subdermal levonorgestrel implant systems, respectively are reliable, reversible contraceptives. The major side-effect of implants is irregular bleeding[68]. While there are no long-term studies that have addressed their effectiveness in reducing MBL in women with menorrhagia, the irregular bleeding due to their use can be managed by administering ethinylestradiol (30–50 µg), NSAIDs taken for 3–5 cycles or the use of levonorgestrel-containing OCs. These measures are effective in minimizing irregular bleeding following progesterone administration[50].

Intrauterine delivery

While menstrual loss is usually increased after the insertion of inert or copper-containing intrauterine contraceptive devices, it is reduced if the device is impregnated with a progestogen or progesterone. Intrauterine administration of progestins, as in the LNG-IUS, results in higher endometrial concentrations of progestin compared with oral administration, with relatively little systemic absorption. This system delivers 20 mg of levonorgestrel every 24 h in a sustained-release formulation that lasts up to 5 years. The LNG-IUS is superior to oral progestogens in reducing menstrual bleeding. Eighty-six per cent reduction in objectively measured MBL is observed 3 months after insertion, and 97% reduction at 12 months, while 20% of women using the LNG-IUS are reported to be amenorrheic after 1 year[69,70]. Provided women are warned to expect irregular, erratic vaginal bleeding in the early months of use[68], and are reassured of the likely improvement in the disruption with time, LNG-IUS offers excellent tolerance and acceptability as well as offering the advantage of highly effective reversible contraception[67].

Continuation rates for LNG-IUS vary, partly depending on the indication for treatment (heavy bleeding or contraception). Treatment compliance generally ranges between 66% and 68%[71,72]. Compared with other forms of treatment the LNG-IUS is much cheaper per menstrual cycle unless it is removed before 5 years[73], and it is at least three times cheaper than hysterectomy[74]. Patient selection plays an important role in determining the success of treatment; some evidence suggests that expulsion rates may be increased in the presence of submucous fibroids.

Progestasert® (Alza Corporation, Mountain View, CA, USA), a progesterone-containing intrauterine contraceptive system is available in the US, and unlike the LNG-IUS needs to be replaced every 12 months. Studies of its contraceptive efficacy indicate that it is equally effective as inert IUCDs[67]. Like the LNG-IUS, Progestasert causes a local reaction, while the antiproliferative action makes the endometrium unresponsive to the effect of estrogen and hostile to implantation[75].

The risk of pelvic inflammatory disease (PID) has generally been cited as a possible reason for the avoidance of IUCDs. However, the association between the two is tenuous and may have been overstated because of poorly designed studies that were affected by bias and did not consider other confounding variables[76,77].

DYSMENORRHEA

Dysmenorrhea, the painful cramping sensation in the lower abdomen often accompanied by other symptoms such as sweating, tachycardia, headaches, nausea, vomiting and diarrhea, occurs just before or during the menses. It is classified as primary dysmenorrhea that usually begins at or shortly after menarche and is usually not accompanied by pelvic pathologic conditions, and secondary dysmenorrhea, that in contrast, arises later and usually is associated with other pelvic pathologies.

Primary dysmenorrhea is believed to affect approximately 50% of menstruating women, and in 10% it is severe enough to limit daily activity[78]. Although the pathogenesis is unclear, the association with uterine hypercontractility, cramping, and other prostaglandin-induced symptoms as well as the demonstration of elevated prostaglandin (PG) $F_{2\alpha}$ and PGE_2 levels in the secretory endometrium, have led to the theory that prostaglandin-induced uterine hypercontractility and vasoconstriction, and the resulting uterine ischemia are associated with the pathogenesis of the symptoms[79]. NSAIDs are the mainstay of treatment, and are effective in alleviating the symptoms in more than 72% of the women. In those patients for whom NSAIDs are either contraindicated or ineffective[80], the oral contraceptives are of proven value. If the patient also requires contraception, oral contraceptive therapy may be the treatment of choice. When used for dysmenorrhea, the exact mode of action of OCs is unclear. They may act by reducing the MBL consequent upon reduction in endometrial growth[78] thus affecting a reduction in prostaglandin output in menstrual blood and ensuing uterine tonicity[81]. However, the role of oral contraceptive therapy in symptom control is limited by the dearth of large randomized controlled studies; the existing studies being limited to cross-sectional comparisons. Furthermore, the efficacy of low-dose oral preparations in symptom relief has also not been established, although there are indications of its effectiveness[82]. In women who fail to respond to NSAIDs or OCPs, it is important to consider secondary causes of dysmenorrhea.

Secondary dysmenorrhea may occur at any age. The pain is usually secondary to some pathological process, the most important of which is endometriosis. Other causes include cervical stenosis, chronic PID, pelvic congestion, conditioned behavior, and stress and tension. The management of most causes of secondary dysmenorrhea is beyond the scope of this chapter as the focus here is management of the primary cause.

Endometriosis is an important cause of morbidity and subfertility in women in their reproductive years[83]. Hormonal contraceptive preparations play a limited role in the symptom alleviation in women with endometriosis. This is discussed in detail in Chapter 4. Given the dearth of randomized placebo-controlled trials, there is little evidence to support the use of ovulation suppression therapy in patients with endometriosis[84]. However, there is promising evidence from case series that the LNG-IUS may have a role to play in reducing the size of rectovaginal endometriotic deposits and alleviating pain in patients with the disorder[85]. LNG-IUS may also have a role to play in symptom alleviation in the related disorder, adenomyosis.

Adenomyosis is an ill-understood disorder and is usually suspected on the basis of menorrhagia, dysmenorrhea and an enlarged uterus. The final diagnosis is, however, histological, following hysterectomy or endometrial resection. The diagnosis may be suspected on the basis of clinical symptoms of pelvic pain, menorrhagia, and enlarged uterus. Magnetic resonance imaging may be helpful in providing confirmatory evidence. Although the treatment is primarily surgical, and the diagnosis is often confirmed from histological examination of the surgical specimen, there is some evidence to suggest the use of LNG-IUS and mifepristone (an antiprogestin) in the management of the symptoms[86,87].

Although the exact mode of action of mifepristone (Mifegyn®, Exelgyn Laboratories, Oxon, UK) is unclear, it may be related to its contraceptive action. In particular, when administered in the follicular phase of the cycle, mifepristone has an inhibitory effect on follicular development and ovulation. In the secretory phase of the menstrual cycle, it has an adverse influence on endometrial development and function. Despite the inconsistent effect on the inhibition of ovulation, mifepristone appears to have a favorable contraception effectiveness when administered weekly, chiefly due to its effect on endometrial receptivity. Furthermore, a high dose of mifepristone (200 mg) administered immediately following ovulation is highly effective in preventing implantation, and thus may be useful as a postcoital contraceptive, with reported failure rates of 3–16%[88]. Mifepristone has been demonstrated to relieve pain in women with symptomatic endometriosis and also to decrease the size of uterine leiomyomata by about 50%[89]. The applicability of the drug for non-contraceptive uses will have to await larger randomized studies exploring its long-term safety and efficacy.

CONCLUSION

Contraceptive preparations play a significant role in the management of women who have an abnormal menstrual cycle, and are an important element in the armamentarium of drugs available to treat this disorder. Judicious use of these compounds demands a thorough understanding of the formulations and an understanding of the mode of actions of the various preparations. Typically, it is prudent to attain familiarity with a small number of preparations and the circumstances in which they are most likely to be beneficial.

REFERENCES

1. Dennerstein L, Gotts G, Brown JB. Effects of age and non-hormonal contraception on menstrual cycle characteristics. Gynecol Endocrinol 1997; 11: 127–33

2. Bhiwandiwala PP, Mumford SD, Feldblum PJ. Menstrual pattern changes following laparoscopic sterilization with different occlusion techniques: a review of 10 004 cases. Am J Obstet Gynecol 1983; 145: 684–94

3. Rebar RW. Hypergonadotropic amenorrhea and premature ovarian failure: a review. J Reprod Med 1982; 27: 179–86

4. Seidenfeld ME, Rickert VI. Impact of anorexia, bulimia and obesity on the gynecologic health of adolescents. Am Fam Physician 2001; 64: 445–50

5. Van Der Spuy ZM, Jacobs HS. Weight reduction, fertility and contraception. IPPF Med Bull 1983; 17: 2–4

6. Franko DL, Blais MA, Becker AE, et al. Pregnancy complications and neonatal outcomes in women with eating disorders. Am J Psychiatry 2001; 158: 1461–6

7. Bulik CM, Sullivan PF, Fear JL, et al. Fertility and reproduction in women with anorexia nervosa: a controlled study. J Clin Psychiatry 1999; 60: 130–5

8. Hsu LK. Outcome of anorexia nervosa. A review of the literature (1954 to 1978). Arch Gen Psychiatry 1980; 37: 1041–6

9. Brinch M, Isager T, Tolstrup K. Anorexia nervosa and motherhood: reproduction pattern and mothering behavior of 50 women. Acta Psychiatry Scand 1988; 77: 611–17

10. Grinspoon SK, Friedman AJ, Miller KK, et al. Effects of a triphasic combination oral contraceptive containing norgestimate/ethinyl estradiol on biochemical markers of bone metabolism in young women with osteopenia secondary to hypothalamic amenorrhea. J Clin Endocrinol Metab 2003; 88: 3651–6

11. Pafumi C, Ciotta L, Farina M, et al. Evaluation of bone mass in young amenorrheic women with anorexia nervosa. Minerva Ginecol 2002; 54: 487–91

12. Seeman E, Szmukler GI, Formica C, et al. Osteoporosis in anorexia nervosa: the influence of peak bone density, bone loss, oral contraceptive use, and exercise. J Bone Miner Res 1992; 7: 1467–74

13. Kauffman RP, Castracane VD. Premature ovarian failure associated with autoimmune polyglandular syndrome: pathophysiological mechanisms and future fertility. J Womens Health (Larchmt) 2003; 12: 513–20

14. Thorneycroft IH. Cycle control with oral contraceptives: a review of the literature. Am J Obstet Gynecol 1999; 180: 280–7

15. DeCherney A. Bone-sparing properties of oral contraceptives. Am J Obstet Gynecol 1996; 174: 15–20

16. Crosignani PG, Vegetti W. A practical guide to the diagnosis and management of amenorrhea. Drugs 1996; 52: 671–81

17. Ferrari C, Piscitelli G, Crosignani PG. Cabergoline: a new drug for the treatment of hyperprolactinaemia. Hum Reprod 1995; 10: 1647–52

18. Vaisrub S. Pituitary prolactinoma and estrogen contraceptives. JAMA 1979; 242: 177–8

19. Testa G, Vegetti W, Motta T, et al. Two-year treatment with oral contraceptives in hyper-prolactinemic patients. Contraception 1998; 58: 69–73

20. Farhi J, Bar-Hava I, Homburg R, et al. Induced regeneration of endometrium following curettage for abortion: a comparative study. Hum Reprod 1993; 8: 1143–4

21. Schenker JG. Etiology of and therapeutic approach to synechia uteri. Eur J Obstet Gynecol Reprod Biol 1996; 65: 109–13

22. Franks S. Polycystic ovary syndrome. N Engl J Med 1995; 333: 853–61

23. ESHRE Capri Workshop Group. Ovarian and endometrial function during hormonal contraception. Hum Reprod 2001; 16: 1527–35

24. Barnes RB. Diagnosis and therapy of hyper-androgenism. Baillieres Clin Obstet Gynaecol 1997; 11: 369–96

25. Botwood N, Hamilton-Fairley D, Kiddy D, et al. Sex hormone-binding globulin and female reproductive function. J Steroid Biochem Mol Biol 1995; 53: 529–31

26. Dewis P, Newman M, Anderson DC. The effect of endogenous progesterone on serum levels of 5 alpha-reduced androgens in hirsute women. Clin Endocrinol (Oxf) 1984; 21: 383–92

27. Cheung AP. Ultrasound and menstrual history in predicting endometrial hyperplasia in polycystic ovary syndrome. Obstet Gynecol 2001; 98: 325–31

28. Perino A, Quartararo P, Catinella E, et al. Treatment of endometrial hyperplasia with levonorgestrel releasing intrauterine devices. Acta Eur Fertil 1987; 18: 137–40

29. Diamanti-Kandarakis E, Baillargeon JP, Iuorno MJ, et al. A modern medical quandary: polycystic ovary syndrome, insulin resistance, and oral contraceptive pills. J Clin Endocrinol Metab 2003; 88: 1927–32

30. Sondheimer S. Metabolic effects of the birth control pill. Clin Obstet Gynecol 1981; 24: 927–41

31. Seed M, Godsland IF, Wynn V, Jacobs HS. The effects of cyproterone acetate and ethinyl oestradiol on carbohydrate metabolism. Clin Endocrinol (Oxf) 1984; 21: 689–99

32. Petitti DB. Clinical practice. Combination estrogen–progestin oral contraceptives. N Engl J Med 2003; 349: 1443–50

33. Crosignani PG, La Vecchia C. Concordant and discordant effects on cardiovascular risks exerted by estrogen and progestogen in women using oral contraception and hormone replacement therapy. ESHRE Capri Workshop Group. Hum Reprod Update 1999; 5: 681–7

34. Falsetti L, Galbignani E. Long-term treatment with the combination ethinylestradiol and cyproterone acetate in polycystic ovary syndrome. Contraception 1990; 42: 611–19

35. Raudrant D, Rabe T. Progestogens with anti-androgenic properties. Drugs 2003; 63: 463–92

36. Vasilakis-Scaramozza C, Jick H. Risk of venous thromboembolism with cyproterone or levonorgestrel contraceptives. Lancet 2001; 358: 1427–9

37. Seaman HE, Vries CS, Farmer RD. The risk of venous thromboembolism in women prescribed cyproterone acetate in combination with ethinyl estradiol: a nested cohort analysis and case–control study. Hum Reprod 2003; 18: 522–6

38. Spitzer WO. Cyproterone acetate with ethinylestradiol as a risk factor for venous thromboembolism: an epidemiological evaluation. J Obstet Gynaecol Can 2003; 25: 1011–18

39. Coulter A, Bradlow J, Agass M, et al. Outcomes of referrals to gynaecology outpatient clinics for menstrual problems: an audit of general practice records. Br J Obstet Gynaecol 1991; 98: 789–96

40. Deligdisch L. Effects of hormone therapy on the endometrium. Mod Pathol 1993; 6: 94–106

41. Iyer V, Farquhar C, Jepson R. Oral contraceptive pill for heavy menstrual bleeding. Cochrane Database of Systematic Reviews. 2000; (2) CD000154

42. Fraser IS, McCarron G. Randomized trial of 2 hormonal and 2 prostaglandin-inhibiting agents in women with a complaint of menorrhagia. Aust NZ J Obstet Gynaecol 1991; 31: 66–70

43. Irvine GA, Cameron IT. Medical management of dysfunctional uterine bleeding. Baillieres Best Pract Res Clin Obstet Gynaecol 1999; 13: 189–202

44. Van Vliet HA, Grimes DA, Helmerhorst FM, et al. Biphasic versus triphasic oral contraceptives for contraception. Cochrane Database Syst Rev 2003; CD003283

45. Hannaford P. Health consequences of combined oral contraceptives. Br Med Bull 2000; 56: 749–60

46. Li DK, Daling JR, Mueller BA, et al. Oral contraceptive use after conception in relation to the risk of congenital urinary tract anomalies. Teratology 1995; 51: 30–6

47. Schwartz SM, Petitti DB, Siscovick DS, et al. Stroke and use of low-dose oral contraceptives in young women: a pooled analysis of two US studies. Stroke 1998; 29: 2277–84

48. Mulders TM, Dieben TO. Use of the novel combined contraceptive vaginal ring Nuva-Ring for ovulation inhibition. Fertil Steril 2001; 75: 865–70

49. Smallwood GH, Meador ML, Lenihan JP, et al. Efficacy and safety of a transdermal contraceptive system. Obstet Gynecol 2001; 98: 799–805

50. Porter C, Rees MC. Bleeding problems and progestogen-only contraception. J Fam Plann Reprod Health Care 2002; 28: 178–81

51. Kovacs G. Progestogen-only pills and bleeding disturbances. Hum Reprod 1996; 11: 20–3

52. Benagiano G, Primiero FM. Seventy-five microgram desogestrel minipill, a new perspective in estrogen-free contraception. Ann NY Acad Sci 2003; 997: 163–73

53. Fraser IS. Treatment of ovulatory and anovulatory dysfunctional uterine bleeding with oral progestogens. Aust NZ J Obstet Gynaecol 1990; 30: 353–6

54. Lethaby A, Irvine G, Cameron I. Cyclical progestogens for heavy menstrual bleeding. Cochrane Database Syst Rev 2000; CD001016

55. Kaunitz AM. Long-acting injectable contraception with depot medroxyprogesterone acetate. Am J Obstet Gynecol 1994; 170: 1543–9

56. Nelson A. Merits of DMPA relative to other reversible contraceptive methods. J Reprod Med 2002; 47: 781–4

57. Belsey EM. Vaginal bleeding patterns among women using one natural and eight hormonal

methods of contraception. Contraception 1988; 38: 181–206

58. Said S, Sadek W, Rocca M, et al. Clinical evaluation of the therapeutic effectiveness of ethinyl oestradiol and oestrone sulphate on prolonged bleeding in women using depot medroxyprogesterone acetate for contraception. World Health Organization, Special Programme of Research, Development and Research Training in Human Reproduction, Task Force on Long-acting Systemic Agents for Fertility Regulation. Hum Reprod 1996; 11: 1–13

59. Paul C, Skegg DC, Williams S. Depot medroxy progesterone acetate. Patterns of use and reasons for discontinuation. Contraception 1997; 56: 209–14

60. Pelkman CL, Chow M, Heinbach RA, Rolls BJ. Short-term effects of a progestational contraceptive drug on food intake, resting energy expenditure, and body weight in young women. Am J Clin Nutr 2001; 73: 19–26

61. Westhoff C. Bone mineral density and DMPA. J Reprod Med 2002; 47: 795–9

62. Orr-Walker BJ, Evans MC, Ames RW, et al. The effect of past use of the injectable contraceptive depot medroxyprogesterone acetate on bone mineral density in normal post-menopausal women. Clin Endocrinol (Oxf) 1998; 49: 615–18

63. Hall P, Bahamondes L, Diaz J, et al. Introductory study of the once-a-month, injectable contraceptive Cyclofem in Brazil, Chile, Colombia, and Peru. Contraception 1997; 56: 353–9

64. Bahamondes L, Lavin P, Ojeda G, et al. Return of fertility after discontinuation of the once-a-month injectable contraceptive Cyclofem. Contraception 1997; 55: 307–10

65. Cuong DT, My Huong NT. Comparative phase III clinical trial of two injectable contraceptive preparations, depot-medroxyprogesterone acetate and Cyclofem, in Vietnamese women. Contraception 1996; 54: 169–79

66. Sivin I. Contraception with NORPLANT implants. Hum Reprod 1994; 9: 1818–26

67. French RS, Cowan FM, Mansour DJ, et al. Implantable contraceptives (subdermal implants and hormonally impregnated intrauterine systems) versus other forms of reversible contraceptives: two systematic reviews to assess relative effectiveness, acceptability, tolerability and cost-effectiveness. Health Technol Assess 2000; 4: 1-107

68. Wan LS, Stiber A, Lam LY. The levonorgestrel two-rod implant for long-acting contraception: 10 years of clinical experience. Obstet Gynecol 2003; 102: 24–6

69. Irvine GA, Campbell-Brown MB, Lumsden MA, et al. Randomised comparative trial of the levonorgestrel intrauterine system and norethisterone for treatment of idiopathic menorrhagia. Br J Obstet Gynaecol 1998; 105: 592–8

70. Andersson K, Odlind V, Rybo G. Levonorgestrel-releasing and copper-releasing (Nova T) IUDs during five years of use: a randomized comparative trial. Contraception 1994; 49: 56–72

71. Baldaszti E, Wimmer-Puchinger B, Loschke K. Acceptability of the long-term contraceptive levonorgestrel-releasing intrauterine system (Mirena): a 3-year follow-up study. Contraception 2003; 67: 87–91

72. Lahteenmaki P, Haukkamaa M, Puolakka J, et al. Open randomised study of use of levonorgestrel releasing intrauterine system as alternative to hysterectomy. BMJ 1998; 316: 1122–6

73. Lethaby AE, Cooke I, Rees M. Progesterone/progestogen releasing intrauterine systems versus either placebo or any other medication for heavy menstrual bleeding. Cochrane Database Syst Rev 2000; CD002126

74. Hurskainen R, Teperi J, Rissanen P, et al. Quality of life and cost effectiveness of levonorgestrel-releasing intrauterine system versus hysterectomy for treatment of menorrhagia: a randomised trial. Lancet 2001; 357: 273–7

75. Luukkainen T, Pakarinen P, Toivonen J. Progestin-releasing intrauterine systems. Semin Reprod Med 2001; 19: 355–63

76. Grimes DA. Intrauterine device and upper-genital-tract infection. Lancet 2000; 356: 1013–9

77. Nelson AL, Sulak P. IUD patient selection and practice guidelines. Dialogues Contracept 1998; 5: 7–12

78. Sundell G, Milsom I, Andersch B. Factors influencing the prevalence and severity of dysmenorrhoea in young women. Br J Obstet Gynaecol 1990; 97: 588–94

79. Creatsas G, Deligeoroglou E, Zachari A, et al. Prostaglandins: PGF2 alpha, PGE2, 6-keto-PGF1 alpha and TXB2 serum levels in dysmenorrheic adolescents before, during and after treatment with oral contraceptives. Eur J Obstet Gynecol Reprod Biol 1990; 36: 292–8

80. Zhang WY, Li Wan Po A. Efficacy of minor analgesics in primary dysmenorrhoea: a systematic review. Br J Obstet Gynaecol 1998; 105: 780–9

81. Lalos O, Joelsson I. Effect of an oral contraceptive on uterine tonicity in women with primary dysmenorrhea. Acta Obstet Gynecol Scand 1981; 60: 229–32

82. Callejo J, Diaz J, Ruiz A, Garcia RM. Effect of a low-dose oral contraceptive containing 20 microg ethinylestradiol and 150 microg desogestrel on dysmenorrhea. Contraception 2003; 68: 183–8

83. Farquhar CM. Extracts from the 'clinical evidence'. Endometriosis. BMJ 2000; 320: 1449–52

84. Farquhar C, Sutton C. The evidence for the management of endometriosis. Curr Opin Obstet Gynecol 1998; 10: 321–32

85. Fedele L, Bianchi S, Zanconato G, et al. Use of a levonorgestrel-releasing intrauterine device in the treatment of rectovaginal endometriosis. Fertil Steril 2001; 75: 485–8

86. Maia H Jr, Maltez A, Coelho G, et al. Insertion of mirena after endometrial resection in patients with adenomyosis. J Am Assoc Gynecol Laparosc 2003; 10: 512–16

87. Spitz IM. Progesterone antagonists and progesterone receptor modulators: an overview. Steroids 2003; 68: 981–93

88. Croxatto HB. Mifepristone for luteal phase contraception. Contraception. 2003; 68: 483–8

89. Steinauer J, Pritts EA, Jackson R, Jacoby AF. Systematic review of mifepristone for the treatment of uterine leiomyomata. Obstet Gynecol 2004; 103: 1331–6

Menstrual migraine   14

E.A. MacGregor

INTRODUCTION

Migraine is a predominantly female disorder. Although it is equally common in both sexes before puberty, there is increased female prevalence following menarche. This difference between the sexes becomes greater with advancing years, peaking during the early 40s and declining thereafter[1]. Some studies suggest that the lifetime prevalence of migraine in women is as great as 25%, compared with only 8% in men[2].

This sex difference during the reproductive years is generally considered to result from the additional trigger of the menstrual cycle, a well-recognized association. Hippocrates noted: 'shivering, lassitude and heaviness of the head denotes the onset of menstruation'. The term 'hysteria' was used, which had physical rather than psychological connotations, simply meaning 'arising from the womb' and the recommended cure was marriage. In 1666, Johannis van der Linden described a particularly severe case of one-sided headache with nausea and vomiting associated with menstruation in the Marchioness of Brandenburg.

Despite evidence for the clinical relationship, the underlying mechanisms remained elusive to researchers over the centuries. In 1873, Liveing posed the questions: 'How are we to interpret the facts; what is the character of the influence exerted and to what extent is it the cause of the malady?'

This chapter aims to provide at least some of the answers to these questions, with practical advice for management.

WHAT IS MIGRAINE?

Migraine is the commonest cause of severe episodic recurrent headache. Accompanying symptoms of heightened sensitivity to light, sound and smell, together with nausea, vomiting and general malaise, restrict normal function.

Migraine headaches typically last between 4 and 72 h and can occur, on average, every 4–6 weeks. However, there is wide variation of attack frequency over a lifetime with periods of increased frequency and periods of freedom, sometimes for several years. Although migraine is a benign condition, the severity and frequency of attacks can result in significant disability and reduced quality of life, even between attacks[3].

The first attack of migraine usually occurs during the teens and early twenties, with 90% of attacks occurring before age 40[4]. Migraine typically disappears in the over 50s[5].

The two most frequently encountered types of migraine differ only in their presence or absence of 'aura'[6]. About 70–80% of migraineurs experience attacks of migraine without aura (formerly known as common or simple migraine); 10% have migraine with aura (formerly known as classical or focal migraine); 15–20% have both types of attacks. Less than 1% of attacks are of aura alone, with no ensuing headache.

Clinically, an attack of migraine can further be divided into five distinct phases[7] (Figure 1).

Prodromal/premonitory phase

Not all migraineurs are aware of prodromal symptoms, which can precede attacks of migraine both with and without aura by 12–24 h. Symptoms are suggestive of hypothalamic disturbance and are distinct from, and unrelated to, the aura. They include: irritability, feeling 'high' or 'low'; extreme lethargy and yawning; dysphasia; anorexia, constipation or diarrhea; craving for sweets or specific foods; urinary frequency, thirst or fluid retention. Friends, family, or work colleagues are more likely to notice these symptoms than the sufferer. Some prodromal symptoms are incorrectly blamed as triggers for the attack. For example, craving for sweet foods may result in a desire to eat chocolate. A few people feel 'on top of the world' before an attack and rush around, later thinking that the attack was caused by overactivity. In fact, these are signs that the attack has already begun. Recognition of these prodromal symptoms can be of enormous benefit since avoiding known trigger factors during this time may be all that is necessary to stop the attack developing further.

Aura

Symptoms of aura probably arise from the cerebral cortex or brain stem and gradually develop over 5–20 min, last under 1 h, and usually completely resolve before the onset of headache. Atypical or permanent symptoms warrant further investigation. Homonymous visual symptoms are most common, experienced in 99% of auras[8]. Sensory disturbance is less common (31%) and is usually associated with visual symptoms. Speech disturbance and

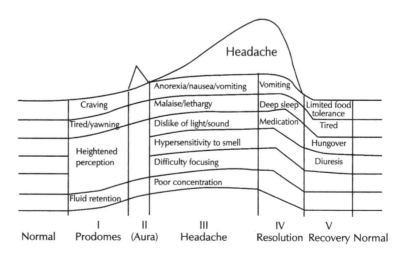

Figure 1 The five phases of a migraine attack. Adapted from reference 7

motor symptoms can also be present (18% and 6%, respectively) but only in association with visual and/or sensory symptoms. Symptoms usually follow one another in succession beginning with visual, followed by sensory symptoms, dysphasia and weakness.

Visual symptoms

These are usually symmetrical, affecting one hemifield of both eyes, although subjectively they may appear to affect only one eye. A migrainous scotoma is typically positive (bright), starting as a small spot gradually increasing in size to assume the shape of a letter 'C', developing scintillating edges which appear as zigzags or fortifications – a term coined in the late 18th century because the visual disturbances resembled a fortified town surrounded by bastions. The aura usually starts at or near the center of fixation, gradually spreading laterally, increasing in size over a period of 5–30 min. In contrast, thrombotic symptoms do not generally have the scintillating and spreading features of the visual aura of migraine and the visual loss usually described as a monocular negative scotoma (black). Transient monocular blindness is *not* typical of migraine and prompts urgent investigation. Generalized 'spots before the eyes', 'flashing lights', blurring of vision, photophobia affecting the whole visual field of both eyes and of variable duration before or with headache often occur during migraine and are not suggestive of focal ischemia.

Sensory symptoms

These are positive, i.e. a sensation of pins and needles rather than numbness. In an ischemic episode, a sense of numbness or 'deadness' is described. Migraine symptoms have a characteristic unilateral distribution affecting one arm, often spreading over several minutes proximally from the hand to affect the mouth and tongue – 'cheiro-oral distribution'. The leg is rarely affected in migraine.

Headache and associated symptoms

The throbbing headache is typically unilateral, sometimes swapping sides during an attack, but may be bilateral. It is aggravated by movement of the head and accompanied by nausea or vomiting, photophobia and/or phonophobia. Although some sufferers can continue limited activities, many have to retire to bed in a darkened room until symptoms subside.

Resolution

Other than with effective medication, the natural course of migraine is to resolve with sleep[9]. Some attacks, particularly in children, improve after vomiting.

Recovery/postdromal phase

After the headache has gone, most migraineurs feel drained and washed-out for a further day. Rarely, they feel very energetic and even euphoric.

DIAGNOSING MIGRAINE

The International Headache Society published a comprehensive headache classification, which has recently been revised[6,10]. However, although the criteria are invaluable for clinical research, they are not suited to routine clinical use.

Migraine can be diagnosed by history and examination. Most cases can be identified by a positive response to questions: 'Have you ever had a migraine?'; 'Have you ever had a 'sick' headache?'; 'Do your headaches stop you from doing things?' A cardinal feature of migraine is complete freedom from symptoms between attacks; daily headaches are not migraine although migraine and daily headaches may coexist.

Aura can be screened by a positive response to the question: 'Have you ever had visual disturbances lasting 5–60 min followed by headache?' The diagnosis is confirmed by the description of typical aura evolving over several minutes. Some patients find it hard to describe auras. Common mistakes include reports of sudden onset when it is gradual, of monocular disturbances when they are homonymous, and incorrect duration of aura. If there is any uncertainty, encourage patients to record their symptoms prospectively. Migraine auras usually follow a similar pattern with each attack although the duration of aura may alter. Therefore, a long history of similar attacks, particularly if onset is in childhood or early adult life, is reassuring. If aura symptoms suddenly change, further investigation may be warranted.

MIGRAINE AND MENSTRUATION

Migraine is a fluctuating condition. A longitudinal study of 73 migraineurs over 40 years showed that attack frequency was variable with time, sometimes with long episodes of remission[11]. Similarly, the association with menstruation is inconsistent with time. Although a few women report a constant association between migraine and menstruation since menarche, the majority report a gradual association between migraine and menstruation developing from their late 30s, with increasing prevalence in the years leading to menopause. Following the menopause, prevalence of all migraine declines.

Prevalence

More than 50% of women with migraine, both in the general population and presenting to specialist clinics, report an association between migraine and menstruation[12]. Data from prevalence studies of menstrual migraine report that anything from 4% to over 70% of women are affected[13]. The reason for this discrepancy is that most studies were undertaken before the development of an agreed definition for menstrual migraine. Further studies are necessary to identify the prevalence.

Definition

'Menstrual' migraine is a loose term encompassing the association between migraine and menstruation. The second edition of International Headache Society classification includes specific definitions for pure menstrual migraine and menstrually related migraine (Table 1)[6]. This definition was based on published studies of diary cards. They showed that migraine was most likely to occur on or between 2 days before menstruation and the first 3 days of bleeding.

Menstrual attacks are almost invariably without aura, even in women who have attacks with aura at other times of the cycle. Of note is that despite many women reporting an association with ovulation, no link between

Table 1 Classification of menstrual migraine[6]

Pure menstrual migraine

Diagnostic criteria

A. Attacks, in a menstruating woman, fulfilling criteria for *Migraine without aura*

B. Attacks occur exclusively on day 1 ± 2 (i.e. days −2 to +3) of menstruation in at least two out of three menstrual cycles and at no other times of the cycle

Menstrually related migraine

Diagnostic criteria

A. Attacks, in a menstruating woman, fulfilling criteria for *Migraine without aura*

B. Attacks occur on day 1 ± 2 (i.e. days −2 to +3) of menstruation in at least two out of three menstrual cycles and additionally at other times of the cycle

Notes

1. The first day of menstruation is day 1 and the preceding day is day −1; there is no day 0.

2. For the purposes of this classification, menstruation is considered to be endometrial bleeding resulting from either the normal menstrual cycle or from the withdrawal of exogenous progestogens, as in the case of combined oral contraceptives and cyclical hormone replacement therapy.

migraine and ovulation has been noted in prospective studies.

Etiology

In order to understand the etiology of menstrual migraine it is important to distinguish between attacks that *solely* occur around the time of menstruation, i.e. pure menstrual migraine, and attacks that *mostly* occur at the time of menstruation in women who have additional attacks at other times of the cycle, i.e. menstrually related migraine. This is because a pure hormonal mechanism is likely to be involved only in women with pure menstrual migraine. In contrast, additional non-hormonal factors are likely to be acting in women with additional non-menstrual attacks. If studies are to uncover the mechanisms responsible for menstrual migraine, it is necessary to study women in whom hormonal events are the sole association.

With this in mind, studies have considered how normal or abnormal hormonal function

might be associated with migraine. Estrogen and progesterone are the main hormones that have been studied in relation to migraine but studies comparing levels of these hormones in women with menstrual migraine versus controls have not found any convincing differences. It also seems that ovulation is not necessary to provoke menstrual attacks since some women using combined oral contraceptives (COCs) may notice migraine occurring during the pill-free interval in association with the bleed that follows withdrawal of ethinylestradiol and progestogen. Research has therefore focused on the naturally declining levels of estrogen and progesterone during the luteal phase of the menstrual cycle, coinciding with the onset of menstrual migraine.

The role of progesterone

Insufficient progesterone in the luteal phase was originally considered to be responsible for the occurrence of menstrual migraine on the basis

201

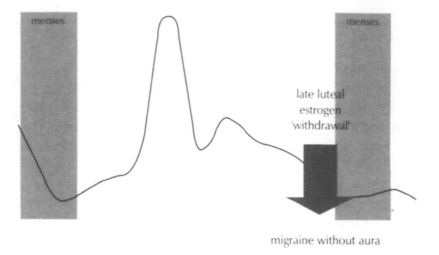

Figure 2 The role of estradiol and progesterone in menstrual migraine

of several studies that supported use of progesterone as a treatment for headache associated with menstruation[14]. However, more recent studies have failed to show efficacy. Somerville used progesterone to treat six women who had attacks of migraine during the late luteal phase[15]. Menstruation was delayed in four of these women but, in spite of this, five experienced migraine at their customary time, unrelated to plasma progesterone levels (Figure 2).

The role of estrogen

In contrast to the lack of an association with falling levels of progesterone, menstrual attacks appear to be associated, at least in some women, with falling levels, or 'withdrawal', of estrogen. The clinical evidence for this includes hormonal situations when estrogen levels falls. For example, women taking COCs who experience migraine during the pill-free week, when estrogen falls after 21 days of high levels[16]. In women using hormone replacement therapy

(HRT), migraine occurred during the week free from estrogen in the old regime of 21 days on treatment, 7 days off[17]. In a placebo-controlled double-blind crossover study of hysterectomized women with bilateral oophorectomies, increased frequency of headache was reported following courses of estrogen[18]. Migraine also recurs directly postpartum, a time when estrogen levels plummet[19].

Somerville undertook several studies in a small group of women who had a history of pure menstrual migraine in the preceding six menstrual cycles. He noted that a period of estrogen 'priming' with several days of exposure to high estrogen levels is necessary for migraine to result from estrogen 'withdrawal', such as occurs in the late luteal phase of the menstrual cycle (see for example reference 20). This would explain why migraine is not associated with ovulation. In contrast to sustained higher estrogen levels in the luteal phase, estrogen levels are relatively low in the follicular phase and do not 'prime' the system sufficiently for the drop in estrogen immediately post ovulation to have an effect.

Several other studies support Somerville's estrogen withdrawal theory. Epstein and colleagues noted that the extent of decline from peak to trough estrogen was greater in all 14 women with migraine in their study compared with eight women in the control group who did not have migraine[21]. They concluded that variation in hormonal activity might be a potentially relevant factor in all women with migraine; factors additional to the hormonal environment could account for the development of 'menstrual' attacks. Lichten and associates studied 28 postmenopausal women challenged with estrogen confirming that in women with a history of premenopausal menstrually related migraine, a drop in serum estrogen could precipitate migraine and that a period of estrogen priming was a necessary prerequisite[22].

MacGregor and co-workers studied 40 women with pure menstrual or menstrually related migraine aged 29–49 (mean 43) years. Urine was collected daily for assay over three menstrual cycles and analyzed for luteinizing hormone (LH), estrone-3-glucuronide, pregnanediol-3-glucuronide and follicle stimulating hormone (FSH)[23]. Migraine was inversely associated with urinary estrogen levels, across the menstrual cycle: attacks were significantly more likely to occur in association with falling estrogen in the late luteal/early follicular phase of the menstrual cycle and significantly less likely to occur during the subsequent part of the follicular phase during which estrogen levels rose. This association was not seen between migraine and urinary progestogen levels.

If the estrogen withdrawal theory is correct, stabilizing estrogen fluctuations by maintaining high, stable levels should prevent migraine. In favor of this, Somerville showed that migraine could be postponed by maintaining high plasma estradiol levels with an intramuscular injection of long-acting estradiol valerate in oil; migraine subsequently occurred when the plasma estradiol fell[20]. This finding also supports the lack of effect of progesterone on migraine since if progesterone was an important factor, the timing of menstrual attacks would have been unaffected by the use of estrogen supplements. The fact that administration of a short-acting estrogen did not produce the same results as the long-acting supplements confirms the hypothesis that prolonged estrogen exposure is necessary for 'withdrawal' to trigger migraine.

More recent trials using more stable routes of delivery have shown efficacy. De Lignières and associates studied 18 women with strictly defined menstrual migraine who completed a double-blind placebo-controlled crossover trial using 1.5 mg estradiol gel, which allows a mean estradiol plasma level of 80 pg/ml to be reached, or placebo daily for 7 days during three consecutive cycles.[24] Treatment was started 48 h before the earliest expected onset of migraine. Only eight menstrual attacks occurred during the 26 estrogen-treated cycles (30.8%) compared with 26 attacks during the 27 placebo cycles (96.3%). Further, attacks during estrogen treatment were considerably milder and shorter than those during placebo. Eighteen women also completed a similar trial by Dennerstein and colleagues in which 1.5 mg estradiol gel or placebo was used daily for 7 days, beginning at least 2 days prior to the expected migraine, for four cycles[25]. The difference between estradiol gel and placebo was highly significant, favoring the estradiol gel, and less medication was used during active treatment. However, the results were not as impressive as the study by De Lignières and co-workers[24]. Dennerstein and colleagues comment that this might be because women in their study had menstrually related migraine rather than pure menstrual migraine. Therefore, their migraine was only partially hormone dependent.

MacGregor and associates used 1.5 mg estradiol gel in a double-blind placebo-controlled study to prevent perimenstrual migraine attacks in 27 women with regular menstrual cycles and menstrual migraine or menstrually related migraine[23]. Each woman was treated in up to six menstrual cycles (three cycles percutaneous estradiol; three placebo). Women identified ovulation, conducting an early morning urine test each day with a commercial monitor. Estradiol gel or placebo was first applied on the tenth day following the first day that the monitor signified ovulation and continued daily until, and including, the second day of menstruation. Use of percutaneous estradiol was associated with a significant reduction in the duration and severity of migraine. No clinically relevant adverse events were reported during the study. However, as Somerville had found, there was a significant increase in the migraine immediately following cessation of active gel compared with placebo. Possible reasons for this post-gel estrogen withdrawal migraine, which will be addressed in further studies, include that the dose of estradiol was inadequate; the duration of treatment was too short; or perhaps that exogenous estrogen prevents the normal secretion of endogenous estrogen.

Estrogen patches have not been found to be as successful as estrogen gel in preventing migraine. Pfaffenrath studied 41 patients completing a trial of 50 μg estradiol patches versus placebo used daily from 2 days prior to the suspected onset of migraine, during a 4-month treatment phase[26]. No significant differences were seen between the two treatments although estradiol was slightly better than placebo in all parameters. Smits and colleagues also studied 50 μg patches versus placebo over three cycles in 20 women and also found no difference between estradiol and placebo[27]. Pradalier and associates studied two groups of 12 women using either 25 μg or 100 μg patches on day 4 and day 1 (two patches per cycle) over two cycles, and compared the results with a pretreatment cycle[28]. They found that the 100 μg dose gave a better clinical result than the 25 μg patches, raising the question of a critical level.

The suggestion from these studies is that the 25 μg and 50 μg patches are not effective in preventing menstrual migraine as they result in suboptimal doses, achieving serum estradiol levels of 25 pg/ml and 40 pg/ml, respectively. In contrast, the 100 μg patch effectively produces higher serum estradiol levels of 75 pg/ml, similar to the levels attained using 1.5 mg percutaneous estradiol.

A study of migraine in the pill-free interval of combined oral contraceptives using an estrogen patch on the last day of the pill cycle, replaced on the fourth day of the pill-free interval, also suggested that 50 μg patches are a suboptimal dose to prevent estrogen withdrawal attacks[29].

Other mechanisms[30]

Although the estrogen withdrawal mechanism is compelling, the reality is more complex since ovarian steroids play a limited role in the overall regulation of the menstrual cycle. It is more likely that menstrual cycle hormone changes play a secondary rather than primary role in 'menstrual' migraine and that hormonal changes trigger some alteration in activity of the hypothalamic–pituitary–adrenal axis, exposing susceptible women to a migraine attack. For example, estrogens are neurosteroids, known to raise levels of endorphins; aberrant opioid control of the hypothalamic–pituitary–adrenal axis has been reported in menstrual migraine. Close inter-relationships between estrogens and other brain neurotransmitters have also been confirmed, especially the catecholamines, noradrenaline, serotonin and dopamine. Fluctuating estrogen levels are associated with impaired glucose tolerance in the luteal phase of the menstrual cycle. This leads to reactive hypoglycemia at the start of menstruation, which could trigger migraine.

Other differences reported in menstrual migraine versus control groups include changes in aldosterone levels, intracellular magnesium, and platelet homeostasis.

Prostaglandins have also been implicated in menstrual migraine. In particular, entry of prostaglandins into the systemic circulation can trigger throbbing headache, nausea and vomiting. In the uterus prostaglandins are synthesized primarily by the endometrium. There is a three-fold increase in prostaglandin levels in the uterine endometrium from the follicular to the luteal phase, with a further increase during menstruation. As a result of the withdrawal of estrogen and progesterone the endometrium breaks down and prostaglandins are released. In support of this mechanism, inhibitors of prostaglandin synthesis are effective for the prevention of menstrual attacks of migraine (see below).

Clinicians will be aware that some postmenopausal women, not taking hormonal treatments, continue to have regular monthly migraine attacks. Migraine attacks can also be cyclical in men, suggesting that some central phenomenon is responsible for these cycles[31].

Presentation

A typical patient is a woman in her late 30s or early 40s reporting migraine since her teens or 20s but only noting a link with menstruation in recent years. Women with other menstrual complaints often do not recognize that the accompanying headaches are actually migraine. This is particularly the case for women who have migraine with aura, who do not recognize attacks without aura. This under-recognition of migraine by patients is compounded by a similar under-recognition of migraine by doctors.

Diagnosis

A description of attacks, coupled with a normal brief physical and neurological examination, is sufficient to diagnose migraine. Diary cards kept prospectively over a minimum of three cycles are necessary to confirm the relationship between migraine and menstruation; many women already keep a note of this in their personal diaries. Relying on the history to make the diagnosis of menstrual migraine is not recommended. An example of this problem is well illustrated by a prospective trial of oral sumatriptan 100 mg in the treatment of menstrual migraine[32]. Women who stated that more than 80% of their attacks occurred between −3 to +5 days from the onset of menstruation participated in a double-blind, placebo-controlled crossover study, conducted over four menstrual cycles. Prospective diaries revealed, however, that only 11% of participants actually met the trial criteria for menstrual migraine.

Investigations

Many women expect some sort of investigation to be undertaken, either a test of their hormones or a brain scan. However, there is no place for specific investigations in clinical practice, other than those indicated to exclude suspected secondary headache resulting from underlying pathology.

Management

Management strategies for the initial and follow-up consultations are shown in Table 2.

For the majority of women reporting menstrual attacks management does not differ from standard treatment recommendations.

Table 2 Management of menstrual migraine

First visit
Optimize attack therapy
Provide diaries
Discuss hormonal and non-hormonal predisposing factors and triggers
If taking combined oral contraceptives (COCs):
    Migraine without aura in pill-free interval: confirm with diaries and consider three to four consecutive packets (reducing
        PFI to 4-5 per year) or continuous COC use
    Migraine with aura: change to progestogen-only or non-hormonal contraception
    Worsening migraine since starting COCs: consider change to progestogen-only or non-hormonal contraception
Arrange review (usually after three menstrual cycles)

Second visit
Review efficacy of attack therapy and change as necessary
Review diaries
    Non-menstrual migraine
        Consider standard prophylaxis if abortive therapy alone inadequate
    Menstrually related migraine
        Consider anovulant hormonal contraceptives if contraception also required
        Consider hormone replacement therapy if symptoms suggestive of perimenopause
    Pure menstrual migraine
        Consider specific perimenstrual prophylaxis if periods regular and if abortive therapy alone inadequate
        Consider anovulant hormonal contraception if periods irregular and/or contraception also required
        Consider hormone replacement therapy if symptoms suggestive of perimenopause

Follow-up visits
Review efficacy of abortive therapy and change as necessary
Review diaries
Consider prophylaxis as indicated by symptoms and diaries
If estrogen supplements are used for more than three cycles and periods become irregular ovulation, and hence the
    production of endogenous progesterone, can be confirmed with blood levels of progesterone taken 7 days before
    expected menstruation, i.e. day 21 of a 28-day cycle. The level should be greater than 30 nmol/l

---

Initial strategies should include acute medication and the provision of diary cards. Effective acute treatment is usually all that is necessary, particularly if attacks only occur once or twice a month.

Symptomatic treatment

The treatment of menstrual attacks of migraine is the same as that of non-menstrual attacks. Acute treatment regimens usually include a combination of analgesics with or without prokinetic anti-emetics, non-steroidal anti-inflammatory drugs, ergot derivatives and triptans[33]. Of the triptans, both rizatriptan and sumatriptan list 'menstrually associated' migraine in their data sheets (or SmPC).

Of specific relevance to clinical practice is that compared with non-menstrual migraine, attacks occurring at the time of menstruation are more severe, last longer and are less responsive to symptomatic medication[12,34,35]. In a small study of women with menstrually related migraine, sumatriptan was less effective for the menstrual attacks (56% improvement from moderate or severe headache at baseline to mild/no headache 4 h post dose) compared with non-menstrual attacks (81% improvement)[32] (Figure 3). In both cases sumatriptan was significantly more effective than placebo.

On a practical note it is worth considering different routes of delivery to bypass gastric stasis, for example the nasal or subcutaneous route, if menstrual attacks are particularly severe. If repeated recurrence of symptoms is a problem, drugs with a longer duration of action and lower recurrence such as ergotamine or frovatriptan should be considered but clinical trial data are lacking.

Identification of non-hormonal triggers

Assuming the concept of multiple factors acting in combination to trigger migraine, hormonal factors combine with non-hormonal triggers to increase the overall susceptibility to attacks at

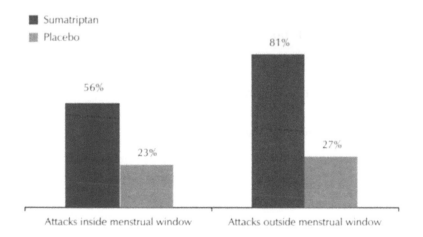

Figure 3 Efficacy of sumatriptan at 4 h post-treatment in 'menstrually associated' migraine versus non-menstrual attacks. From reference 32

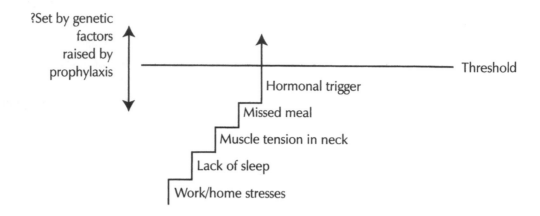

Figure 4 The 'threshold' theory for migraine. From reference 13

the time of menstruation[36] (Figure 4). Therefore, every effort should be made to identify and eliminate non-hormonal triggers. In some cases, this may reduce the frequency and severity of all attacks. In others, non-hormonal attacks are eliminated while menstrual attacks persist.

Diary cards

By the time the diary cards are reviewed at follow-up, a percentage of patients will have their attacks under control, with no need for further intervention. Another group will have attacks throughout the cycle, which are not obviously related to menstruation (Figure 5a). These women may benefit from standard prophylactic therapy, if considered necessary.

Specific prophylaxis for menstrual migraine

Only a small percentage of women will have menstrual migraine and wish to consider specific prophylaxis (Figure 5b). Depending on each woman's wishes, the regularity of the menstrual cycle, timing of attacks in relation to bleeding, presence of dysmenorrhea or menorrhagia, presence of menopausal symptoms, or need for contraception, several options can be tried, both non-hormonal and hormonal.

Although many patients favor non-drug approaches, non-drug prophylaxis of menstrual migraine appears to be ineffective[37,38].

None of the drugs and hormones recommended below are licensed for management of menstrual migraine because, although effective in clinical trials, evidence is limited. Given that there are no investigations to identify the most effective prophylactic, an empirical approach is necessary, prescribing on a named-patient basis (Table 3). Because of the fluctuating nature of migraine, it is sensible to try a method for at least two to three cycles before considering alternative prophylaxis.

Non-steroidal anti-inflammatory drugs

Non-steroidal anti-inflammatory drugs (NSAIDS), which are effective prostaglandin

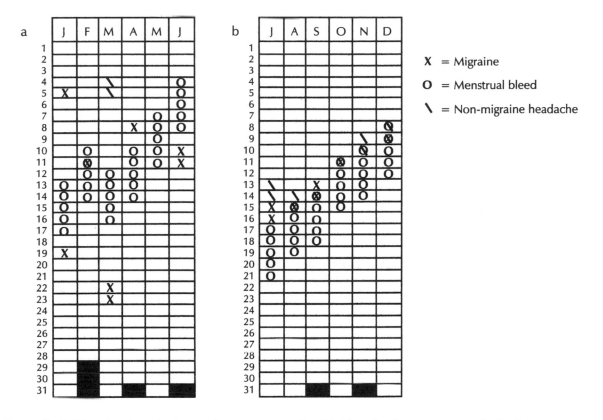

Figure 5 (a) Diary showing migraine unrelated to menstruation. (b) Diary showing pure menstrual migraine

Table 3 Use of licensed products in an unlicensed way[39]

The prescribing physician must:
Adopt an evidence-based practice, endorsed by a responsible body of professional opinion
Ensure good practice including follow-up, to comply with professional indemnity requirements. *N.B. This will often mean providing dedicated written materials because the manufacturer's insert does not apply*
Explain to the individual that it is an unlicensed prescription
Give a clear account of the risks and benefits
Obtain informed (verbal) consent and record this and the discussion in full
Finally, keep a separate record of the patient's details

inhibitors, should be tried as first-line agents for migraine attacks that start on the first to third day of bleeding, particularly in the presence of dysmenorrhea and/or menorrhagia[40]. Side-effects of NSAIDs include gastrointestinal disturbance. Misoprostol 800 μg or omeprazole 20–40 mg daily may give some gastroduodenal protection[41]. Contraindications include peptic ulcer and aspirin-induced allergy. Interactions include anticoagulants and antihypertensive agents.

Mefenamic acid is an effective migraine prophylactic and has been reported to be particularly helpful in reducing migraine associated with menorrhagia and/or dysmenorrhea[40]. A dose of 500 mg, three to four times daily, may be started either 2 or 3 days before the expected onset of menstruation, but is often effective even when started on the first day of bleeding; this is useful if periods are irregular. Treatment is usually only necessary for the first 2–3 days of bleeding.

Naproxen has also been found to be effective in the management of headache associated with dysmenorrhea. Studies using 550 mg once or twice daily perimenstrually have shown efficacy[42–44]. Fenoprofen 600 mg has been tried, taken twice daily from 3 days before the onset of menstruation until the last day of bleeding[45].

There is no evidence that the new COX-2 inhibitors (celecoxib, valdecoxib) are more effective than traditional NSAIDs. They are more costly but may provide a relative safety advantage for patients who need to use these agents for long periods of time and are especially prone to gastrointestinal complications.

Magnesium and vitamin therapy

Magnesium prolidone carboxylic acid 360 mg decreased the duration and intensity of premenstrually occurring migraine in a placebo-controlled, double-blind study of 24 women with premenstrual syndrome and migraine[46]. This study was principally aimed at identifying the effect of magnesium on a number of premenstrual problems, not just headache. The generalizability of the results to women whose menstrual headaches do not occur in association with other premenstrual symptoms is unclear. Diarrhea is the major side-effect and can sometimes be controlled by changing preparation.

Estrogen supplements

Perimenstrual estrogen can be used only when menstruation is regular and predictable. Although this regimen uses treatments normally given for HRT, it is important to note that for 'menstrual' migraine, hormones are given as supplements. This means that if the woman has an intact uterus, no additional progestogens are necessary provided that she is ovulating regularly. This is because she will be producing adequate amounts of her own progesterone to counter the effects of unopposed estrogen, which could otherwise lead to endometrial proliferation. If cycles become irregular, ovulation and hence the production of endogenous progesterone can be confirmed with blood levels of progesterone taken 7 days before expected menstruation, i.e. day 21 of a 28-day cycle. The level should be greater than 30 nmol/l.

Supplemental estrogens are not recommended for women who have estrogen-dependent tumors or other estrogen-dependent conditions, including a history of venous thromboembolism.

The recommended strategy for perimenstrual prophylaxis is estradiol gel 1.5 mg applied daily from 2–3 days before expected menstruation for 7 days[47]. This regimen may be more effective than transdermal patches as the gel produces higher, more stable levels of estrogen. Alternatively, transdermal estrogen

$100\,\mu g$ can be used from 2–3 days before expected menstruation up to the fourth or fifth day of menstruation, i.e. two twice-weekly patches or one 7-day patch, although an additional patch may be necessary if menstruation is late[47].

If side-effects are a problem (bloating, breast tenderness, leg cramps, nausea) a lower dose should be tried for the next cycle.

There is evidence that some women responding to estrogen supplements experience delayed attacks when the supplements are discontinued[23]. In these women, the duration of supplement use can be extended until day 7 of the cycle, by which time endogenous estrogen should be rising.

Continuous hormonal strategies

Suppression of cyclical ovarian activity is generally effective for the management of menstrual migraine. Notably, women who experience amenorrhea report improvement in migraine. However, even when ovulation is suppressed breakthrough bleeding can occur, often associated with migraine. Somerville and Carey hypothesized that since fluctuations in estrogen levels can occur even when ovulation is suppressed, estrogen withdrawal will still act as a migraine trigger[48].

Continuous hormonal methods are particularly useful if cycles are irregular, or when the above strategies prove ineffective despite a convincing hormonal link.

Continuous combined hormonal contraceptives

Continuous hormones, in place of the usual regime of 3 weeks of active, followed by 1 week of inactive, pills or no therapy, have been recommended based on evidence that estrogen withdrawal provokes migraine in susceptible women. No double-blind placebo-controlled trials, or even open-label trials, of this strategy in menstrual migraine have been performed. However, continuous hormonal contraceptive regimens are becoming increasingly popular and accepted for other indications, so there is extensive clinical experience of their use in this way. For women who desire contraception or have endometriosis and whose headaches are clearly linked to estrogen withdrawal, this regimen may be reasonable. If women find that continuous estrogens are associated with unacceptable breakthrough bleeding or they prefer to have a regular withdrawal 'period' there is some evidence that supplemental estrogen used in the pill-free interval can prevent migraine at this time[29].

Contraceptive doses of ethinylestradiol should not be used by women with migraine with aura because of the synergistic increased risk of ischemic stroke[49]. This is not a concern with physiological doses of estradiol.

Levonorgestrel intrauterine system (Mirena®)

This is highly effective at reducing menstrual bleeding and associated pain. It can be considered for migraine related to menorrhagia. Systemic effects are usually minor but erratic bleeding and spotting is common in the early months of use. Most women are amenorrheic within 1 year due to the effects of local progestogen on the endometrium. The treatment is not effective for women who are sensitive to estrogen withdrawal as a migraine trigger, as the majority of women still ovulate with the system in situ.

Injectable depot progestogens

These inhibit ovulation, similar to the mode of action of COCs. Although irregular bleeding can occur in early months of treatment, amenorrhea is usual with continued use. Inhibition of the normal menstrual cycle should alleviate menstrual migraine. It is therefore important to warn women who use this method that they should persevere until amenorrhea is achieved, having repeat injections earlier than is required for contraception, if necessary.

Estradiol implants or patches

These are the most effective methods of obtaining high stable estrogen levels, inhibiting ovulation. Magos and colleagues showed that implant doses large enough to suppress ovulation and produce constant plasma estrogen levels achieved a 96% response rate in 24 patients studied[50]. However, in unhyst-erectomized women, progestogen opposition is necessary to protect the endometrium, which can mimic premenstrual symptoms, including headache[51]. Although there are no clinical trials for migraine, suppression of ovulation with 100 μg patches used continuously together with continuous progestogen are likely to be effective with fewer progestogenic side-effects.

Oral progestogen-only contraceptives

In general, standard contraceptive oral pro-gestogens have little place in the management of menstrual migraine since most do not inhibit ovulation and are associated with a disrupted menstrual cycle[52]. In contrast, unlicensed higher doses of oral progestogen, sufficient to inhibit ovulation, have shown benefit[53]. On this basis

Cerazette®, a new anovulatory progestogen-only pill may have advantages over standard progestogen-only pills for women with migraine.

Gonadotropin releasing hormone analogs

These have been tried but adverse effects of estrogen deficiency, e.g. hot flushes, restrict their use[54]. The hormones are also associated with a marked reduction in bone density and should not usually be used for longer than 6 months without regular monitoring and bone densitometry. 'Add-back' continuous combined estrogen and progestogen can be given to counter these difficulties[55]. Given these limitations, in addition to increased cost, such treatment should be instigated only in specialist departments.

Hormone replacement therapy

The menopause marks a time of increased migraine. HRT can help, not only by stabilizing estrogen fluctuations associated with migraine, but also by relieving night sweats which disturb sleep.

Estrogen Studies suggest that non-oral routes of delivery of estrogen are more likely to improve migraine than oral estrogens[56,57]. Oral estrogens are associated with wide day-to-day variations in serum concentrations that could play a part in triggering migraine, particularly if coupled with a background of fluctuating endogenous estrogens in perimenopausal women. Conversely, non-oral routes such as transdermal or percutaneous routes are associated with more stable estrogen levels at physiological doses.

Tailoring treatment is particularly difficult for perimenopausal women as too high a dose, coupled with surges of endogenous estrogen, can trigger migraine aura, as well as causing symptoms of estrogen excess including nausea, fluid retention, breast tenderness and leg cramps. Kaiser and Meienberg reported on ten women seen in an ophthalmology clinic who were using transdermal estrogen patches delivering 50 μg daily[58]. Six women had a history of migraine (three migraine with aura, three migraine without aura) prior to using replacement therapy. All six women developed increased headache severity and accompanying visual scintillations. One patient with no previous history of migraine developed visual scintillations with no accompanying headache. Withdrawal of estrogens and additional prophylactic antimigrainous therapy led to marked improvement in all women, with complete loss of migraine in four patients. MacGregor reported similar case studies of development of aura associated with use of HRT[59]. Loss of aura followed reduction in the dose of estrogen.

Progestogens   Additional progestogen is necessary to prevent endometrial cancer in unhysterectomized women using estrogen replacement. This is usually given as a 12–14-day course each month. However, adverse effects are common, including perimenstrual symptoms, headaches and migraine[50,60]. Changing route from oral to transdermal progestogen can be effective. Alternatively, change the type of progestogen as side-effects are fewer with progesterone derivatives such as dydrogesterone than with testosterone derivatives such as norethisterone[61].

Progesterone is another option, available as suppositories and, in some countries, as micronized tablets. However, sedation is a common adverse effect when progesterone is given orally. Local progesterone vaginal gel can be useful in these situations. Continuous progestogen is often better tolerated that cycles of progestogen. The Mirena system can provide continuous progestogen with minimal systemic effects. Continuous oral or transdermal progestogen use is generally recommended for premenopausal women as it is often associated with erratic bleeding, which can lead to unnecessary investigations.

Other prophylactic treatments

Triptans

One open study used prophylactic oral sumatriptan in 20 women who reported a predictable association between migraine and menstruation or withdrawal bleeding from COCs, and who had shown a past response to sumatriptan[62]. Sumatriptan 25 mg t.d.s. was started 2–3 days before expected onset of perimenstrual headache and taken for 5 days. In 126 sumatriptan-treated cycles, headache was absent in 52.4% and reduced in severity by ≥ 50% in 42%.

In a double-blind, placebo-controlled trial using naratriptan 1 mg b.d. and 2.5 mg b.d. given from 2 days before the expected onset of menses for 5 days, the difference between the 1 mg dose and placebo just reached statistical significance, with 23% of patients headache-free in all treated menstrual cycles, compared with 8% of placebo-treated patients, for a therapeutic gain of 15%[63]. The 2.5 mg dose was not superior to placebo.

Results from studies using frovatriptan for perimenstrual prophylaxis, unpublished at the time of writing, appear promising.

Triptan prophylaxis of menstrual migraine is costly, and trials to date suggest a modest benefit in a relatively small population. As yet, there are no trials that compare triptan prophylaxis of menstrual migraine with other lower-cost regimens. Further, use of triptans for prophylaxis limits the choice for effective abortive therapy. No prophylactic strategy is 100% effective all of the time; abortive therapy remains the mainstay of treatment. Thus, perimenstrual prophylaxis with triptans is not a choice for the majority of women with menstrual or menstrually related migraine but may be considered for the subset of women with refractory menstrual migraine in whom other therapies fail; certainly triptan prophylaxis should be tried before resorting to other regimens that have even less evidence of safety and effectiveness.

Bromocriptine

Bromocriptine is a dopamine agonist that inhibits gonadotropin releasing hormone and LH. Use of bromocriptine can result in reduced peak luteal estradiol levels and consequent reduced premenstrual estrogen withdrawal. Further, dopamine agonists inhibit the secretion of prolactin, which has been implicated in the pathogenesis of menstrual migraine. Two studies have suggested the efficacy of bromocriptine in migraine although larger double-blind placebo-controlled studies are necessary before it can be recommended[64,65]. Further, its use is limited by side-effects of light-headedness and nausea.

Antiestrogens

Danazol, an antiestrogen, has been used with some effect, but adverse effects again restrict its use[66,67].

Tamoxifen, also an antiestrogen, has been associated with improvement in migraine[68,69]. However, a recent case study reported exacerbation of migraine associated with tamoxifen administration in a woman who had a history of menstrual migraine but who was menopausal following chemotherapy for breast cancer[70].

Surgery

Many women (and some doctors) believe that removal of the offending organs with oophorectomy and/or hysterectomy must be effective. Perhaps this is not surprising given the profound influence of the menstrual cycle on migraine. However, studies show that migraine is more likely to deteriorate after surgical menopause with bilateral oophorectomy[71]. If other medical problems require surgical menopause the effects on migraine are probably lessened by subsequent estrogen replacement therapy, as for natural menopause.

WHAT TO DO WHEN TREATMENT FAILS?

In most cases, menstrual migraine can be effectively controlled by following the above strategies. However, a few cases may be refractory, even to total suppression of the menstrual cycle. The usual reason for such treatment failure is incorrect diagnosis. Therefore, if migraine remains refractory, despite trials of several different strategies given in an adequate dose for an adequate duration, reconsider the diagnosis.

One common cause for refractory migraine is medication overuse[6]. Symptomatic drugs such as painkillers, 'triptans' or ergotamine, are effective provided that they are used intermittently and certainly no more often than 2 or 3 days a week. Frequent use of these drugs for headache can have the opposite effect, perpetuating the cycle of pain rather than relieving it.

The exact mechanism of this type of headache is unknown but it is generally believed that a disturbance of central pain systems is involved. Interestingly, only those who are prone to headaches develop this syndrome and it is not often seen in people taking daily painkillers for reasons other than headache, such as arthritis or back pain.

The only effective treatment is to stop the drugs, either immediately or by gradually reducing the amount over several weeks. Clinical studies show that up to 60% of sufferers who are withdrawn from drugs improve although it can take up to 3 months before full improvement is seen.

CONCLUSION

Many women report an association between migraine and menstruation. Most attacks can be controlled with symptomatic treatment without further intervention. Diary cards are essential to confirm pure menstrual migraine or menstrually related migraine. A variety of prophylactic options are available for these conditions, which can be tailored to individual needs.

REFERENCES

1. Stewart W, Lipton R, Celentano D, Reed M. Prevalence of migraine headache in the United States. Relation to age, income, race, and other sociodemographic factors. JAMA 1992; 267: 64–9

2. Rasmussen B, Jensen R, Schroll M, Olesen J. Epidemiology of headache in a general population: a prevalence study. J Clin Epidemiol 1991; 44: 1147–57

3. World Health Organization. Mental Health: New Understanding, New Hope. Geneva: WHO, 2001

4. Selby G, Lance J. Observations on 500 cases of migraine and allied vascular headache. J Neurol Neurosurg Psychiatry 1960; 23: 23–32

5. Blau J. Loss of migraine: when, why and how. J R Coll Physicians Lond 1987; 21: 140–2

6. Headache Classification Subcommittee of the International Headache Society. The International Classification of Headache Disorders, 2nd edn. Cephalalgia 2004; 24: 1–151

7. Blau J. Migraine: theories of pathogenesis. Lancet 1992; 339: 1202

8. Russell M, Olesen J. A nosographic analysis of the migraine aura in the general population. Brain 1996; 119: 355–61

9. Wilkinson M, Williams K, Leyton M. Observations on the treatment of an acute attack of migraine. Res Clin Stud Headache 1978; 6: 141–6

10. Headache Classification Committee of the International Headache Society. Classification and diagnostic criteria for headache disorders, cranial neuralgias and facial pain. Cephalalgia 1988; 8(Suppl 7): 1–96

11. Bille B. A 40-year follow-up of school children with migraine. Cephalalgia 1997; 17: 488–91

12. Couturier EG, Bomhof MA, Neven AK, van Duijn NP. Menstrual migraine in a representative Dutch population sample: prevalence, disability and treatment. Cephalalgia 2003; 23: 302–8

13. MacGregor EA. 'Menstrual migraine': towards a definition. Cephalalgia 1996; 16: 11–21

14. Singh I, Singh I. Progesterone in the treatment of migraine. Lancet 1947; 1:745–7

15. Somerville B. The role of progesterone in menstrual migraine. Neurology 1971; 21: 853–9

16. Whitty CW, Hockaday JM, Whitty MM. The effect of oral contraceptives on migraine. Lancet 1966; 1: 856–9

17. Kudrow L. The relationship of headache frequency to hormone use in migraine. Headache 1975; 15: 36–40

18. Dennerstein L, Laby B, Burrows G, et al. Headache and sex hormone therapy. Headache 1978; 18: 146–53

19. Stein G. Headaches in the first post partum week and their relationship to migraine. Headache 1981; 21: 201–5

20. Somerville B. The role of estradiol withdrawal in the etiology of menstrual migraine. Neurology 1972; 22: 355–65

21. Epstein M, Hockaday J, Hockaday T. Migraine and reproductive hormones throughout the menstrual cycle. Lancet 1975; 1: 543–8

22. Lichten EM, Lichten JB, Whitty A, Pieper D. The confirmation of a biochemical marker for women's hormonal migraine: the depo-estradiol challenge test. Headache 1996; 36: 367–71

23. MacGregor E, Frith A, Ellis J, Aspinall L. Estrogen 'withdrawal': a trigger for migraine? A double-blind placebo-controlled study of estrogen supplements in the late luteal phase in women with menstrually-related migraine. Cephalalgia 2003; 23: 684

24. De Lignières B, Vincens M, Mauvais-Jarvis P, et al. Prevention of menstrual migraine by percutaneous oestradiol. BMJ 1986; 293: 1540

25. Dennerstein L, Morse C, Burrows G, et al. Menstrual migraine: a double-blind trial of percutaneous estradiol. Gynecol Endocrinol 1988; 2: 113–20

26. Pfaffenrath V. Efficacy and safety of percutaneous estradiol vs. placebo in menstrual migraine. Cephalalgia 1993; 13 (Suppl 13): 244

27. Smits M, van der Meer Y, Pfeil J, et al. Perimenstrual migraine: effect of Estraderm TTS and the value of contingent negative variation and exteroceptive temporalis muscle suppression test. Headache 1994; 34: 103–6

28. Pradalier A, Vincent D, Beaulieu P, et al. Correlation between estradiol plasma level and therapeutic effect on menstrual migraine. In Rose F, ed. New Advances in Headache Research. London: Smith-Gordon, 1994: 129–32

29. MacGregor EA, Hackshaw A. Prevention of migraine in the pill-free week of combined oral contraceptives using natural estrogen supplements. J Fam Plann Reprod Healthcare 2002; 28: 27–31

30. Silberstein SD, Merriam GR. Sex hormones and headache. J Pain Symptom Manage 1993; 8: 98–114

31. Medina J, Diamond S. Cyclical migraine. Arch Neurol 1981; 38: 343–4

32. Gross M, Barrie M, Bates D, et al. The efficacy of sumatriptan in menstrual migraine. Eur J Neurol 1995; 2: 144–5

33. Steiner T, MacGregor E, Davies P. British Association for the Study of Headache. Guidelines for all doctors in the diagnosis and management of migraine and tension-type headache. Management Guidelines, 2nd edn. 2004. www.bash.org.uk

34. Visser WH, Jaspers NM, de Vriend RH, Ferrari MD. Risk factors for headache recurrence after sumatriptan: a study in 366 migraine patients. Cephalalgia 1996; 16: 264–9

35. MacGregor EA, Hackshaw A. Prevalence of migraine on each day of the natural menstrual cycle. Neurology 2004; 63: 351–3

36. Amery W, Vandenbergh V. What can precipitating factors teach us about the pathogenesis of migraine? Headache 1987; 27: 146–50

37. Solbach P, Sargent J, Coyne L. Menstrual migraine headache: results of a controlled, experimental, outcome study of non-drug treatments. Headache 1984; 24: 75–8

38. Szekely B, Botwin D, Eidelman B, et al. Nonpharmacological treatment of menstrual headache: relaxation-biofeedback behavior therapy and person-centred insight therapy. Headache 1986; 26: 86–92

39. Mann R. Unlicensed medicines and the use of drugs in unlicensed indications. In Goldberg A, Dodds-Smith I, eds. Pharmaceutical Medicine and the Law. London: Royal College of Physicians, 1991: 103–10

40. Johnson R, Hornabrook R, Lambie D. Comparison of mefenamic acid and propranolol with placebo in migraine prophylaxis. Acta Neurol Scand 1986; 73: 490–2

41. Gøtzsche P. Non-steroidal anti-inflammatory drugs. BMJ 2000; 320: 1058–61

42. Sargent J, Solbach P, Damasio H, et al. A comparison of naproxen sodium to propranolol hydrochloride and a placebo control for the prophylaxis of migraine headache. Headache 1985; 25: 320–4

43. Szekely B, Meeryman S, Post G. Prophylactic effects of naproxen sodium on perimenstrual headache: a double-blind, placebo-controlled study. Cephalalgia 1989; 9: 452–3

44. Nattero G, Allais G, De Lorenzo C, et al. Biological and clinical effects of naproxen sodium in patients with menstrual migraine. Cephalalgia 1991; 11(Suppl 11): 201–2

45. Diamond S. Menstrual migraine and non-steroidal anti-inflammatory agents. Headache 1984; 24: 52

46. Facchinetti F, Montorsi S, Borella P, et al. Magnesium prevention of premenstrual migraine: a placebo controlled study. In Rose FC, ed. New Advances in Headache Research. London: Smith-Gordon, 1991: 329–32

47. MacGregor E. Migraine in Women, 3rd edn. London: Martin Dunitz, 2003

48. Somerville B, Carey M. The use of continuous progestogen contraception in the treatment of migraine. Med J Aust 1970; 1: 1043–5

49. MacGregor E, Guillebaud J. Recommendations for clinical practice. Combined oral contraceptives, migraine and ischaemic stroke. Br J Fam Plann 1998; 24: 53–60

50. Magos A, Zilkha K, Studd J. Treatment of menstrual migraine by estradiol implants. J Neurol Neurosurg Psychiatry 1983; 46: 1044–6

51. Magos A, Brewster E, Singh R, et al. The effects of norethisterone in postmenopausal women on estrogen replacement therapy: a model for the premenstrual syndrome. Br J Obstet Gynaecol 1986; 93: 1290–6

52. Chumnijaraki T, Sunyavivat S, Onthuam Y, Udomprasetgurl V. Study on the factors associated with contraception discontinuation in Bangkok. Contraception 1984; 29: 241–8

53. Davies P, Fursdon-Davies C, Rees M. Progestogens for menstrual migraine. J Br Menopause Soc 2003; 9: 134

54. Holdaway I, Parr C, France J. Treatment of a patient with severe menstrual migraine using the depot LHRH analogue Zoladex. Aust N Z J Obstet Gynaecol 1991; 31: 164–5

55. Murray S, Muse K. Effective treatment of severe menstrual migraine headaches with gonadotropin-releasing hormone agonist and 'add-back' therapy. Fertil Steril 1997; 67: 390–3

56. MacGregor EA. Effects of oral and transdermal estrogen replacement on migraine. Cephalalgia 1999; 19: 124–5

57. Nappi R, Cagnacci A, Granella F, et al. Course of primary headaches during hormone replacement therapy. Maturitas 2001; 38: 157–63

58. Kaiser H, Meienberg O. Deterioration of onset of migraine under estrogen replacement therapy in the menopause. J Neurol Neurosurg Psychiatry 1993; 240: 195–7

59. MacGregor EA. Estrogen replacement: a trigger for migraine aura? Headache 1999; 39: 674–8

60. Vestergaard P, Pernille Hermann A, Gram J, et al. Improving compliance with hormonal replacement therapy in primary osteoporosis prevention. Maturitas 1997; 28: 137–45

61. Panay N, Studd J. Progestogen intolerance and compliance with hormone replacement therapy in menopausal women. Hum Reprod Update 1997; 3: 159–71

62. Newman L, Lipton R, Lay C, Solomon S. A pilot study of oral sumatriptan as intermittent prophylaxis of menstruation-related migraine. Neurology 1998; 51: 307–9

63. Newman L, Mannix L, Landy S, et al. Naratriptan as short-term prophylaxis of menstrually associated migraine: a randomized, double-blind, placebo-controlled study. Headache 2001; 41: 248–56

64. Hockaday J, Peet K, Hockaday T. Bromocriptine in migraine. Headache 1976; 16: 109–14

65. Herzog A. Continuous bromocriptine therapy in menstrual migraine. Neurology 1997; 48: 101–2

66. Calton G, Burnett J. Danazol and migraine. N Engl J Med 1984; 310: 721–722

67. Lichten E, Bennett R, Whitty A, Daoud Y. Efficacy of danazol in the control of hormonal migraine. J Reprod Med 1991; 36: 419–24

68. Powles T. Prevention of migrainous headaches by tamoxifen. Lancet 1986; 2: 1344

69. O'Dea J, Davis E. Tamoxifen in the treatment of menstrual migraine. Neurology 1990; 40: 1470–1

70. Mathew P, Fung F. Recapitulation of menstrual migraine with tamoxifen. Lancet 1999; 353: 467–8

71. Dalton K. Discussion on the aftermath of hysterectomy and oophorectomy. Proc R Soc Med 1956; 50: 415–18

The perimenopause · 15

V. Ravnikar and M. Rees

INTRODUCTION

Menopause is a natural phenomenon that occurs in all women as they age and enter their sixth decade of life. It is often preceded by irregular menstruation or perimenopause with great variability in cycle length[1]. While population studies with objective measurement of menstrual blood loss have shown that menstrual flow does not increase significantly nor does it get less as women get older, a common complaint in the perimenopausal years is that of unpredictable excessive bleeding[2]. This may be due to a greater frequency of anovular cycles. The term 'perimenopausal menstrual chaos' may be usefully applied.

Estrogen deficiency occurs naturally with the menopause due to oocyte depletion resulting from follicular atresia. Menopausal symptoms, usually hot flushes and vaginal dryness, often start in the perimenopause. Replacement with estrogen combined with progestogen is well recognized to treat these symptoms, but duration of use is controversial. It is also uncertain as to whether estrogen started in the perimenopause can prevent major disease entities such as heart disease, osteoporosis and dementia as randomized trials such as the Women's Health Initiative (WHI) have mainly studied women over the age of 60[3,4].

Assessment and treatment of the perimenopause with an evaluation of the current controversies in management are covered in this chapter.

DEFINITIONS

The menopause is defined as the cessation of the menstrual cycle, and is derived from the Greek *menos*, month and *pausos*, an ending. Various definitions are in use and those based on the Stages of Reproductive Aging Workshop (STRAW) are detailed below[5]:

(1) *Menopause* is defined as the absence of menses for at least 1 year in the fifth or sixth decade of life. In the United States, the average age of menopause is 51 years. Current smoking, lower educational attainment, being separated/widowed/divorced, non-employment, and history of heart disease are all independently associated with earlier natural menopause, while parity, prior use of oral contraceptives, and Japanese race/ethnicity were associated with later age at natural menopause[6].

(2) The *perimenopause*, or transition, is defined as the 2–8 years preceding the menopause and the 1 year after the last menstrual period which usually occurs in the sixth

decade of life in the United States. Thus, the perimenopause can last for several years and is defined by lack of consistent ovulation and, therefore, of relative or absolute progesterone deficiency. As a result, patients have irregular cycles either with shortened follicular phases or with intermittent oligomenorrhea.

(3) *Premature menopause* is defined as menopause occurring before the age of 40 and can be associated with chromosome abnormalities, autoimmune endocrine disease and metabolic disorders such as galactosemia. This is covered in Chapter 8.

INVESTIGATIONS

Endocrine

Follicle stimulating hormone (FSH) levels are only helpful if the diagnosis of ovarian failure is in doubt and the levels are reported in the menopausal range (over 30 IU/l). In the perimenopause the daily variation in FSH levels renders this parameter of limited value. There is little need to check FSH levels in women with vasomotor symptoms over the age of 45. A blood test indicating a FSH level > 30 μIU/ml is diagnostic of poor ovarian activity but will not predict the date of the last menstrual period[7].

Endometrial assessment

There is no need to assess the endometrium routinely before starting hormone replacement therapy (HRT) in women with no abnormal bleeding since the incidence of endometrial cancer is < 0.1%[8]. However, it is essential in those with abnormal bleeding, e.g. a sudden change in menstrual pattern, intermenstrual bleeding or postcoital bleeding. When taking HRT, women with abnormal bleeding again need investigation. With sequential HRT (the treatment modality used in perimenopausal women), abnormal bleeding is denoted by a change in pattern of withdrawal bleeds or breakthrough bleeding. Relevant risk factors for endometrial cancer should be sought in the history, e.g. nulliparity, late menopause, diabetes, obesity, chronic anovulation, use of unopposed estrogens and a family history of endometrial cancer.

The main methods of assessment are transvaginal ultrasound, endometrial biopsy and hysteroscopy and are detailed in Chapter 5 on menorrrhagia.

Skeletal assessment

The perimenopause is a time when the need for skeletal assessment should be made. Risk factors for osteoporosis include systemic corticosteroid use, a family history especially with a first-degree relative, premature menopause and low body mass index. The gold standard for assessment of bone status is the bone mineral density measurement. Bone mineral density predicts fracture and can be used in combination with age to predict absolute rates of fracture[9]. The main sites for measurement are the spine (L_1 or L_2 to L_4) and various regions at the hip. There are some difficulties in measuring the spine as kyphosis, scoliosis and aortic calcification can lead to falsely elevated values of bone mineral density. Therefore it is now recommended that the best site to measure for diagnosis is the hip. Total hip or neck of femur bone mineral density are the most commonly used measurements.

The World Health Organization has developed criteria for interpreting bone densitometry tests. The T score compares the individual bone density (g/m^2) with the young normal mean value and expresses the difference as a standard deviation score. The definition of normal is therefore a T score of not more than -1.0 SD below the young adult mean, osteopenia between -1.0 and -2.5 below, osteoporosis as -2.5 below the mean and severe osteoporosis, the latter with a fracture. A bone density measurement of between 0 to -1.0 SD below the mean is considered normal.

SYMPTOMS OF ESTROGEN DEFICIENCY IN PERIMENOPAUSAL WOMEN

The most common symptoms are hot flushes, night sweats and vaginal dryness (Table 1).

Hot flushes and night sweats

One of the prime early features of the menopausal transition is the vasomotor episode

better known as the hot flush and can occur prior to the cessation of menstrual bleeding[10].

Hot flushes can occur at any time of the day and at night, when normal sleep patterns may be disturbed. They affect about 50% of perimenopausal women[10]. Chronically disturbed sleep can in turn lead to insomnia, irritability and difficulties with short-term memory and concentration[11].

The actual hypothalamic thermoregulatory event is poorly understood. Serotonin and its receptors in the central nervous system have been implicated[12].

Vaginal dryness

A common symptom of estrogen deficiency in the perimenopause is vaginal dryness starting before periods cease[10,13]. It may affect about one-third of women and will lead to dyspareunia in 16%[10].

TREATMENT OF ESTROGEN DEFICIENCY SYMPTOMS IN THE PERIMENOPAUSE

Systemic hormone replacement therapy

Systemic HRT is highly effective in alleviating hot flushes and night sweats[14]. HRT consists of an estrogen, combined with a progestogen in non-hysterectomized women[15]. Progestogens are given sequentially with the estrogen in perimenopausal women resulting in a withdrawal bleed. Continuous administration of estrogen and progestogen is only suitable for postmenopausal women because of the high risk of irregular bleeding if used in the perimenopause. Different routes of admin-

Table 1 Frequency of 27 complaints at three different climacteric phases in 1250 Dutch Caucasian perimenopausal women. Adapted from reference 10

Complaints	n	%
Flushing	607	49
Night-time sweating	631	51
Daytime sweating	556	45
Vaginal dryness	366	29
Vaginal itching	293	23
Pain during intercourse	204	16
Insomnia	592	47

istration are employed: oral, transdermal, subcutaneous, intranasal and vaginal. There is extensive current debate over the relative merits of the oral versus the non-oral route. Currently there appears to be no clear advantage of the transdermal over the oral route. Furthermore, all estrogens, regardless of the route of administration, eventually pass through the liver and are recycled by the enterohepatic circulation. Thus in routine clinical practice the oral route is the usual first line of treatment unless there is a pre-existing medical condition. Some practitioners, however, prefer to embark on transdermal therapy.

Estrogens

Two types of estrogen are available: synthetic and natural. Synthetic estrogens such as ethinylestradiol and mestranol are less suitable for HRT because of their greater metabolic impact. Natural estrogens include estradiol, estrone and estriol mainly chemically synthesized from soya beans or yams. Conjugated equine estrogens contain about 50–65% estrone sulfate and the remainder consists of equine estrogens, mainly equilin sulfate. These may also be classified as 'natural'.

Progestogens

The progestogens used in HRT are almost all synthetic, are structurally different to progesterone and are also derived from plant sources. Currently they are mainly administered orally, though norethisterone and levonorgestrel are available in transdermal patches combined with estradiol, and levonorgestrel can be delivered directly to the uterus. Progesterone is formulated as a 4% vaginal gel and is licensed

for use in HRT, but availability varies worldwide.

Progestogens are divided into two main groups:

(1) 17-hydroxyprogesterone derivatives (dydrogesterone, medroxy/progesterone acetate);

(2) 19-nortestosterone derivatives (norethisterone, norgestrel).

Other gestagens such as dienogest, drospirenone, trimegestone and norgestimate, are also being used in HRT.

Progestogens are added to estrogens to reduce the increased risk of endometrial hyperplasia and carcinoma which occurs with unopposed estrogen. Progestogen can either be given for 10–14 days every 4 weeks, or for 14 days every 13 weeks[15,16]. The first leads to monthly bleeds and the second to 3-monthly bleeds. Progestogen must be given to women who have undergone endometrial ablative techniques since it cannot be assumed that all the endometrium has been removed, even if prolonged amenorrhea has been achieved (see Chapter 10).

The intrauterine system (Mirena) delivers levonorgestrel to the endometrium, and can provide the progestogen component of HRT[17]. The estrogen can then be given by whatever route is acceptable to the individual woman. It also provides a solution to the problems of erratic and heavy bleeding and contraception in the perimenopause. It is also the only way in which a 'no-bleed' regimen can be achieved in perimenopausal women.

Local estrogen therapy

Some women do not wish, or cannot tolerate, systemic HRT and simply require relief of vaginal symptoms. Synthetic estrogens should be avoided since they are well absorbed from the vagina. The options available are low-dose natural estrogens such as vaginal estriol by cream or pessary, or estradiol by tablet or ring. Long-term treatment is required since symptoms return on cessation of therapy. With the recommended dose regimens no adverse endometrial effects should be incurred and a progestogen need not be added for endometrial protection with such low-dose preparations[15].

Non-estrogen based treatments for estrogen-deficiency symptoms

Progestogens such as norethisterone 5 mg/day or megestrol acetate 40 mg/day can be effective in controlling hot flushes and night sweats[15]. In such doses norethisterone affords some limited protection to the skeleton, but there are no data at present regarding megestrol acetate. Furthermore, in doses that achieve vasomotor symptom control the risk of venous thrombo-embolism is increased[18].

There is increasing evidence that selective serotonin re-uptake inhibitors (SSRIs) such as venlafaxine, paroxetine and fluoxetine are effective in treating hot flushes, increasing the range of options where estrogen is contra-indicated[19,20].

Propanolol is now little used because studies of its effects have produced conflicting results. Clonidine 50–75 mg twice daily is also of limited value apart from its effectiveness for hot flushes.

Vaginal bioadhesive moisturisers are long acting compared to simple lubricants and help restore the protective acidic pH and may be useful for vaginal dryness[21].

PREVENTION AND TREATMENT OF OSTEOPOROSIS IN PERIMENOPAUSAL WOMEN

There is evidence from randomized controlled trials (including WHI) that HRT reduces the risk of both spine and hip as well as other osteoporotic fractures[22]. The 'standard' bone-conserving doses of estrogen were considered to be estradiol 2 mg, conjugated equine estrogens 0.625 mg and transdermal 50 μg patch. However, it is now evident that half these doses also conserve bone mass[23]. The most recent epidemiological studies suggest that for HRT to be an effective method of preventing fracture continuous and life-long use is required[24]. Regulatory authorities such as those in the UK have advised that HRT should not be used as a first-line treatment for osteoporosis prevention as the risks outweigh the benefits. While alternatives to HRT use are available for the prevention and treatment of osteoporosis in elderly women, estrogen may still remain the best option particularly in perimenopausal and/or symptomatic women. Few data are available on the efficacy of alternatives such as bisphosphonates in perimenopausal women.

We have long-term data showing lower fracture rates and bone loss in women who used estrogen for two decades[25,26]. Studies of alternatives for preventing fractures are mainly limited to elderly postmenopausal women either at risk of osteoporosis or with established disease. Little is known for perimenopausal women in their 50s and their long-term safety over 20 years is not known. Most data for bisphosphonates were obtained in women who already had osteoporosis[27,28]. In perimenopausal women bisphosphonates have shown stabil-ization of bone density but no difference in fracture rate compared with placebo[29]. The long-term (> 10 years) use of bisphosphonates might be beneficial, but they could possibly make bone more brittle due to profound suppression of bone formation rates[30]. The data for teriparatide (parathyroid hormone) are also limited to postmenopausal women with osteoporosis and although fractures are reduced at the spine, this has not been demonstrated at the hip[31]. Raloxifene has been studied also in osteoporotic women and only reduces the risk of vertebral not hip fracture[32]. Similarly evidence for calcium and vitamin D is also confined to elderly women[33]. Thus, until data are available to show that alternatives to HRT are suitable for preventing fractures 20 years in the future estrogen remains the best option for perimenopausal women.

CLINICAL STUDIES OF HORMONE REPLACEMENT THERAPY THAT HAVE INFLUENCED PRACTICE

Three studies published since 1998 have greatly affected gynecological practice and prescribing of HRT. Previously there had been a tendency to believe that HRT was a universal panacea. There were two randomized placebo-controlled trials, Heart and Estrogen/progestin Replacement Study (HERS) and the WHI[3,34,35]. In both of these the majority of women were aged over 60. It is therefore debatable as to whether the findings from an asymptomatic postmenopausal cohort can be applied to symptomatic perimenopausal women. The third, the Million Women Study (MWS), is an observational study and the first publication presented data on breast cancer risk in 2003[36]. These studies have led to more focused prescribing.

Heart and Estrogen/progestin Replacement Study

The effect of hormones on the secondary prevention of heart disease in women was examined in the HERS. Performed on 2763 postmenopausal women with established coronary heart disease (CHD), the two arms of the study were conjugated equine estrogens 0.625 mg combined with medroxyprogesterone acetate 2.5 mg, and placebo. The trial ended at 4.1 years since, instead of showing protection against heart disease, there was an increase in events in the first year with a subsequent null effect the following years (relative risk (RR) 0.99; 95% confidence interval (CI) 0.80–1.22)[34]. There were no differences between non-fatal myocardial infarction, CHD death, unstable angina or coronary revascularization between the two groups. Since there was a question as to whether or not the trial was ended too early, an open-label arm of the HERS II study was continued, for 2.7 years, and this again showed a null effect[35]. Therefore, HERS and HERS II proved that after 6.8 years estrogen/progestin therapy did not reduce the risk of recurrent coronary disease.

Women's Health Initiative

The early 1990s saw the evolution of the WHI, designed to examine various strategies for the prevention and control of some of the most common causes of morbidity and mortality among postmenopausal women[3]. Postmenopausal women ranging in age from 50 to 79 years were enrolled into either a clinical trial (CT) that would eventually include about 64 500 women, or an observational study (OS) that would involve about 100 000 women. The

CT was designed to allow randomized controlled evaluation of three distinct interventions:

(1) A low-fat eating pattern, hypothesized to prevent breast cancer and colorectal cancer and, secondarily, CHD;

(2) HRT, hypothesized to reduce the risk of CHD and other cardiovascular diseases and, secondarily, to reduce the risk of hip and other fractures, with increased breast cancer risk as a possible adverse outcome;

(3) Calcium and vitamin D supplementation, hypothesized to prevent hip fractures and, secondarily, other fractures and colorectal cancer.

Overall benefit-versus-risk assessment was a central focus in each of the three CT components. Women who proved to be ineligible for, or who were unwilling to enrol in the CT components were invited to enrol in the OS. At their 1-year anniversary of randomization, CT women were invited to be further randomized into the calcium and vitamin D (CaD) trial, which was projected to include 45 000 women. Both hormone therapy arms have been stopped; the combined arm in 2002 and the estrogen-only arm in 2004.

Although the reason for stopping the combined arm was primarily because the risk of invasive breast cancer exceeded the pre-determined cut-off point for this adverse effect, it was the lack of benefit with regard to cardiovascular disease prevention that attracted the most attention. In industrialized countries cardiovascular disease accounts for about a quarter of total mortality in women over 50 (Table 2 and Figure 1)[37]. However, the excess risk of adverse outcomes in women aged 50–59 were small: 5 for CHD, 4 for stroke and 5 for breast cancer per 10 000 women per year of use.

Million Women Study

The aim of the MWS is to investigate the effects of HRT on the health of women attending the National Health Service Breast Screening Programme (NHSBSP) in the UK. Between 1996 and 2001, 1 084 110 women aged between 50 and 64 years who were invited to attend 66 of the 100 UK breast screening units completed a questionnaire about their lifestyle, socio-economic background, reproductive and medical history and HRT use.

Analysis was restricted to postmenopausal women ($n = 828 923$) whose mean age was 55.9 years. Overall, 50% of women had used HRT at some time; 33% were current HRT users at the time of questionnaire completion with a mean duration of use of 5.8 years. During the average follow-up for cancer incidence of 2.6 years, 9364 incident breast cancers were diagnosed (at

Table 2 The main causes of death in women over the age of 50 in England and Wales in 2000. The numbers for osteoporosis and Alzheimer's disease are probably underestimates because these are often not accurately reported on death certificates. From reference 37

Disease	Number of women
Heart disease	47 887
Stroke	35 528
Breast cancer	10 035
Colon cancer	4 597
Osteoporosis	968
Alzheimer's disease	1 542
Endometrial cancer	852
Blood clots (VTE)	1 115
Road traffic accidents	372
All reasons	268 300

VTE, venous thromboembolism

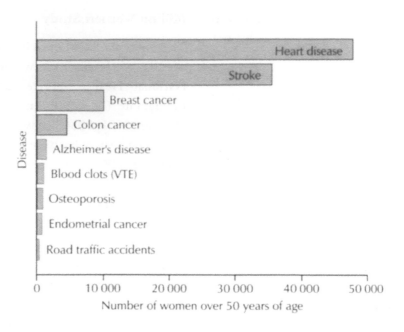

Figure 1 Diagrammatic presentation of Table 2 showing main causes of death. VTE, venous thromboembolism

a mean of 1.2 years from recruitment). The RR of breast cancer for current HRT users was 1.66 (95% CI 1.58–1.75); risk increased with increasing total duration of use but past use had no significant effect. Estimates varied by the HRT type (i.e. unopposed estrogen RR 1.30 (95% CI 1.21–1.40); combined HRT RR 2.00 (95% CI 1.88–2.12); tibolone RR 1.45 (95% CI 1.25–1.68)) but were unaffected by the specific estrogen or progestogen prescribed, pattern of progestogen administration or route of administration (vaginal preparations were not evaluated). The only factor reported to modify (i.e. increase) risk was a body mass index of $< 25\,kg/m^2$ but no specific details were given in the paper.

Five-hundred and seventeen women who were diagnosed with breast cancer during the mean 4.1 year follow-up died from their disease; the average time between diagnosis and death

was 1.7 years. Compared with past HRT users, current use at baseline was reported to increase breast cancer mortality (RR 1.22; 95% CI 1.00–1.48) but this was of borderline statistical significance ($p = 0.05$).

The MWS design, analysis and conclusions have been questioned[38]. The higher-risk estimates reported in comparison with the randomized WHI study, especially the estrogen-alone arm which found no increased risk, probably reflect the observational nature of the MWS[39]. The reported increase in breast cancer risk with the MWS after an apparently short duration of exposure (i.e. < 1–2 years) can be attributed to an underestimation of the total duration of HRT exposure as the risk estimates presented were based on HRT use at recruitment. The study investigators did not adjust the total duration of use to account for the likely continued use of HRT in the period between recruitment and cancer diagnosis (i.e. mean of 1.2 years). The results of the MWS should be interpreted in the context of completed/ongoing placebo-controlled HRT trials and the knowledge that the data provided are probably representative of about 25% of all women in the UK in the 50–64-year age group (based on uptake for the first, prevalent NHSBSP round of 75%, MWS questionnaire completion in attendees of 50% and the number of UK screening centers that participated in the study, 66 out of 94)[40,41]. Differences between women attending or not attending the NHSBSP and between attendees who agreed or declined to participate in the study cannot be easily controlled for. The contrasting findings of the WHI estrogen-alone arm to those of MWS suggest that the latter study has grossly overestimated the risk of breast cancer.

EFFECTS OF HERS, WHI AND MWS ON PRESCRIPTIONS OF HORMONE REPLACEMENT THERAPY

Since publication of these studies many women have stopped HRT often without consulting their doctors. In the USA annual hormone therapy prescriptions had increased from 58 million in 1995 to 90 million in 1999, representing approximately 15 million women per year, then remained stable until June 2002[42]. Following the publication of the WHI results in July 2002, hormone therapy prescriptions declined in successive months. Small increases were observed in vaginal formulations and in new prescriptions for low-dose estrogen-alone therapy. In the UK a survey in one general practice found that 43% of women who had stopped HRT had done so without consulting their family doctor[43].

ALTERNATIVE AND COMPLEMENTARY THERAPIES

Many women use alternative and complemenatary therapies believing them to be safer and 'more natural' especially in the light of adverse publicity regarding the standard pharmacopeia. In the USA a survey undertaken in 1998 estimated that out-of-pocket expenditure on alternative therapies totaled $27 billion per year[44]. In the UK one survey found that about 11% of the adult population had visited at least one therapist in the past 12 months. Further, a survey of women attending a menopause clinic in the West Midlands in the UK showed that 43% were using over-the-counter supplements[46]. However, the evidence from randomized trials that complementary and alternative therapies improve menopausal symptoms or conserve bone mass is poor. A major concern is those which may interact with other therapies.

Phytoestrogens

Phytoestrogens are plant substances that are structurally or functionally similar to estradiol and which are found in many foods. The preparations used vary from enriched foods such as bread and drinks (soy milk) to tablets. They consist of a number of classes of which the isoflavones and lignans are the most important in humans. Isoflavones occur in high concentrations in soybeans, chick peas and possibly other legumes as well as clovers. Lignans are found in cereal bran, whole cereals, vegetables, legumes and fruits but oilseeds such as flaxseed contain the highest concentrations. The major isoflavones are genistein and daidzein (Figure 2).

The major lignans are enterolactone and enterodiol.

The role of phytoestrogens has stimulated considerable interest since populations consuming a diet high in isoflavones such as the Japanese appear to have a lower incidence of menopausal vasomotor symptoms, cardiovascular disease, osteoporosis, breast, colon, endometrial and ovarian cancers. However, epidemiological studies need to be supported by data with analyses of the isoflavone content of foods and measures of their bioavailability[47].

Randomized placebo-controlled trials, are required. With regard to menopausal symptoms the evidence is conflicting for both soy and derivatives from red clover (see for example references 48 and 49). Similarly there are also debates about the effects on lipoproteins, endothelial function and blood pressure. Nevertheless, in the USA, the Food and Drug Administration has approved food or food substances containing specific amounts of soy protein to reduce the risk of heart disease.

Soy phytoestrogens and the synthetic isoflavone ipriflavone may maintain bone mass but the evidence is conflicting[50]. Additionally, ipriflavone in one study induced lymphocytopenia in a significant number of women[51]. Further studies are underway, including a European Union study (PHYTOS) which should help to further quantify the relative importance of these compounds and define optimal dose for bone-preserving effects[50].

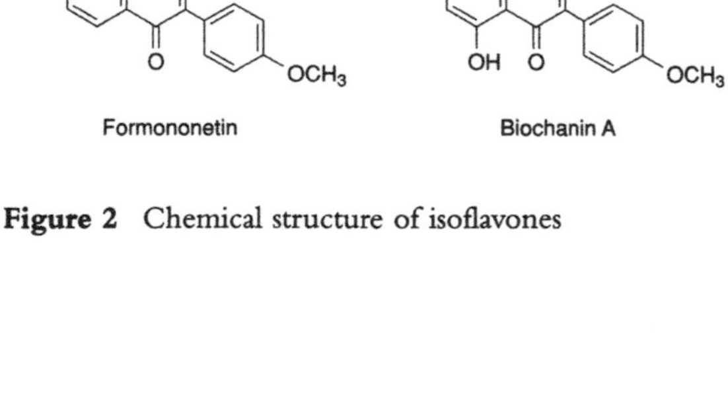

Herbalism

Herbalism needs to be used with caution in women with a contraindication to estrogen since some herbs, e.g. ginseng, have estrogenic properties. There can be interactions with anticoagulants, serotonin re-uptake inhibitors and antiepileptics. Furthermore, there is little control over the quality of the products; thus it is unusual to know what is actually in herbal preparations and dietary supplements[52]. Severe adverse reactions including renal and liver failure and cancer have recently been reported[53]. Moreover, some preparations contain high levels of heavy metals such as arsenic, lead, and mercury. The safety of some herbs such as aloe vera, kava kava and milk thistle are being tested.

Black cohosh has been certified by the German Commission E to have a favorable risk–benefit ratio for use in 'climacteric neurovegetative complaints'. It has also been found to be beneficial for menopausal complaints. The precise mechanism of action is unclear, but some of the constituents bind to estrogen and serotonin receptors[54].

St John's Wort can be used successfully to treat depression and has been tested in randomized controlled trials and may also help with menopausal complaints. There are concerns that it is a liver enzyme inducer, and could potentially interact with HRT[55].

Figure 2 Chemical structure of isoflavones

Ginseng is another popular therapy. However, it does not appear to improve vasomotor symptoms[56].

Progesterone and wild yam transdermal creams

Progesterone creams are being advocated for the treatment of menopausal symptoms and skeletal protection. They have been recently examined in a randomized controlled trial. Although no protective effect on bone density was found after 1 year, a significant improvement in vasomotor symptoms was seen in the treated group[57]. There are concerns that women may use progesterone creams for endometrial protection. Studies so far are short term and results are conflicting[58,59]. On current evidence women using such a combination are increasing their risk of endometrial cancer, and the practice should be discouraged. Wild yam cream is also popular, but no evidence shows any effect on menopausal symptoms and no evidence shows that it is safe. Claims have been made that steroids such as diosgenin in yams (*Dioscorea villosa*) are converted in the body to progesterone, but this is biochemically impossible in humans.

Other complementary therapies

Other complementary therapies include acupressure, acupuncture, Alexander technique, Ayurveda, osteopathy and Reiki. These have been covered in recent reviews, and need further examination in relation to the perimenopause[60].

CONCLUSION

The perimenopause is a time where women may experience menstrual chaos as well as symptoms of estrogen deficiency leading to concerns regarding osteoporosis. There has been significant controversy about the use of HRT in management of the perimenopause. However, it still remains the best option since non-estrogen based therapies for osteoporosis have mainly been studied in older women and those for hot flushes have only been examined in short-term trials. Alternative and complementary therapies have proved attractive but data are lacking regarding safety and efficacy and well-designed studies are required.

PRACTICE POINTS

Common perimenopausal complaints

- Hot flushes and night sweats affect 50% of women
- Vaginal dryness affects 29% of women
- Erratic menstruation will encompass both long and short menstrual cycles
- Excessive menstrual bleeding may be related to anovular cycles

Treatment of menopausal symptoms

Hormonal

- Systemic sequential estrogen and progestogen therapy
- Vaginal estrogen
- Intrauterine levonorgestrel

Non-hormonal

- Selective serotonin re-uptake inhibitors
- Vaginal lubricants

REFERENCES

1. Vollman RF. The Menstrual Cycle. Philadelphia: WB Saunders, 1977

2. Hallberg L, Hogdahl AM, Nilsson L, Rybo G. Menstrual blood loss – a population study. Variation at different ages and attempts to define normality. Acta Obstet Gynecol Scand 1966; 45: 320–51

3. Writing Group for the Women's Health Initiative Investigators. Risks and benefits of estrogen plus progestin in healthy postmenopausal women: principal results from the Women's Health Initiative randomized controlled trial. JAMA 2002; 288: 321–33

4. Naftolin F, Taylor HS, Karas R, et al; Women's Health Initiative. The Women's Health Initiative could not have detected cardio-protective effects of starting hormone therapy during the menopausal transition. Fertil Steril 2004; 81: 1498–501

5. Soules MR, Sherman S, Parrot E, et al. Executive summary: Stages of Reproductive Aging Workshop (STRAW). Fertil Steril 2001; 76: 874–8

6. Gold EB, Bromberger J, Crawford S, et al. Factors associated with age at natural menopause in a multiethnic sample of midlife women. Am J Epidemiol 2001; 153: 865–74

7. Burger HG, Dudley EC, Robertson DM, Dennerstein L. Hormonal changes in the menopause transition. Recent Prog Horm Res 2002; 57: 257–75

8. Korhonen MO, Symons JP, Hyde BM, et al. Histologic classification and pathologic findings for endometrial biopsy specimens obtained from 2964 perimenopausal and postmenopausal women undergoing screening for continuous hormones as replacement therapy (CHART 2 Study). Am J Obstet Gynecol 1997; 176: 377–80

9. Cummings SR, Bates D, Black DM. Clinical use of bone densitometry. JAMA. 2002; 288: 1889–97

10. Maartens LW, Leusink GL, Knottnerus JA, et al. Climacteric complaints in the community. Fam Pract 2001; 18: 189–94

11. Polo-Kantola P, Erkkola R, Irjala K, et al. Climacteric symptoms and sleep quality. Obstet Gynecol 1999; 94: 219–24

12. Berendsen HH. The role of serotonin in hot flushes. Maturitas 2000; 36: 155–64

13. Dennerstein L, Dudley EC, Hopper JL, et al. A prospective population-based study of menopausal symptoms. Obstet Gynecol 2000; 96: 351–8

14. MacLennan A, Lester S, Moore V. Oral estrogen replacement therapy versus placebo for hot flushes: a systematic review. Climacteric 2001; 4: 58–74

15. Rees M, Purdie DW. Management of the Menopause: the Handbook of the British Menopause Society. Marlow, UK: British Menopause Society Publications Ltd., 2002

16. Erkkola R, Kumento U, Lehmuskoski S, et al. No increased risk of endometrial hyperplasia with fixed long-cycle estrogen–progestogen therapy after five years. J Br Menopause Soc 2004; 10: 9–13

17. Raudaskoski T, Tapanainen J, Tomas E, et al. Intrauterine 10 microg and 20 microg levonorgestrel systems in postmenopausal women receiving oral estrogen replacement therapy: clinical, endometrial and metabolic response. Br J Obstet Gynaecol 2002; 109: 136–44

18. Vasilakis C, Jick H, del Mar Melero-Montes M. Risk of idiopathic venous thromboembolism in users of progestagens alone. Lancet 1999; 354: 1610–11

19. Loprinzi CL, Kugler JW, Sloan JA, et al. Venlafaxine in management of hot flashes in survivors of breast cancer: randomized controlled trial. Lancet 2000; 356: 2059–63

20. Stearns V, Isaacs C, Rowland J, et al. A pilot trial assessing the efficacy of paroxetine hydrochloride (Paxil) in controlling hot flashes in breast cancer survivors. Ann Oncol 2000; 11: 17–22

21. Bygdeman M, Swahn ML. Replens versus dienoestrol cream in the symptomatic treatment of vaginal atrophy in postmenopausal women. Maturitas 1996; 23: 259–63

22. Cauley JA, Robbins J, Chen Z, et al. Women's Health Initiative Investigators. Effects of estrogen plus progestin on risk of fracture and bone mineral density: the Women's Health Initiative randomized trial. JAMA 2003; 290: 1729–38

23. Lees B, Stevenson JC. The prevention of osteoporosis using sequential low-dose hormone replacement therapy with estradiol-17 beta and dydrogesterone. Osteoporos Int 2001; 12. 251–8

24. Royal College of Physicians. Osteoporosis: Clinical Guidelines for Prevention and Treatment. Update on Pharmacological Interventions and an Alogorithm for Management. London: Royal College of Physicians, 2000

25. Cauley JA, Zmuda JM, Ensrud KE, et al. Timing of estrogen replacement therapy for optimal osteoporosis prevention. J Clin Endocrinol Metab 2001; 86: 5700–5

26. Ahlborg HG, Johnell O, Karlsson MK. Long term effects of estrogen therapy on bone loss in postmenopausal women: a 23 year prospective study. Br J Obstet Gynaecol 2004; 111: 335–9

27. McClung MR, Geusens P, Miller PD, et al. Effect of risedronate on the risk of hip fracture in elderly women. Hip Intervention Program Study Group. N Engl J Med 2001; 344: 333–40

28. Marcus R, Wong M, Heath H 3rd, Stock JL. Antiresorptive treatment of postmenopausal osteoporosis: comparison of study designs and outcomes in large clinical trials with fracture as an endpoint. Endocr Rev 2002; 23: 16–37

29. Ravn P, Bidstrup M, Wasnich RD, et al. Alendronate and estrogen–progestin in the long-term prevention of bone loss: four-year results from the early postmenopausal intervention cohort study. A randomized, controlled trial. Ann Intern Med 1999; 131: 935–42

30. Chavassieux PM, Arlot ME, Reda C, et al. Histomorphometric assessment of the long-term effects of alendronate on bone quality and remodeling in patients with osteoporosis. J Clin Invest 1997; 100: 1475–80

31. Neer RM, Arnaud CD, Zanchetta JR, et al. Effect of parathyroid hormone (1–34) on fractures and bone mineral density in postmenopausal women with osteoporosis. N Engl J Med 2001 10; 344: 1434–41

32. Ettinger B, Black DM, Mitlak BH, et al. Reduction of vertebral fracture risk in postmenopausal women with osteoporosis treated with raloxifene: results from a 3-year randomized clinical trial. Multiple Outcomes of Raloxifene Evaluation (MORE) Investigators. JAMA 1999; 282: 637–45

33. Willis MS. The health economics of calcium and vitamin D_3 for the prevention of osteoporotic hip fractures in Sweden. Int J Technol Assess Health Care 2002; 18: 791–807

34. Hulley S, Grady D, Bush T, et al. Randomized trial of estrogen plus progestin for secondary prevention of coronary heart disease in postmenopausal women. Heart and Estrogen/progestin Replacement Study (HERS) Research Group. JAMA 1998; 280: 605–13

35. Grady D, Herrington D, Bittner V, et al. Cardiovascular disease during 6.8 years of hormone therapy: Heart and Estrogen/

progestin Replacement Study follow-up (HERS II). JAMA 2002; 288: 49–57

36. Beral V; Million Women Study Collaborators. Breast cancer and hormone-replacement therapy in the Million Women Study. Lancet 2003; 362: 419–27

37. Office for National Statistics. Mortality Statistics: Cause: Review of the Registrar General on deaths by cause, sex and age, in England and Wales, 2000. Series DH2 no.27. London: Office of National Statistics, 2001. www.statistics.gov.uk

38. Garton M. Breast cancer and hormone-replacement therapy: the Million Women Study. Lancet 2003; 362: 1328–31

39. The Women's Health Initiative Steering Committee. Effects of conjugated equine estrogen in postmenopausal women with hysterectomy: the Women's Health Initiative randomized controlled trial. JAMA 2004; 291 1701–12

40. NHS Breast Screening Review 2002; www.cancerscreening.nhs.uk

41. The Million Women Study Collaborators. The Million Women Study: design and characteristics of the study population. Breast Cancer Res 1999; 1: 73–80

42. Hersh AL, Stefanick ML, Stafford RS. National use of postmenopausal hormone therapy: annual trends and response to recent evidence. JAMA 2004; 291: 47–53

43. Gray S. Influence of the media and the Women's Health Initiative results. J Br Menopause Soc 2003; 9: 178

44. Eisenberg DM, Davis RB, Ettner SL, et al. Trends in alternative medicine use in the United States, 1990–1997: results of a follow-up national survey. JAMA 1998; 280: 1569–75

45. Thomas KJ, Nicholl JP, Coleman P. Use and expenditure on complementary medicine in England: a population based survey. Complement Ther Med 2001; 9: 2–11

46. Gokhale L, Sturdee DW, Parsons AD. The use of food supplements among women attending menopause clinics in the West Midlands. J Br Menopause Soc 2003; 9: 32–5

47. Rowland I, Faughnan M, Hoey L, et al. Bioavailability of phyto-oestrogens. Br J Nutr 2003; 89 (Suppl 1): S45–58

48. van der Weijer PHM, Barentsen R. Isoflavones from red clover (Promensil®) significantly reduce menopausal hot flush symptoms compared with placebo. Maturitas 2002; 42: 187–93

49. Tice JA, Ettinger B, Ensrud K, et al. Phytoestrogen supplements for the treatment of hot flashes: the Isoflavone Clover Extract (ICE) Study: a randomized controlled trial. JAMA 2003; 290: 207–14

50. Cassidy A. Dietary phytoestrogens and bone health. J Br Menopause Soc 2003; 9: 17–21

51. Alexandersen P, Toussaint A, Christiansen C, et al. Ipriflavone in the treatment of postmenopausal osteoporosis: a randomized controlled trial. JAMA 2001; 285: 1482–8

52. Rees M, Mander T, eds. Managing the Menopause without Oestrogen. London: BMS and RSM Press, 2004

53. Nortier JL, Martinez MC, Schmeiser HH, et al. Urothelial carcinoma associated with the use of a Chinese herb (Aristolochia fangchi). N Engl J Med 2000; 342: 1686–92

54. Burdette JE, Liu J, Chen SN, et al. Black cohosh acts as a mixed competitive ligand and partial agonist of the serotonin receptor. J Agric Food Chem 2003; 51: 5661–70

55. Barnes J, Anderson LA, Phillipson JD. St John's wort (Hypericum perforatum L.): a review of its chemistry, pharmacology and clinical properties. J Pharm Pharmacol 2001; 53: 583–600

56. Wiklund IK, Mattsson LA, Lindgren R, Limoni C. Effects of a standardized ginseng extract on quality of life and physiological

parameters in symptomatic postmenopausal women; a double-blind, placebo-controlled trial. Swedish Alternative Medicine Group. Int J Clin Pharmacol Res 1999; 19: 89–99

57. Leonetti HB, Longo S, Anasti JN. Transdermal progesterone cream for vasomotor symptoms and postmenopausal bone loss. Obstet Gynecol 1999; 94: 225–8

58. Leonetti HB, Wilson J, Anasti JN. Topical progesterone cream has an antiproliferative effect on estrogen-stimulated endometrium. Fertil Steril 2003; 79: 221–2

59. Wren BG, McFarland K, Edwards L, et al. Effect of sequential transdermal progesterone cream on endometrium, bleeding pattern, and plasma progesterone and salivary progesterone levels in postmenopausal women. Climacteric 2000; 3: 155–60

60. Ernst E. Alternative and complementary therapies. In Rees M, Keith L, eds. The Year in Postmenopausal Health. Oxford: Clinical Publishing, 2004: 211–22

Index

T - #0609 - 071024 - C0 - 254/190/12 - PB - 9780367392277 - Gloss Lamination